NUTRITION AND THE BRAIN

Volume 6

Nutrition and the Brain Series

Series Editors: Richard J. Wurtman
Judith J. Wurtman

Nutrition and the Brain

Volume 6

Physiological and Behavioral Effects of Food Constituents

Editors

Richard J. Wurtman, M.D.

Professor of Neuroendocrine Regulation
Department of Nutrition and
Food Science
Massachusetts Institute of Technology
Cambridge, Massachusetts

Judith J. Wurtman, Ph.D.

Research Associate
Department of Nutrition and
Food Science
Massachusetts Institute of Technology
Cambridge, Massachusetts

Raven Press ■ New York

Raven Press, 1140 Avenue of the Americas, New York, New York 10036

Made in the United States of America

Library of Congress Cataloging in Publication Data

Main entry under title:

Physiological and behavioral effects of food constituents.

    Nutrition and the brain ; v. 6)
    Includes bibliographical references and index.
    1. Nutrition—Addresses, essays, lectures. 2. Food—
Composition—Addresses, essays, lectures. 3. Human be-
havior—Nutritional aspects—Addresses, essays, lectures.
I. Wurtman, Richard J. II. Wurtman, Judith J.
III. Series. [DNLM: 1. Nutrition. 2. Brain—Physiology.
W1 MU8632 v.6 / WL 300 P578]
QP376.N86 vol. 6   599′.01′88s   [615′.78]   83-9690
[QP141]
ISBN 0-89004-733-2

Preface

The brain requires a number of substances that it cannot make. The study of brain nutrition must therefore encompass all metabolic and physiologic processes that make these nutrients available to it.

Nutrients are delivered to brain cells by the blood stream and transported across the blood-brain barrier by specific uptake mechanisms that are probably localized within capillaries or adjacent membranes. These nutrients may have entered the blood as a result of (1) the consumption of food, and its digestion in and absorption by the gut; (2) its synthesis in, and secretion from, such organs as the liver; or (3) both processes. Classically, the field of nutrition has concerned itself only with the first such group of compounds, i.e., those that cannot be synthesized anywhere in the body, and whose presence in the blood results from their presence in particular foods. Actually, however, the nutritional state of the brain is just as dependent on the availability of compounds such as adenine (which the liver secretes into the blood stream) or choline and glucose (which enter the blood both from dietary sources and from hepatic synthesis).

Brain cells also require trace amounts of hormones, which, like some nutrients, are secreted by other organs into the circulation. These compounds are not included here among the brain's nutrients; rather, this term is reserved for compounds that the brain utilizes in relatively large amounts as (1) substrates or cofactors for its enzymes, (2) constituents of its macromolecules, or as (3) precursors for its secretions, such as the neurotransmitters.

Prior volumes in this series have examined the brain's requirements for particular nutrients; the behavioral and physiological mechanisms that it uses to satisfy these requirements; the evidence that certain food constituents can be toxic to the brain; and the possible utility of one set of food chemicals, choline and lecithin, in the treatment of brain disorders involving cholinergic neurons.

This volume presents critical summaries of several currently debated topics that relate to nutrients and the brain. The effects and pharmacologic disposition of caffeine are discussed, as well as the regulation by the U.S. Food and Drug Administration of food constituents that might affect brain function and behavior. The tests currently available for assessing effects of foods on behavior, especially in children, are surveyed. Discussions are included on the effects of particular dietary amino acids, such as tyrosine, tryptophan, and threonine, on brain neurotransmission. Also discussed are the brain mechanisms underlying appetites for particular food constituents.

This volume will be of interest to neuroscientists, neurologists, psychiatrists and psychologists, physiologists and pharmacologists, and people working on nutrition and metabolism.

Cambridge, Massachusetts RICHARD J. WURTMAN
April 1983 JUDITH J. WURTMAN

Contents

Contributors

Marvin J. Bleiberg
Division of Toxicology, Bureau of Foods, Food and Drug
Administration, Washington, D.C. 20204

John E. Blundell
Department of Psychology, The University of Leeds,
Leeds LS2 9JT, U.K.

P. Michael Bolger
Division of Toxicology, Bureau of Foods, Food and Drug
Administration, Washington, D.C. 20204

Reid W. von Borstel
Laboratory of Neuroendocrine Regulation, Department of Nutrition and
Food Science, Massachusetts Institute of Technology,
Cambridge, Massachusetts 02139

David G. Hattan
Division of Toxicology, Bureau of Foods, Food and Drug
Administration, Washington, D.C. 20204

Sara H. Henry
Division of Toxicology, Bureau of Foods, Food and Drug
Administration, Washington, D.C. 20204

Stephen B. Montgomery
Division of Toxicology, Bureau of Foods, Food and Drug
Administration, Washington, D.C. 20204

Allen H. Neims
Department of Pharmacology and Therapeutics, University of Florida
College of Medicine, Gainesville, Florida 32610

Judith L. Rapoport
Unit on Childhood Mental Illness, Biological Psychiatry Branch, National Institute of Mental Health, Bethesda, Maryland 20205

Alan M. Rulis
Division of Food and Color Additives, Bureau of Foods, Food and Drug Administration, Washington, D.C. 20204

Judith M. Rumsey
Unit on Childhood Mental Illness, Biological Psychiatry Branch, National Institute of Mental Health, Bethesda, Maryland 20205

Alan F. Sved
Department of Neuroscience, New Jersey Medical School, University of Medicine and Dentistry of New Jersey, Newark, New Jersey 07103

Nutrition and the Brain, Vol. 6 edited by
R. J. Wurtman and J. J. Wurtman.
Raven Press, New York © 1983.

Caffeine: Metabolism and Biochemical Mechanisms of Action

*Allen H. Neims and **Reid W. von Borstel

*Department of Pharmacology and Therapeutics, University of Florida College of Medicine, Gainesville, Florida 32610; and **Laboratory of Neuroendocrine Regulation, Department of Nutrition and Food Science, Massachusetts Institute of Technology, Cambridge, Massachusetts 02139

Caffeine [1,3,7-trimethylxanthine (1,3,7-TMX); Fig. 1] is one of the most widely consumed pharmacologically active substances. It occurs naturally in several plant components including the coffee bean, tea leaf, kola nut, cacao seed, and ilex leaf. Most of us have ingested the caffeine from these plants, usually as a constituent of beverages. The average American consumes 2 to 3 mg/kg of caffeine daily (47); many people consume more than 10 mg/kg/day. About 75% of this caffeine derives from coffee, a cup of which contains between 50 and 150 mg of the alkaloid. For simplicity, it may be assumed that one cup of coffee delivers about 1 mg/kg of caffeine to an adult; this dose leads to a peak plasma concentration of 1 to 2 μg/ml (5 to 10 μM). As much as 3 mg/kg can be consumed in a short time under everyday circumstances. For comparison, a cup of tea contains about 50 mg of caffeine whereas a 12-ounce cola beverage contains about 35 mg of caffeine. Caffeine is also present in several over-the-counter medications including analgesics, appetite suppressants, and central stimulants.

The biological actions of caffeine depend on its dose and on the duration of exposure. At doses less than 50-fold those typically consumed, functional changes can be detected in a variety of systems and processes, e.g., the central nervous system (CNS), the cardiovascular system, the respiratory system, smooth and skeletal muscle, gastrointestinal secretion, the rate of urine formation, basal metabolic rate and intermediary metabolism, DNA repair, and reproduction (47,102). The brain seems to be the organ most sensitive to caffeine (37). Sleep latency is nearly doubled in some subjects by a single serving of 1 to 2 mg/kg. The "alerting" effects of caffeine, namely those that maintain functions in the face of fatigue, can be detected in regular caffeine consumers after a single dose of about 2 to 3 mg/kg (causing peak plasma concentrations of 10 to 15 μM). In nonconsumers of caffeine, such doses can produce irritability and nervousness (37,104). Conversely, caffeine deprivation can provoke the same undesired effects in regular consumers (37,105). At slightly higher caffeine doses (3 to 5 mg/kg) various respiratory (stimulation), cardiovascular (hypertension, transient bradycardia, then tachycardia; increase in plasma renin and epinephrine), gastrointestinal (secretion), and diuretic actions can be discerned (105). The cardiovascular effects are not observed when the same dose is given to regular coffee drinkers (106) and, like respiratory stimulation, may be in part mediated centrally (37). Most other effects of caffeine are seen only after consumption of unusually high doses.

Several recent reviews have dealt with the use and actions of caffeine: The American Council of Science and Health (83) has summarized the health effects of caffeine; Dews (37) and Friedman (56) have reviewed its psychopharmacologic and biochemical effects, respectively; and Eichler (43) has discussed its pharmacology. Our chapter deals specifically with two aspects of this extensive subject: (a) the comparative metabolism of caffeine, with emphasis on its fate in humans; and (b) a critical discussion of the biochemical mechanisms underlying the actions of caffeine, with particular reference to adenosine receptors.

I. COMPARATIVE METABOLISM OF CAFFEINE

Caffeine is moderately soluble in water, yet sufficiently hydrophobic to traverse biological membranes with ease. It is not ionized at physiological pH (30). These physicochemical properties are largely responsible for several of caffeine's most

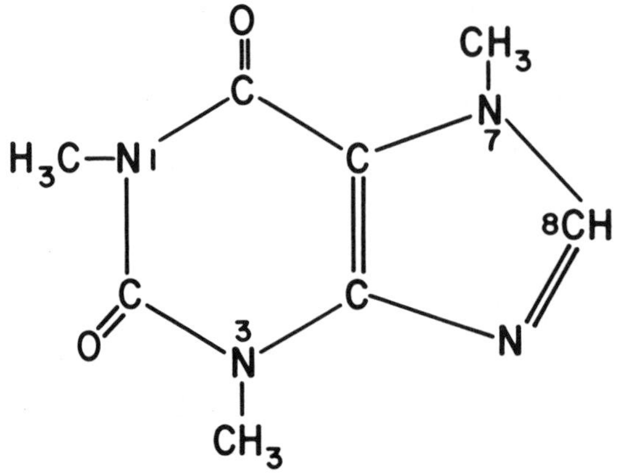

FIG. 1.   The structure of caffeine (1,3,7-trimethylxanthine).

important metabolic characteristics: (a) rapid and complete absorption from the gastrointestinal tract; (b) rapid, yet passive, distribution to all organs including brain, testes, and those of the fetus; (c) inefficient excretion by the kidneys; and (d) a dependence on biotransformation for efficient elimination from the body. These generalizations apply to all mammals studied to date. In contrast, the rate and route of caffeine's biotransformation are highly dependent on species.

A. Absorption and Distribution

Caffeine is rapidly and completely absorbed from the gastrointestinal tract after oral consumption (15,25). There is no appreciable first-pass effect in rats (5) or humans. Although the material in which caffeine is ingested may have some influence on its absorption rate, the effects are small (14). After consumption, peak plasma concentrations are usually attained within minutes to an hour or two (14,21,33,91).

Once absorbed, caffeine is widely distributed in the body. Most evidence suggests that distribution, albeit rapid, is passive (15,25). Caffeine's apparent volume of distribution in several mammals studied was 0.5 to 0.7 liters/kg—about equal to total body water volume (15,92). Even "protected" regions such as brain, testes, and fetus are readily accessible to caffeine. During a single passage through the cerebral circulation, 80% equilibration between plasma and brain is obtained (81a). Diffusion into the CNS may be partly carrier facilitated, since competition for transport between adenine and caffeine has been demonstrated (81a). This combination of facile absorption and distribution to brain probably explains the consumer's rapid perception of caffeine's central actions.

Caffeine is poorly bound to plasma protein; only about 25% binds in humans when total plasma caffeine concentrations are between 2 and 20 μg/ml (10 and 100 μM). Perhaps predictably, the concentration of caffeine in saliva ranges from 55 to 95% of that present in plasma. An hour or two after oral consumption of caffeine, its concentration in saliva can be used as a convenient index of plasma caffeine in humans (33,91).

B. Excretion

The capacity of caffeine to permeate biological membranes with ease underlies the characteristics of its excretion by the kidney. Caffeine entering the tubule by glomerular filtration is reabsorbed almost as rapidly as is filtered water. The process of reabsorption seems passive. We have found that the urine/plasma concentration ratio for caffeine is about 1.4 in rat, beagle, and human. This applies also under conditions of varying pH and diuresis, and implies that more than 98% of filtered caffeine is reabsorbed before excretion. It follows that the rate of caffeine clearance without biotransformation would be only slightly greater than the rate of urine flow. The half-life of caffeine in plasma under such circumstances would be several days, and clearance would be only a few milliliters per kilogram per hour. This, indeed, is observed in newborn infants (1) and in adults with severe liver failure (115). However, in healthy adults, caffeine's clearance is about 80 ml/kg/hr, and its $t_{1/2}$ is about 5 to 6 *hr*; less than 2% of caffeine doses administered to such subjects is recovered as unchanged caffeine in the urine (14,25,28). In newborns, where metabolism is slow, the average clearance rate for caffeine is 8 to 9 ml/kg/hr, its $t_{1/2}$ is 4 *days*, and not surprisingly, more than 80% of an administered caffeine dose is recovered as such in the urine (1).

C. Biotransformation

Caffeine is biotransformed primarily in liver to several metabolites through a complex set of sequential and parallel (or competing) reactions. These metabolites are, for the most part, excreted in urine much more efficiently than is caffeine. Since the rate at which each reaction occurs varies markedly among species, the profile of urinary caffeine metabolites is also species-specific (25,57).

In all animals studied to date caffeine is initially converted to one or another dimethylxanthine [theophylline (1,3-DMX); paraxanthine (1,7-DMX); theobromine (3,7-DMX)], to 1,3,7-trimethyluric acid (1,3,7-TMU), and/or to 6-amino-5[*N*-formylmethylamino]-1,3-dimethyluracil (12,14). The demethylations of caffeine to the various dimethylxanthines are oxidative in nature and yield formaldehyde; these reactions are almost certainly catalyzed by the cytochrome P-450 monooxygenase system (5,49,67,134). The oxidation of caffeine to trimethylurate is also thought to be catalyzed by the P-450 monooxygenase. Xanthine oxidase is not active toward caffeine. The conversion of caffeine to its diaminouracil derivative is fundamentally a hydration reaction, but the metabolic pathway remains unresolved and may involve a combination of oxidation and reduction reactions. These five possibilities for the initial biotransformation of caffeine are summarized in Fig. 2.

Some of the primary metabolites of caffeine, especially the dimethylxanthines, also serve as substrates for further biotransformation by demethylation, oxidation to the respective urate, and/or hydration to the respective diaminouracil. Several different forms of cytochrome P-450 seem to be involved in the various reactions. Xanthine oxidase probably plays a role in the conversion of 1-methylxanthine to 1-methylurate (20). Most of the various metabolic possibilities are summarized in Fig. 3. The rate of each step, the circulating concentration of each metabolite, and the mode of urinary excretion of each derivative all contribute to caffeine's metabolic profile. A few metabolites, such as trimethylallantoin and those containing sulfur, have been described only in rodent urine and are not discussed further here. Since caffeine metabolites are for the most part excreted in urine more rapidly than is caffeine, urinary metabolite profiles tend to be more species-specific than those of plasma or tissue. Indeed, *significant* quantities of only a few metabolites (mainly dimethylxanthines) are found in plasma (14,28,57,117). Finally, the *rate* and *pathway* of biotransformation can vary independently. Two different animals can have the same clearance (or $t_{1/2}$) for caffeine, yet produce different sets of metabolites.

In the sections that follow, we review caffeine metabolism in humans and selected laboratory animals. For most of the species, data are available only with regard to

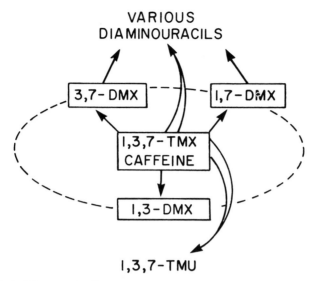

FIG. 2. The initial routes of caffeine biotransformation. DMX, Dimethylxanthine; TMU, trimethylurate.

the disposition of caffeine by healthy young adult animals, usually males. If results in humans and a limited number of animal experiments are any indication, rather striking differences will be found depending on factors such as age, sex, pregnancy, disease, exposure to other foreign compounds, etc.

1. Humans

Several studies suggest that in healthy young adults the disappearance of caffeine from plasma or saliva is first-order after single oral doses of up to 10 mg/kg. The mean $t_{1/2}$ is about 5 to 6 hr in nonsmokers. The mean clearance rate is about 80 ml/kg/hr. The apparent volume of distribution is about 0.7 liters/kg, so that the peak concentration in plasma in μg/ml is usually less than 1.4 times the dose in mg/kg. Thus if a typical adult consumes a cup or two of coffee containing 140 mg of caffeine (2 mg/kg), the peak plasma concentration will be about 2.5 μg/ml (or 12.5 μM). Six hours later the plasma concentration will be about 1.25 μg/ml.

Cumulative urinary metabolite profiles (14,28) indicate that about 70% of a serving of caffeine initially undergoes 3-N-demethylation to yield paraxanthine (1,7-DMX). Paraxanthine is the primary metabolite of caffeine found in plasma, and a large fraction of the urinary metabolites represents further metabolic derivatives of paraxanthine. Although all three dimethylxanthines can be detected in plasma after a dose of caffeine (117), the area-under-the-plasma-concentration-time curves (AUCs) for theophylline and theobromine are less than 10% of caffeine's AUC, but that for paraxanthine is 34% that of caffeine (57).

The situation with regard to the formation of diaminouracil derivatives in humans is not completely resolved. About 1 to 2% of a dose of caffeine is recovered in

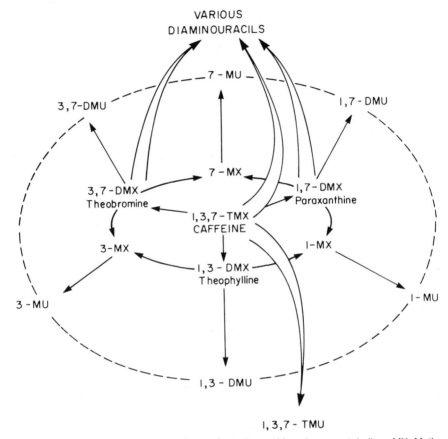

FIG. 3. Potential routes of caffeine biotransformation and its primary metabolites. MX, Methylxanthine; MU: methylurate; DMU: dimethylurate.

urine as 6-amino-5-(*N*-formylmethylamino)-1,3-dimethyluracil (28). Callahan and colleagues (28), however, have recovered about 10 to 30% of the dose in urine of various individuals as an acetylated diaminouracil derivative of paraxanthine (5-acetylamino-6-amino-3-methyluracil) (Table 1). This compound is derived from a less stable metabolite bearing a formyl substituent on the 6-amino group; individual variation in the yield of acetylated metabolites reflects genetic polymorphism in the rate of acetylation (D. M. Grant, W. Kalow, and B. K. Tang, *personal communication*).

The rate of caffeine elimination, which is determined primarily by its rate of biotransformation, varies considerably between different groups of humans. We will consider separately the effects of age, smoking, pregnancy, disease, and the interaction of caffeine with other foreign compounds.

Premature (7,58) and full-term (92) newborns eliminate caffeine slowly because biotransformation is immature (1). The newborns exhibit a mean plasma half-life and caffeine clearance of 3 to 4 days and 8 to 9 ml/kg/hr, respectively. These values

TABLE 1. *Metabolites in human urine arising from an*
oral dose of caffeine, 5 mg/kg[a]

Metabolites	% of administered dose	Metabolites	% of administered dose
A$_1$	14.70	3,7-DMX	1.88
A$_2$	3.10	1,3,7-TMX	1.24
1-MX	18.14	1-MU	14.81
3-MX	4.11	1,3-DMU	1.80
7-MX	9.88	1,7-DMU	5.36
1,3-DMX	0.89	1,3,7-TMU	1.30
1,7-DMX	5.86		

[a]Modified from Callahan et al. (28). Urine was collected for 48 hr; the values represent the means of four subjects. For abbreviations, see legends to Figs. 2 and 3. A$_1$ is 5-acetylamino-6-amino-3-methyluracil.

are substantially lower than the half-life of 5 to 6 hr and the clearance of 80 ml/kg/hr found in adults. As much as 80% of a caffeine dose is excreted unchanged in newborns' urine (1). There are certain potentially important consequences of this circumstance. The typical infant in North America is born with an umbilical cord plasma caffeine concentration of between 0.5 and 2 μg/ml. Because of caffeine's prolonged half-life, several days are required after birth for its elimination and the disappearance of any actions it might have. The infant will not experience the peaks and troughs of concentration typical of the adult under usual circumstances of consumption and elimination. Finally, the low rate of caffeine clearance allows for repetitive doses to accumulate to much higher steady-state concentrations in newborns than in adults given the same quantity of caffeine in mg/kg. This is significant when caffeine is used as a drug to treat apnea in premature infants (7). Caffeine concentration in breast milk is roughly equal to its concentration in the mother's plasma. It can be computed that the suckling infant is exposed to only a small percentage of the caffeine that his mother consumes. Fortunately, the infant's ability to eliminate caffeine seems to mature sufficiently rapidly to prevent excessive accumulation of the compound on breast feeding. Nonetheless, several studies reveal that such infants may achieve plasma caffeine concentrations up to 1 or 2 μg/ml, not unlike those present in the adult after drinking a cup of coffee (6).

As the metabolic process matures during the first several months after birth, the caffeine metabolites that appear in urine are not different from those found in the adult (1). The infant comes to eliminate caffeine more rapidly than the adult per unit body weight before age 1 year (1). Although children of ages 1 to 5 years have not yet been evaluated, older children continue to eliminate caffeine quite rapidly. The average half-life of 2.3 hr and clearance of 250 ml/kg/hr in 6- to 13-year-olds (A. H. Neims, *unpublished results*) are surprisingly greater than the respective values of 5 to 6 hr and 80 ml/kg/hr found in nonsmoking adults. Although these data do not directly address the question of different sensitivities of the brain to the central actions of caffeine at different ages, they do document that, relative to the adult, the youngster is exposed (in terms of AUC) to less caffeine than the adult, assuming each takes the same serving in mg/kg. The elderly dispose of caffeine at virtually the same rates as do young adults (124; A. H. Neims, *unpublished results*).

Cigarette smoking is associated with a substantial increase in the rate of caffeine clearance (91). Caffeine's half-life in smokers is 3 to 4 hr instead of 5 to 6 hr, and clearance doubles from 80 to 155 ml/kg/hr. This phenomenon has been studied by following caffeine's disappearance from plasma or saliva (21) and by following isotopically labeled caffeine in a breath test (11). Presumably one or more component(s) of cigarette smoke is acting to induce the enzymes involved in caffeine's biotransformation. Direct studies of the inductive action on caffeine's metabolism of one set of components, the polycyclic aromatic hydrocarbons (PAH), have been conducted in rats (5,134). The known association between increased caffeine consumption and cigarette smoking in humans could depend in part on increased caffeine clearance, i.e., more caffeine is needed to obtain a given plasma level and a given behavioral effect.

There is no appreciable sexual dimorphism in the rate of caffeine elimination. Pregnancy is, however, associated with an increase in the half-life and a decrease in clearance of caffeine, but only during the second and, especially, third trimesters. Toward the end of the third trimester, the half-life of caffeine increases to about 18 hr and its clearance decreases to 23 ml/kg/hr (2). There is a striking return of the kinetic profile to nonpregnant values within a few days just before, or more likely, after birth. This phenomenon is probably the result of changes in the hormonal milieu: Oral contraceptives also significantly decrease the rate of caffeine elimination (93). The fetus *probably* metabolizes caffeine inefficiently, but the rapid permeation of caffeine across the placenta allows the mother to function as the locus of biotransformation for herself and her fetus. The placenta might catalyze the biotransformation of caffeine, especially in smokers; however, the biological significance of this phenomenon is unknown.

Caffeine itself induces the enzymes involved in the metabolism of certain drugs in rats (82). Chronic caffeine consumption may act to induce its own biotransformation in humans, but the effect is likely to be small (91). Cimetidine (36) and theobromine or other xanthine derivatives (39) appear to act as inhibitors of substituted xanthine biotransformation. Finally, patients with severe liver failure also dispose of caffeine slowly (115).

Much less is known about possible group differences in caffeine's metabolite profile than about differences in its rate of elimination. Kinetic data indicate that the significance of a given caffeine dose must be interpreted in light of the characteristic rate of caffeine clearance for that particular group of consumers. Kinetic differences between groups have much more impact on AUC (a measure of total exposure) and on steady-state caffeine concentrations than on peak plasma concentrations attained after a single dose.

2. Nonhuman Primates

The kinetic profile of caffeine in plasma of *Macaca* resembles that of humans in that its $t_{1/2}$ is 6 hr and its clearance about 100 ml/kg/hr; no dose dependency is seen at a dose of 10 mg/kg (57). But the route of caffeine's biotransformation is quite different from that in humans. Theophylline, not paraxanthine, is the major metabolite seen in plasma; indeed its AUC in plasma is 146% that of caffeine. The relative figures for theobromine and paraxanthine are 16.8 and 9.4%, respectively. Thus paraxanthine, the major dimethylxanthine metabolite in human plasma, is less important in this monkey. The urinary metabolite profile of caffeine in *Macaca* also suggests that 7-N-demethylation to theophylline is the most important initial metabolic reaction. As in humans, only a small fraction of caffeine is recovered in urine as diaminouracil derivatives, but full recovery of the administered dose has not been accomplished.

Striking differences in caffeine biotransformation are apparent among the different nonhuman primates. Caffeine is more toxic to the squirrel monkey than might have been anticipated, and its elimination rate in that species is quite slow (25). A direct comparison of caffeine biotransformation in three different nonhuman primates revealed different urinary metabolite profiles in each (27). The metabolite profile of caffeine in the baboon does resemble that of *Macaca*. Interestingly, the rate of caffeine disposition decreases during pregnancy in the baboon (31).

3. Beagle

Untreated adult beagles given caffeine intravenously (20 mg/kg) dispose of it in first-order fashion, with a plasma $t_{1/2}$ of 4 hr. Clearance is 133 ml/kg/hr. All three DMXs and 3-MX can be discerned in plasma. Evaluation of the urinary metabolite pattern reveals that the predominant route of caffeine's metabolism in the beagle involves an initial 7-N-demethylation to theophylline with subsequent metabolism of the theophylline to 3-MX, 1,3-DMU, and 1-MU (presumably through 1-MX). Thus the beagle more resembles *Macaca* than man.

Shortly after birth, when the metabolism of caffeine is deficient in puppies (4,133), the metabolic route is less defined. During the first postnatal month, the canine adult pattern of metabolites emerges coincident with acquisition of an adult-like pharmacokinetic profile (4).

Pretreatment of the beagle with phenobarbital or with β-naphthoflavone stimulates caffeine elimination, with the plasma $t_{1/2}$ decreasing to 1.5 hr in both cases (3). Phenobarbital pretreatment does not have a prominent effect on metabolite profile, but pretreatment with PAH increases the likelihood of an initial 3-N-demethylation to paraxanthine. In this sense, the PAH-induced beagle more closely resembles humans than does the untreated beagle or *Macaca*. Nonetheless, appreciable differences persist in metabolite patterns between the species.

4. Rat

Little is known about strain differences, so our discussion focuses primarily on the Sprague-Dawley rat. First-order kinetics, which prevail in humans up to single servings of caffeine of 10 mg/kg, imply that a constant fraction or percentage of the dose is eliminated per unit time. Saturation kinetics, which can be detected in the rat at doses less than 5 mg/kg and plasma concentrations of caffeine as low as 2 to 4 µg/ml (10 to 20 µM) (5,25,57,75), imply that this proportionality no longer exists. At its extreme (zero-order kinetics), only a constant *amount* of compound is eliminated per unit time regardless of how much is given to the animal. The "$t_{1/2}$" of caffeine in the rat at doses less than 10 mg/kg is about 1.5 to 2.0 hr. Saturation analysis reveals a V_{max} of 0.106 µg/ml/min and a K_m of 8.2 µg/ml (5).

The consequences of saturation kinetics in the rat are multiple: (a) although the rat clears most chemicals more rapidly than do humans, this is true for caffeine only when its dose is less than about 40 mg/kg. At higher doses, the AUC "exposure" to caffeine in the rat increases disproportionately (57); (b) steady-state or plateau concentrations of caffeine associated with repetitive dosing increase disproportionately more in rats when the dose is increased than in humans within the usual range of caffeine consumption; and (c) metabolite profiles in the rat can change with dose (57). It should be noted also that 1-year-old rats dispose of caffeine appreciably more slowly than do 3-month-olds (57).

Caffeine's initial mode of degradation in the rat seems quite diffuse, with oxidation at the 8-position, demethylation at 3-N, 7-N, and 1-N positions, and hydrolytic ring splitting to the 5-amino-6-(N-formylmethylamino)-1,3-dimethyluracil all important. The rat also produces an array of other metabolites (9). Certain metabolites, such as trimethylallantoin, are not found in humans. Others, such as trimethyluric acid and 6-amino-5-[N-formylmethylamino]-1,3-dimethyluracil, are major metabolites in the rat, but comprise less than a few percent of the recovered urinary components in humans (28). Pathways that do not involve demethylation account for more than 40% of caffeine metabolites in the rat but less than 5% of caffeine metabolites in humans (14).

The newborn rat is relatively more effective in metabolizing caffeine than is the human infant (10). Phenobarbital does increase the rat's capacity to metabolize caffeine but does not influence dose dependency (5). Pretreatment with PAH greatly stimulates caffeine metabolism and eliminates saturation kinetics, even with caffeine doses exceeding 25 mg/kg. The $t_{1/2}$ of caffeine in such pretreated rats is only about 15 min (5).

5. Other Animals

The mouse disposes of caffeine efficiently through biotransformation to several metabolites. Plasma disappearance curves are first-order even after a dose of 100 mg/kg. Plasma $t_{1/2}$ is about 1.5 hr and clearance about 325 ml/kg/hr. AUCs for theophylline, theobromine, and paraxanthine in plasma relative to that for caffeine are 3.5, 47, and 20%, respectively (57). 1-, 3-, and 7-N-demethylation, as well as

8-oxidation, appear almost equally likely as the initial direction for caffeine's degradation. Secondary metabolism occurs but is less striking than that seen in humans. The initial 8-oxidation generates a substantial amount of 1,3,7-TMU, a metabolite seen only in small concentrations in humans.

On the basis of its urinary metabolite profile (57), the guinea pig probably disposes of caffeine slowly. But documentation is lacking. The urinary metabolite pattern is striking in that caffeine represents 21% of identified excretion products. This is 10-fold higher than seen in most other species and presumably reflects slow biotransformation. Interestingly, the three dimethylxanthines—1,3-DMX, 3,7-DMX, and 1,7-DMX—comprise an additional 75% of recovered metabolites. Relative to the other species investigated, the guinea pig seems to have substantial difficulty not only in metabolizing caffeine, but also in further metabolizing the primary dimethylxanthine metabolites.

Caffeine is eliminated from the plasma of adult rabbits by first-order kinetics after a 10 mg/kg dose. Prominent dose-dependent kinetics are seen at doses greater than or equal to 50 mg/kg (57). At the lower doses, the $t_{1/2}$ for caffeine is 69 min and clearance is about 420 ml/kg/hr. Theophylline and theobromine exhibit AUCs in plasma of about 32 and 15%; respectively, relative to that of caffeine. Paraxanthine, on the other hand, has an AUC that is 228% that of caffeine. Paraxanthine is also a major urinary metabolite. Thus, like humans, the rabbit seems to initiate caffeine's breakdown by 3-N-demethylation. Unlike humans, however, the rabbit further degrades the paraxanthine slowly. Major human metabolites such as 1-MX, 1-MU, and 7-MX are substantially less prominent in rabbit's urine. The potential production of diaminouracil derivatives and the possible changes in metabolite pattern with dose are unexplored.

6. In Vitro *Studies*

Caffeine biotransformation has been studied *in vitro* using liver perfusion, liver slices, and microsomal preparations. Microsomes from uninduced animals are less effective at catalysis than might have been anticipated (13,49,132). Both the influence of inducers and saturation kinetics in the rat have been confirmed.

In summary, the rate and route of caffeine's biotransformation and thus its rate of elimination vary considerably with species. Animals exposed to caffeine are also exposed to its metabolites. Because of seemingly efficient renal excretion of most metabolites, appreciable exposure of tissues is usually limited to one or more of the dimethylxanthines. In humans and rabbits, paraxanthine is the major metabolite found in plasma; in many nonhuman primates and the beagle, theophylline is primary. Initial biotransformation not involving demethylation seems most significant in the rat. In humans, age, habits, pregnancy, and other chemicals influence caffeine's kinetics. When assessing the biological actions of caffeine in the laboratory or in life situations, the impact of these differences on the presence of caffeine and its metabolites in terms of concentration and time should not be ignored.

II. BIOLOGICAL ACTIONS IN RELATION TO ADENOSINE

In spite of the widespread use of methylxanthines—caffeine, theophylline, and theobromine—as food constituents and as drugs, the biochemical events mediating their pharmacological actions are not well understood. On the basis of experiments performed mainly on isolated tissue or organ preparations *in vitro*, several detailed mechanisms have been proposed whereby methylxanthines might act on neural, cardiovascular, renal, and respiratory processes; however, the precise actions and potencies of methylxanthines observed *in vivo* have often been particularly difficult to reconcile with information obtained from *in vitro* studies. Thus the hypothesis that caffeine and theophylline act *in vivo* mainly by inhibiting the cyclic AMP (cAMP)-degrading enzyme, phosphodiesterase (PDE), is untenable given caffeine's relatively low potency as an inhibitor of the enzyme, compared with its potency in modulating physiological processes *in vivo*. Even relatively high doses of methylxanthines generally fail to increase tissue cAMP levels in intact animals (26). Similarly, differences between the *in vivo* and *in vitro* potencies of methylxanthines diminish the likelihood that caffeine acts as a cardiac and CNS stimulant by direct effects on calcium storage and translocation (102).

Over the past decade, considerable evidence has been marshalled that supports the hypothesis that the physiologically most important molecular action for methylxanthines involves competitive antagonism at extracellular adenosine receptors (52): Free adenosine is present in extracellular spaces of tissues in concentrations that may be sufficient to exert a tonic influence on many physiological processes. Adenosine administration to animals can produce sedation, bradycardia, hypotension, hypothermia, and attenuation of the responses of the heart, vasculature, and adipose tissues to sympathetic stimulation (40,54,77). These effects (apparently mediated by specific adenosine receptors located on the external surfaces of plasma membranes) are generally opposite those produced by caffeine or theophylline alone. Indeed, methylxanthines competitively antagonize these and other adenosine actions at concentrations similar to those found in plasma after the consumption of 1 to 3 cups of coffee (5 to 30 μM; 102). No other single known molecular interaction of methylxanthines seems as likely as antagonism of adenosine receptors to be able to explain the multiplicity of caffeine's effects upon biological systems. However, as will be discussed, substantial indirect evidence suggests that adenosine-receptor antagonism might not fully explain all of caffeine's physiological effects in humans. Nonetheless, in the absence of other plausible proposals for mechanisms that might mediate the effects of low methylxanthine doses, main interest attends the adenosine-receptor-blocker hypothesis. If caffeine acts via adenosine receptors and if more than a single group of such receptors exists, then it might be possible, by modifying the caffeine molecule, to produce agents that will mimic some of caffeine's actions, perhaps with greater potency, without producing other effects (113). A drug, enprofylline (3-propylxanthine), has already been developed that is more potent than theophylline or caffeine as a bronchodilator, yet lacks stimulatory actions on the CNS and does not cause diuresis. However, it is apparently ineffective as an adenosine antagonist (94,95).

The remainder of this chapter addresses the experimental evidence and hypotheses currently used to explain the effects of methylxanthines on the brain, kidney, respiratory apparatus, and heart. For each organ system, a brief summary is provided of the methylxanthine effects most relevant to human pharmacology, as well as a discussion of the possible cellular loci where methylxanthines might act to produce these effects. Occasionally, results from experiments involving caffeine or theophylline are intermingled, based on the generally accepted (102) supposition that the differences between the physiologically important actions of low doses of these compounds are more quantitative than qualitative.

A. Methylxanthine Effects on the CNS

Caffeine is perhaps best known as a stimulant of the CNS; certain aspects of this action, e.g., abatement of drowsiness and fatigue, and restoration of capacity for work, undoubtedly account for the popularity of methylxanthine-containing beverages. The antisoporific and alertness-enhancing effects of caffeine are apparent at low doses (~2 mg/kg) that have few, if any, discernible effects on other physiological systems (37); higher doses (10 to 15 mg/kg) of caffeine or theophylline can produce nervousness and insomnia and very much higher doses (200 mg/kg) seizures and death (102).

Many investigations aimed at elucidation of the biochemical mechanisms underlying the effects of methylxanthines use locomotor activity or similar behavioral measures as indices of stimulation (114,123). However, it is not clear that locomotor activity in animals is adequate as a correlate to the enhanced subjective alertness reported by humans after caffeine consumption. The cortical electroencephalogram (EEG) seen after caffeine administration is similar to that seen during normal physiological arousal and to that produced by direct stimulation of the reticular formation (111), a brain stem neuronal network believed to play a major role in the regulation of wakefulness. Caffeine-induced EEG activation apparently reflects enhanced neuronal activity in the reticular formation, and in rats this brain region is uncommonly sensitive to caffeine (50). In other brain regions, such as the cortex, relatively high doses of caffeine (10 to 100 mg/kg) given intravenously generally lead to a modest (less than twofold) increase in spontaneous neuronal activity (cf. 97). The main action of systemically administered caffeine in visual cortical neurons, for example, is not so much increased basal activity, but rather enhanced cellular response to receptive field stimulation, similar to that observed after direct reticular stimulation (50). Spontaneous neuronal firing frequency in the reticular formation is particularly sensitive to caffeine. Oral caffeine (2.8 mg/kg) increased the spontaneous firing rate of reticular formation neurons (single units) from a basal frequency of 10 spikes/sec to 50 impulses/sec (50). When this dose of caffeine is given to otherwise untreated rats by intraperitoneal injection, no increase is discerned in spontaneous locomotor activity (123); in mice, activity actually decreases at this caffeine dose (114).

1. Mechanisms for CNS Stimulation by Methylxanthines

PDE inhibition can almost certainly be ruled out as a significant contributor to the *stimulatory* effects of physiologically relevant caffeine doses; caffeine treatment *in vivo* (25 mg/kg/day) neither increases cerebral cAMP content nor reduces the specific activity of cAMP PDE in brain (26). Theophylline does not increase brain cAMP even at near-lethal doses (200 mg/kg) and, in fact, *prevents* the increase in brain cAMP otherwise seen after electroshock convulsions; this cAMP increase in seizures is apparently caused by enhanced adenosine output secondary to hypoxia, and is not seen in animals kept in an oxygen-enriched environment during seizure activity (109). Adenosine is a potent stimulator of adenylate cyclase in many tissues including brain (110); in other tissues including some CNS cell types, adenosine can attenuate the stimulation of adenylate cyclase by β-adrenergic agonists (127); there are at least two pharmacologically distinguishable adenosine receptor subtypes. In addition, 3-propylxanthine, which is more potent than theophylline as a PDE inhibitor but ineffective as an adenosine antagonist (95), does not enhance locomotor activity; indeed the main CNS effect of sublethal doses of this compound is sedation. Other potent PDE inhibitors, such as papaverine, RO201724, and ICI63197 also tend to act as sedatives rather than as stimulants (34).

The possibility that the central stimulatory effects of caffeine and theophylline result from competitive antagonism of the tonic depressant effect of endogenous adenosine is attractive for several reasons. Intraventricular adenosine injection has been shown to cause behavioral and electrocortical sleep in dogs, cats, and chickens (48,60,80). In humans, the therapeutic administration of the adenosine deaminase inhibitor deoxycoformycin (as an antileukemia agent), which increases circulating (and presumably cerebral) adenosine levels, has the side effect of inducing lethargy and somnolence (78). Most of the pharmacological effects of adenosine in nervous tissue (modulation of adenylate cyclase activity, depression of spontaneous or trans-synaptically evoked neuronal firing, inhibition of neurotransmitter release, inhibition of depolarization-induced enhancement of synaptic calcium influx) can be antagonized by caffeine and theophylline in low (less than 100 μM) concentrations (which have no apparent direct effects on cAMP metabolism or on intracellular calcium dynamics) (34). The behavioral depression induced by slowly metabolized adenosine receptor agonists, such as 1-phenylisopropyladenosine (1-PIA) and cyclohexyladenosine (CHA), can be reversed by low doses of caffeine or theophylline (114). The relative potencies of a number of xanthine derivatives in stimulating spontaneous motor activity correspond to their relative affinities for adenosine receptors, as assessed by their capacity to inhibit the binding of [³H]CHA to the "A_1" adenosine receptor subtype in brain membrane preparations (114). Significantly, the brain levels of these xanthine compounds after the administration of behaviorally effective doses are consonant with their affinities at adenosine receptors (114).

This evidence favors adenosine-receptor blockade as a mechanism for methylxanthine-induced CNS stimulation, although this hypothesis presently lacks rigorous confirmation. Adenosine is rapidly metabolized when administered either systemically or intracranially (51), and it is therefore difficult to study the behavioral effects of physiological levels of the compound. When given intracranially to dogs, cats, and chickens, adenosine induces electrocortical and behavioral sleep patterns (48,60,80); these animals adopt their normal sleeping postures under such circumstances. However, only one case in the literature reports the effect of a peripherally administered methylxanthine, aminophylline (theophylline-ethylene diamine), on the *behavioral* effect of intracranially administered adenosine, and this was in chickens. Adenosine alone, when injected into the hypothalamus or, at higher doses, into the third ventricle, induced sleep lasting 10 to 30 min; after intramuscular injection of aminophylline at a dose (110 μmoles/kg) that produced neither behavioral nor EEG effects on its own, adenosine administration quite anomalously evoked immediate behavioral and electrocortical sleep lasting 3 to 4 hr (60).

Again, because adenosine is rapidly metabolized, relatively stable adenosine analogs are generally used in studies purporting to assess centrally mediated behavioral effects of adenosine and their inhibition by caffeine (41,114). The most commonly used of these, 1-PIA and CHA, unlike centrally administered adenosine, are apparently not hypnotic agents (41,57), although they do produce a behavioral depression in rats and mice in which the animal maintains an upright hunched position with eyes open (41). Because they are metabolically stable and presumably enter the brain, these adenosine analogs are usually administered peripherally, although they are very potent in eliciting hypotension by direct action on the cardiovascular system is lower than effective behavioral-depressant doses (96; R. W. von Borstel, *unpublished observations*); it is therefore possible that some of their behavioral effects may be secondary to a drop in blood pressure or hypothermia. Significantly, *peripherally* administered adenosine produces behavioral depression in mice, similar to that produced by peripherally given 1-PIA or CHA, but results in an EEG pattern characteristic of a waking state (77).

The behavioral-depressant effects of stable adenosine derivatives do correlate well with their relative affinities for brain adenosine receptors of the "A_1" subtype as assessed in [^{3}H]CHA binding assays (114), with the exception of cyclopropyl-carboxamidoadenosine, which is anomalously potent as a behavioral depressant; its affinity for central "A_1" adenosine binding sites is substantially lower than the affinity of 1-PIA (23). The threshold dose for hypotensive effects of this compound is approximately two orders of magnitude lower than that for 1-PIA (96). The sedative action of some of these allegedly specific adenosine agonists wears off after approximately 3 hr, and is often followed by several hours of hyperactivity and occasional hyperphagia (23); similar behavioral activation has not been reported after central or peripheral adenosine administration, although intraperitoneal injection of adenosine (but not of adenine, inosine, or 2-deoxyadenosine) does cause premature arousal of hibernating ground squirrels (126). Administration of low methylxanthine doses during the early sedative phase of the behavioral action of 1-PIA increases spontaneous locomotor activity up to 300% above control levels (114). While it is proposed that central stimulation by methylxanthines may result from adenosine receptor antagonism, this phenomenon might equally well represent an unmasking or potentiation of a latent behavioral activation caused by 1-PIA via mechanisms not necessarily directly related to adenosine receptors. The effects of methylxanthines in the late-appearing phase of behavioral hyperactivity after administration of some adenosine derivatives, such as 1-PIA, have not yet been reported. In addition, although isobutylmethylxanthine (IBMX) is more potent than theophylline as an adenosine-receptor blocker (24), and although peripherally administered IBMX is reported to increase slightly the spontaneous firing frequency of cortical neurons (97), and markedly attenuates the depressant effects of iontophoretically applied adenosine on these neurons [as does theophylline or caffeine (97)], IBMX does not stimulate locomotor activity in mice, except during 1-PIA-induced behavioral depression (57). In this instance, IBMX enhances locomotor activity above that seen in animals not treated with 1-PIA.

Despite these apparent inconsistencies, an action at adenosine receptors is currently the most plausible mechanism for the central stimulatory effects of low to moderate doses of caffeine and theophylline (34). Research less susceptible to artifactual interference by peripheral adenosine-agonists effects might include: (a) behavioral and EEG studies in animals given either a slow infusion of adenosine or very low doses of certain adenosine derivatives directly into intracranial cannulas ending in specific brain regions, particularly the reticular formation; (b) studies of the behavioral effects of xanthine derivatives (8-phenyltheophylline, diethylphenylxanthine) that exhibit much higher affinities for adenosine receptors than do caffeine or theophylline; (c) study of 8-parasulfophenyltheophylline, a compound approximately as potent as theophylline as an adenosine antagonist (24), whose charge may prevent it from gaining access to the intracellular spaces where nonpolar xanthines such as caffeine and theophylline would presumably act were they working via modulation of intracellular calcium translocation, PDE inhibition, or other possible molecular mechanisms. Examination of the possible behavioral action of *p*-sulfophenyltheophylline administered directly into the brain [since its charge also probably prevents free passage across the blood–brain barrier (114)] might provide strong evidence for or against the adenosine hypothesis of methylxanthine action.

The caffeine-induced increase in spontaneous firing frequency of reticular formation neurons could be effectively antagonized by nicotinic acid (niacin) doses of 0.2 to 0.4 mg/kg (50). This observation has not been fully considered in the context of elucidating the mechanism of the effect of caffeine alone, although nicotinamide potentiates the capacity of adenosine to protect mice against audiogenic seizures (77). In addition, niacin reduces the lethality of large doses (300 mg/kg) of caffeine; adenosine analogs are ineffective in this regard (41).

Another mechanism that is sometimes proposed as the basis for methylxanthine effects upon neuronal processes involves changes in cellular calcium dynamics (29). In another excitable tissue, skeletal muscle, high caffeine concentrations (0.5 to 1 mM) augment the twitch response to electrical stimulation; this is apparently the result of the sensitization of calcium release mechanisms in the terminal cisternae of the sarcoplasmic reticulum (102). Higher caffeine concentrations can directly induce muscle contracture, even in the absence of extracellular calcium; this may stem from methylxanthine-induced increases in the calcium permeability of the sarcoplasmic reticulum, which sequesters intracellular calcium in the process of terminating muscular contraction (102).

In nervous tissue, methylxanthine concentrations in excess of 1 mM are needed to demonstrate significant effects on calcium uptake, storage, or release as determined by direct assessment of the dynamics of the calcium isotope $^{45}Ca^{2+}$ in synaptosomes and synaptic vesicles (38). However, some indirect evidence suggests that methylxanthines might facilitate calcium release and/or translocation in nervous tissue; both caffeine and calcium, injected intraventricularly, can antagonize opiate analgesia (65) as well as the opiate-induced reduction in acetylcholine release from the cortical surface (70). Opiate effects may be mediated by changes in calcium disposition in the brain (107). The inhibitory effects of methylxanthines on opiate actions might, however, be ultimately tied to an action at adenosine receptors: Morphine enhances adenosine release from cortical tissue *in vitro* and *in vivo* by a naloxone-reversible mechanism (55,98); adenosine can inhibit cortical acetylcholine release (69); and intracranial administration of adenosine and some of its stable derivatives has been reported to produce analgesia (138). [Curiously, intraperitoneal administration of adenosine *antagonizes* morphine analgesia (59)]. In addition, the stimulatory effect of adenosine on adenylate cyclase and the inhibition of trans-synaptic potentials by the nucleotide can both be attenuated by modest elevations of extracellular calcium concentration (74).

B. Diuretic Effects of Methylxanthines

The three major food-related methylxanthines—caffeine, theophylline, and theobromine—are all effective as diuretic agents, causing increased water, sodium, potassium, and chloride excretion (102). Tolerance and cross-tolerance to all three of these drugs appears during chronic administration (42), suggesting a common mechanism of action.

Theophylline is believed to act as a diuretic via more than one distinct mode of action. It can increase renal blood flow (RBF) and glomerular filtration rate (GFR), apparently as the combined result of enhanced cardiac output and specific renal vascular effects (128). Enhanced RBF is not essential for methylxanthine-induced diuresis, as experiments with isolated kidneys perfused at constant flow rates have shown; methylxanthines also inhibit tubular reabsorption of water and electrolytes (99). The enhancement of RBF and GFR by theophylline is a short-lived (about 15 min) phenomenon whereas peak urine output occurs several hours after methylxanthine administration; thus, depression of tubular reabsorption is probably the dominant physiological basis for methylxanthine diuresis, but increased GFR, when present, is a contributing factor (99).

1. Possible Mechanisms for Methylxanthine-Induced Diuresis

Theophylline concentrations of at least 500 μM are required for 50% inhibition of rabbit kidney cAMP PDE, and the effects of theophylline on isolated rabbit kidney are not mimicked by other PDE inhibitors (63). In addition, enprofylline, which is more active than theophylline as a PDE inhibitor and as a tracheal smooth muscle relaxant, has no diuretic effects in humans or rats (94). These findings argue against the notion that methylxanthines exert their renal effects via PDE inhibition. The apparent inactivity of enprofylline as an antagonist at adenosine receptors strengthens the possibility that adenosine might be involved in the diuretic effect of methylxanthines. This possibility has been proposed on the basis of adenosine's depressant action on RBF (52,88). Adenosine infusion into renal circulation, either *in vivo* (88) or in isolated kidneys (63), causes transient vasoconstriction, potentiates the constrictor response to renal sympathetic nerve stimulation, and induces a marked decrease in GFR; these actions are partially antagonized by low concentrations of theophylline.

Adenosine infusion also can reduce urine volume substantially; however, this particular effect is *not* attenuated by concomitant infusion of theophylline, at least in dogs (88). Further, adenosine reduces RBF and GFR in rats only when the animal's renin–angiotensin system is stimulated by manipulations such as sodium restriction, hemorrhage, or angiotensin infusion; adenosine had very little effect in sodium-loaded rats, and rats consuming "normal" amounts of sodium were not tested in this study (90). The biochemistry of this dependence of renal vascular sensitivity to adenosine on the activity of the renin–angiotensin system is obscure (89); the responsiveness of systemic blood pressure to adenosine was not different in sodium-restricted and sodium-loaded rats. Adenosine inhibits renin release from kidney, and this action is competitively antagonized by theophylline (62).

It is difficult to reconcile these features of adenosine's renal actions with the hypothesis that methylxanthines exert their diuretic effects exclusively via blockade of adenosine receptors. Further, theobromine is not significantly less potent than caffeine as a diuretic in rats (121), whereas theobromine is three to ten times less potent than caffeine as an adenosine antagonist (34,26). Effective diuretic doses of theobromine cause less CNS stimulation than do equally effective diuretic doses of theophylline (99). It would be particularly useful in this case to examine the diuretic potencies of low doses of xanthine derivatives that exhibit a much higher affinity for adenosine receptors (such as 8-phenyltheophylline or diethylphenyltheophylline) than do theophylline, caffeine, or theobromine.

Some evidence suggests that the diuretic effect of methylxanthines may in large part be mediated by prostaglandins (PGs), specifically PGE. Indomethacin administered intravenously in a dose (5 mg/kg) that inhibits prostaglandin synthesis by over 95% significantly attenuated theophylline-induced natriuresis in rabbits (87). In rats, the relative potencies of theophylline, caffeine, and theobromine as diuretic agents correlated well with their respective potencies as stimulators of urinary PGE excretion, and the time course of this increased urinary PGE output corresponded to the time course of increases in urine volume and sodium excretion after theophylline administration (120). Indomethacin (10 mg/kg) almost completely abolished the theophylline-induced increases in PGE, water, sodium, chloride, and potassium excretion. In slices of rat renal medulla, theophylline concentrations as low as 1 μM significantly enhanced the rate of PGE, but not PGF, synthesis (121). PGE inhibits tubular sodium reabsorption and causes dilation of the renal vasculature in several species, including the rat (61). Since tolerance to the diuretic effect of methylxanthines occurs after their administration for a prolonged period (42), it might be important to determine whether chronic methylxanthine administration reduces either the capacity of theophylline to stimulate PGE synthesis or the sensitivity of the kidney to PGE. Since chronic caffeine administration enhances the hypotensive potency of adenosine (129), it might also be useful to examine adenosine's antidiuretic potency in animals subjected to long-term caffeine administration. The biochemical events mediating the stimulation of renal prostaglandin synthesis by methylxanthines are unknown; the potency of theobromine in relation to caffeine in this context suggests that adenosine-receptor antagonism is not involved.

C. Actions of Methylxanthines on the Respiratory Apparatus

The most important uses for methylxanthines in contemporary medical practice are in the treatment of two particular respiratory disorders: bronchial asthma and intermittent apnea of premature infants.

Theophylline and, to a lesser extent, caffeine, are effective as bronchodilators and stimulants of medullary respiratory centers; the application of these pharmacological properties in clinical practice has recently been reviewed (102). However, since relatively high methylxanthine levels (approximately 50 μM in plasma) are required for the treatment of apnea and, in particular, bronchial asthma, undesirable side effects, such as CNS stimulation and cardiovascular effects, can be avoided only by careful monitoring of plasma methylxanthine concentration (102). In addition, theophylline reduces cerebral blood flow in hypoxic rats (136) and reduces anoxic survival time in newborn mice (122); both of these effects are most undesirable, particularly under conditions of impaired respiratory function.

Thus clarification of the mechanism(s) by which methylxanthines exert their beneficial effects on the respiratory apparatus might have real clinical importance: such knowledge might facilitate the design of xanthine derivatives that selectively act on the bronchiole and/or the medullary respiratory centers with minimal effects on other physiologic functions. This strategy has in fact yielded enprofylline (94,95), a drug that is effective as a bronchodilator in humans as well as laboratory animals, and yet seems to lack CNS stimulatory and diuretic effects. The compound is, however, more potent as a cardiac stimulant than is theophylline *in vitro*.

It is likely that no single biochemical mechanism underlies the effects of methylxanthines on respiratory dynamics. Interpretations of the influences of methylxanthines, PDE inhibitors, and adenosine on respiratory processes have largely centered on studies on isolated tracheal preparations *in vitro*. Although this a logical and useful approach, results thus obtained can be misleading, particularly in the case of adenosine, unless appropriate complementary studies are done in relatively intact animals.

1. Bronchodilation by Methylxanthines

Many PDE inhibitors induce relaxation of tracheal smooth muscle *in vitro*, and there is generally a reasonable correlation between their rank order of potency at inhibiting cAMP PDE and their effectiveness at relaxing isolated tracheal preparations (101). Inhibitors with greater specificity for inhibition of cGMP hydrolysis with respect to cAMP are less effective as tracheal relaxants (53). However, there is a marked tachyphylaxis to the relaxant effects of inhibitors specific for cAMP PDE; tachyphylaxis is not apparent in the repeated treatment of tracheal muscle with theophylline or IBMX (53). There is evidence that cAMP levels sometimes do rise during theophylline-induced tracheal relaxation (125), whereas other reports suggest that changes in cAMP levels are not necessarily linked to the relaxant effects of theophylline (72). Moreover, at the maximum plasma concentrations of theophylline (100 μM) found during asthma therapy, cAMP PDE is inhibited by less than 10% in most tissues (102). Thus, although PDE inhibitors do display an action similar to that of methylxanthines in this instance, the effects of methylxanthines themselves, particularly *in vivo*, do not seem to operate mainly by this mechanism.

In vitro, adenosine can have a contracting effect on relaxed tracheal muscle (53,108); the compound also has a modest enhancing effect on antigen-induced release of histamine (a potent bronchoconstrictor, which may contribute to the pathology of asthma) from chopped guinea pig lung tissue (135) and purified rat pleural-cavity mast cells (118). These observations have led to the suggestion that the pharmacological action of theophylline in bronchial asthma may result from an inhibition of the influences of endogenous adenosine on the trachea and cells that release histamine or other anaphylactic mediators (52).

However, most studies on the receptor-mediated actions of adenosine on isolated tracheal muscle report a potent relaxant or spasmolytic effect (22,32,46,71), which is antagonized by theophylline and caffeine at low methylxanthine concentrations (10 to 50 μM). The methylxanthines themselves, at higher concentrations, have relaxant effects in the same system (71). In guinea pig trachea, the effect of adenosine (e.g., relaxation versus contraction) depends on how the tracheal muscle is prepared; transverse strips generally relax in response to adenosine, whereas in the low-tone spirally cut tracheal strips, adenosine tends to induce contractions (108). This dual effect may be the result of differing actions of adenosine on the different muscular components of the trachea.

These conflicting actions of adenosine *in vitro* still leave open the question of whether theophylline acts as a bronchodilator *in vivo* via adenosine antagonism; however, evidence from studies in whole isolated lung and in intact animals suggests that this is probably not the case. As long ago as 1931, it was shown that adenosine (and adenine nucleotides) administered intravenously has a relaxant effect on histamine-constricted guinea pig bronchioles *in vivo* (17). Adenosine also prevents pilocarpine-induced bronchospasm [H. Florey and A. Q. Wells, *unpublished observations* cited by Bennet and Drury (17)]. A more recent study of the actions of adenosine on the respiratory apparatus confirmed that in guinea pigs and dogs, small amounts of adenosine (50 to 100 μg/kg)—and adenine nucleotides—even below the nucleoside's hypotensive threshold, produced only bronchodilation and consistently resulted in attenuation of the bronchoconstriction induced by histamine or acetylcholine administration (19). Much higher doses (20 to 50 mg/kg, i.v.) of 5′AMP, ADP, and ATP caused clear-cut bronchospasm instead of preventing it, whereas even massive doses of adenosine (250 mg/kg, i.v.) did not induce significant bronchospasm *in vivo*. In the same study, it was shown in isolated guinea pig lungs that, whereas low doses of adenosine infused into the pulmonary artery again had only spasmolytic effects, higher adenosine doses given by the same route did indeed have a constrictive effect, thus highlighting the need for *in vivo* experiments in the assessment of the physiological significance of the results of *in vitro* adenosine studies. The effect of methylxanthines on adenosine's influence on the trachea and bronchioles *in vivo* has apparently not been examined.

The physiological significance of the theophylline-reversible potentiating effect of adenosine on antigen-induced histamine release from lung tissue and mast cells is difficult to evaluate; adenosine, even at unphysiologically high concentrations (10 to 100 μM), did not enhance antigen-stimulated histamine release by more than 30% (118). Further, adenosine has been reported to *reduce* antigen-induced histamine release in human basophils (81).

Enprofylline is an alkylxanthine that exhibits potency greater than or equal to that of theophylline as a bronchodilator and as an inhibitor of anaphylactic reactions, yet neither antagonizes the depressant effects of adenosine on guinea pig tracheal or myenteric plexus preparations nor produces enhanced locomotor activity in mice (94,95). Thus, to the degree that enprofylline, caffeine, and theophylline share a similar mechanism of action on the respiratory apparatus, adenosine antagonism does not seem to be a necessary feature in the antiasthmatic actions of methylxanthines. (This is desirable, in view of adenosine's protective effect in hypoxic tissue). Although enprofylline is slightly more potent than theophylline as a PDE inhibitor, this property probably does not contribute to enprofylline's bronchodilator action (95). Considerable evidence argues against a significant role for cAMP in anaphylactic histamine release in mast cells (119). Therefore, the mechanisms whereby methylxanthines exert their clinically important antiasthmatic actions are still undefined. The evidence just cited suggests that neither adenosine receptor antagonism nor PDE inhibition provides an adequate explanation.

2. Methylxanthines in Apnea

Theophylline and caffeine are effective and rapidly acting therapeutic agents in the treatment of intermittent apnea in preterm infants. This disorder, characterized by episodes of apnea lasting more than 20 sec, can lead to neurological damage secondary to hypoxia (102). The theophylline derivative aminophylline is also effective in stabilizing Cheyne-Stokes respiration (alternating periods of rapid and very slow respiration) by virtue of its ethylene-diamine content; interestingly, theophylline alone is apparently ineffective (79).

The beneficial effect of methylxanthines in apnea is apparently the result of an effect on medullary respiratory centers (102), where they increase the sensitivity of central chemoreceptors to P_{CO_2}. Since this represents a "stimulatory" action on nervous tissues, the mediation of this methylxanthine effect by blockade of adenosine receptors is an attractive possibility. Indeed the intraventricular administration of 1-PIA and 2-chloroadenosine (both slowly metabolized adenosine receptor agonists) in cats (45) and rats (85), respectively, produced a depression of respiratory output that could be reversed in both cases with either intravenous or intraventricular aminophylline or theophylline. A very high dose of 1-PIA (10 μg) given into the third ventricle of cats resulted in apnea; this too was reversed by methylxanthines. As in the case of the other central actions of long-acting adenosine analogs, caution must be exercised in extrapolating their effects to those that might be exerted by adenosine itself, particularly that formed endogenously.

A detrimental effect of endogenous adenosine on respiratory processes, implicit in the hypothesis that beneficial effects of methylxanthines reflect adenosine antagonism, might be difficult to reconcile with the substantial body of evidence suggestive of a protective role of adenosine in tissues receiving inadequate oxygenation. This protective effect presumably results from the nucleoside's capacity to increase blood flow and reduce tissue oxygen utilization, particularly in the heart and the brain (18,137).

Adenosine itself, infused into the carotid artery of dogs, causes an increase in respiratory rate and amplitude (19). This effect is not altered by carotid sinus denervation or vagal transection and, most significantly, is enhanced after ligation of the external carotid artery. Thus adenosine itself may actually have a direct stimulatory effect on central respiratory centers; this possibility warrants further study, perhaps with slow adenosine infusions into intracranial catheters ending near medullary respiratory centers. ATP, administered intracranially or intraperitoneally, markedly increased hypoxic survival time in rats (73); adenosine itself has apparently not been tested. Low doses of theophylline (6 mg/kg) markedly reduced anoxic survival time in newborn mice (122). In addition, respiratory stimulation by theophylline alone was abolished in animals given selective lesions of dopamine or serotonin neurons during neonatal development (84); such lesions did not affect the respiratory depressant effects of 2-chloroadenosine in rats (85).

Caffeine and theophylline are much more potent as respiratory stimulants when respiration is depressed by opiates (102). Caffeine doses that do not affect respiration in control subjects can exert significant stimulatory effects in patients given therapeutic doses (10 mg) of morphine. The mechanism underlying this phenomenon is not known, although in the case of another central opiate effect antagonized by caffeine—the inhibition by morphine of cortical acetylcholine release—intraventricular calcium injection also reverses the opiate action (70).

D. Methylxanthine Actions on the Heart

The bolus oral consumption of 250 mg of caffeine, the amount in 2 to 3 cups of coffee, can produce cardiovascular effects in human subjects. Blood pressure increases by 14/10 mm Hg, and heart rate undergoes a slight fall and then a significant rise (105). This caffeine treatment also produces hormonal changes that may be relevant to cardiovascular regulation: Plasma renin activity and plasma and urinary catecholamine levels increase substantially. Theophylline, at therapeutic plasma concentrations (50 to 100 μM), also causes qualitatively similar cardiovascular effects, and these have been shown to coincide with an increase in cardiac contractile force (86). Higher doses of caffeine or theophylline lead to pronounced tachycardia. However, when the same caffeine dose as above (250 mg) is given to subjects who have consumed caffeine daily for 2 weeks, neither cardiovascular nor hormonal changes were observed (106).

Research on the mechanisms whereby caffeine or theophylline exert their positive inotropic and chronotropic effects often focuses on examining on direct methylxanthine actions in isolated heart preparations. In such experiments, methylxanthines do indeed produce increases in contractility (103) and contraction frequency (116), although relatively high methylxanthine concentrations (0.5 to 5 mM) are needed to elicit significant effects. Methylxanthines appear to exert their *direct* stimulatory actions on the heart by enhancing the accessibility of calcium to the intracellular contractile machinery (35). Lower (but still high in the context of physiological significance) levels of theophylline and caffeine (0.1 to 1 mM) can potentiate the responsiveness of isolated atrial preparations to the positive inotropic effects of norepinephrine (103); this has been interpreted as reflecting enhancement of a cAMP-dependent effect by inhibition of cardiac PDE (103). The role of cAMP as mediator of caffeine's inotropic effects has been called into question; while inotropic responses to catecholamines often coincide with increases in tissue cAMP, the adrenoceptors mediating enhanced contractility can be pharmacologically dissociated from those affecting cAMP levels (16). In the perfused rat heart, the PDE inhibitors papaverine and pentoxyfylline, as well as theophylline, markedly raised cAMP content without significantly enhancing cardiac contractility (8). Adenosine enhances cAMP formation (as do β-adrenergic agonists) in guinea pig ventricular slices (68); adenosine, however, decreases myocardial contractility (66), whereas catecholamines increase contractility. In rats *in vivo*, cardioactive caffeine doses (25 mg/kg) have no effect on heart cAMP levels (26). Thus the relationship between the cardiac effects of methylxanthines and their inhibition of cAMP PDE is questionable (as is, perhaps, the relationship between cAMP and myocardial contractility).

In intact, anesthetized rats, caffeine and theophylline doses as low as 3 mg/kg cause significant increases in blood pressure and heart rate (116). These effects, particularly at the lower methylxanthine doses, can be prevented by pretreatment of the rats with reserpine or hexamethonium, which inactivate the sympathetic nervous system, and also by pretreatment with propranolol, a β-adrenergic antagonist (116). Thus the cardiovascular stimulatory effects of methylxanthines may be caused by enhanced catecholamine release from sympathetic nerves and/or the adrenal medulla. It is not known whether this enhanced release is mediated centrally or peripherally. In the study cited above (105), which examined cardiovascular and hormonal effects of 250-mg caffeine doses in humans, plasma norepinephrine and epinephrine levels were increased by 75 and 207%, respectively, suggesting a major contribution by the adrenal medulla. Caffeine and theophylline enhance catechol-amine release from the isolated, perfused adrenal gland, but very high methylxan-thine concentrations (1.6 to 5.5 mM) are required (100). In rats, moderate caffeine or theophylline doses (20 mg/kg, i.p.) enhance the rate of adrenal catecholamine synthesis by 80 and 50%, respectively; adrenal catecholamine levels do not change, suggesting that the catecholamines are being released at a rate corresponding to their synthesis (112). Cervical spinal cord transection prevented the enhancement of adrenal catecholamine synthesis by methylxanthines, indicating the importance of intact nerve impulse flow; such active neural input is generally absent in perfusion studies of isolated organs.

Adenosine, at physiological concentrations ($\sim$1 μM), is an effective inhibitor of norepinephrine release from sympathetic nerves (131); low levels of theophylline and caffeine ($\sim$50 μM or less) antagonize this adenosine effect *in vitro* (44) and *in vivo* (76). Adenosine is apparently less potent, but still active, as an inhibitor of epinephrine release from electrically stimulated, isolated perfused rat adrenal glands (130). Adenosine (and therefore methylxanthines) might be acting at other sites to alter sympathoadrenal catecholamine output; the nucleoside can alter neurotrans-mission in sympathetic ganglia (64), and might well act on CNS pathways regulating sympathetic outflow. Thus the chronotropic and inotropic effects of low doses of methylxanthines *in vivo* may reflect the antagonism of a tonic inhibitory influence of endogenous adenosine on sympathetic nervous activity. Little direct positive evidence supports this view; however, it is a testable hypothesis that seems a more plausible explanation of the cardiovascular effects of caffeine in quantities com-monly consumed than explanations based on *direct* methylxanthine effects like those demonstrated in isolated heart preparations. The latter, as has been discussed, usually require unreasonably high levels of caffeine or theophylline.

The direct stimulatory effects of caffeine and theophylline on isolated hearts probably do not involve significant interaction with adenosine; 3-propylxanthine is inactive at adenosine receptors and yet is more potent than theophylline in stimu-lating rate and force of contraction in isolated hearts (94). It should be recalled that theophylline concentrations of at least 0.5 mM are needed to elicit significant cardiovascular effects in such experimental systems (103).

In summary, caffeine has demonstrable effects on a number of organs, including the brain, the heart, the kidney, and vascular and respiratory tract smooth muscle. The biochemical mechanism currently believed to mediate most such effects is blockade of adenosine receptors, which are themselves heterogeneous, widely dis-tributed, and of varying sensitivity to the methylxanthines. However, it seems apparent that not all of caffeine's important actions can be attributed to this mech-anism.

ACKNOWLEDGMENTS

We wish to thank Dr. Richard Wurtman and Ms. Marianne Callahan for helpful discussions and advice, and Robyn Fizz for assistance in manuscript preparation.

Reid W. von Borstel was the recipient of a National Science Foundation predoctoral fellowship.

REFERENCES

1. Aldridge, A., Aranda, J. V., and Neims, A. H. (1979): Caffeine metabolism in the newborn. *Clin. Pharmacol. Ther.*, 25:447–453.
2. Aldridge, A., Bailey, J., and Neims, A. H. (1981): The disposition of caffeine during and after pregnancy. *Semin. Perinatol.*, 5:310–314.
3. Aldridge, A., and Neims, A. H. (1979): The effects of phenobarbital and β-naphthoflavone on the elimination kinetics and metabolite pattern of caffeine in the beagle dog. *Drug Metab. Dispos.*, 7:378–382.
4. Aldridge, A., and Neims, A. H. (1980): Relationship between the clearance of caffeine and its 7-N-demethylation in developing beagle puppies. *Biochem. Pharmacol.*, 29:1909–1915.
5. Aldridge, A., Parsons, W. D., and Neims, A. H. (1977): Stimulation of caffeine metabolism in the rat by 3-methylcholanthrene. *Life Sci.*, 21:967–974.
6. Aranda, J. V., Costum, B., Turmen, T., Louridas, T., and Collinge, J. (1980): Caffeine burden in young infants. *Pediatr. Res.*, 14:464 (Abstr.).
7. Aranda, J. V., Gorman, W., Outerbridge, E. W., and Neims, A. H. (1977): Pharmacokinetic disposition of caffeine in premature neonates with apnea. *Pediatr. Res.*, 11:414 (Abstr.).
8. Argel, M. I., Vittone, L., Grassi, A. O., Chiappe, L. E., Chiappe, G. E., and Cingolani, H. E. (1980): Effect of phosphodiesterase inhibitors on heart contractile behavior, protein kinase activity and cyclic nucleotide levels. *J. Mol. Cell Cardiol.*, 12:939–954.
9. Arnaud, M. J. (1976): Identification, kinetic and quantitative study of [2-14C] and [1-Me-14C] caffeine metabolites in rat's urine by chromatographic separations. *Biochem. Med.*, 16:67–76.
10. Arnaud, M. J., and Bracco, I. (1980): Fetal and early postnatal caffeine metabolism in the rat. In: *World Conference on Clinical Pharmacology and Therapeutics, London*. Abstract 0556.
11. Arnaud, M. J., Thelin-Doerner, A., Ravussin, E., and Acheson, K. J. (1980): Study of the demethylation of [1,3,7-Me-13C] caffeine in man using respiratory exchange measurements. *Biomed. Mass Spectrom.*, 7:521–524.
12. Arnaud, M. J., and Welsch, C. (1979): Metabolic pathway of theobromine in the rat and identification of two new metabolites in human urine. *J. Agric. Food Chem.*, 27:524–527.
13. Arnaud, M. J., and Welsch, C. (1980): Comparison of caffeine metabolism by perfused rat liver and isolated microsomes. In: *Microsomes, Drug Oxidations, and Chemical Carcinogenesis, Vol. 2*, pp. 813–816. Academic Press, New York.
14. Arnaud, M. J., and Welsch, C. (1980): Caffeine metabolism in human subjects. In: *Ninth Colloquium on the Science and Technology of Coffee, London*, pp. 385–396.
15. Axelrod, J., and Reichenthal, J. (1953): The fate of caffeine in man and a method for its estimation in biological material. *J. Pharmacol. Exp. Ther.*, 107:519–523.
16. Benfey, B. G., Kunos, G., and Nickerson, M. (1974): Dissociation of cardiac inotropic and adenylate cyclase activating adrenoreceptors. *Br. J. Pharmacol.*, 51:253–257.
17. Bennet, D. W., and Drury, A. N. (1931): Further observations relating to the physiological activity of adenine compounds. *J. Physiol. (Lond.)*, 72:288–320.
18. Berne, R. M. (1980): The role of adenosine in the regulation of coronary blood flow. *Circ. Res.*, 47:807–813.
19. Bianchi, A., DeNatale, G., and Giaquinto, S. (1963): The effects of adenosine and its phosphorylated derivatives upon the respiratory apparatus. *Arch. Int. Pharmacodyn. Ther.*, 145:498–517.
20. Birkett, D. J., Grygiel, J. J., and Miners, J. O. (1980): In: *World Conference on Clinical Pharmacology and Therapeutics, London*.
21. Bonati, M., Litini, R., Galletti, F., Young, J. F., Tognani, G., and Garattini, S. (1982): Caffeine disposition after oral doses. *Clin. Pharmacol. Ther.*, 32:98–106.
22. Brown, C. M., and Collis, M. G. (1982): Evidence for an A_2/Ra adenosine receptor in the guinea-pig trachea. *Br. J. Pharmacol.*, 76:381–387.
23. Browne, R. G. (1982): Behavioral activation produced by adenosine analogs (poster abstract #83). *International Symposium on Adenosine*. Charlottesville, Virginia.
24. Burns, R. F., Daly, J. W., and Snyder, S. H. (1980): Adenosine receptors in brain membranes: Binding of N^6 cyclohexyl[^{3}H]adenosine and 1,3-diethyl-8-[^{3}H]phenylxanthine. *Proc. Natl. Acad. Sci. USA*, 77:5547–5551.
25. Burg, A. W. (1975): Physiological disposition of caffeine. *Drug Metab. Rev.*, 4:199–228.

26. Burg, A. W., and Warner, E. (1975): Effect of orally administered caffeine and theophylline on tissue concentrations of 3',5' cyclic AMP and phosphodiesterase. *Fed. Proc.*, 34:332 (Abstr.).
27. Caldwell, J., O'Gorman, J., and Adamson, R. H. (1981): Urinary metabolites of caffeine in the chimpanzee, rhesus monkey and galago. *Pharmacologist*, 23:212 (Abstr.).
28. Callahan, M. M., Robertson, R., Branfmen, A. R., McComish, M., and Yesair, D. W. (1980): Human metabolism of radiolabeled caffeine following oral administration. In: *Ninth Colloquium on the Science and Technology of Coffee*, London.
29. Cardinali, D. P. (1980): Methylxanthines: Possible mechanisms of action in brain. *Trends Pharmacol. Sci.*, 1:405–407.
30. Cavalieri. L. F., Fox, J. J., Stone, A., and Chang, N. (1954): On the nature of xanthine and substituted xanthines in solution. *J. Am. Chem. Soc.*, 76:1119–1122.
31. Christensen, H. D., Manion, C. V., and Kling, O. R. (1981): Caffeine kinetics during late pregnancy. In: *Drug Metabolism in the Immature Human*, edited by L. F. Soyka and G. P. Redmond, pp. 163–181. Raven Press, New York.
32. Coleman, R. A. (1980): Purine antagonists in the identification of adenosine receptors in guinea pig trachea and the role of purines in non-adrenergic inhibitory neurotransmission. *Br. J. Pharmacol.*, 69:359–366.
33. Cook, C. E., Tallent, C. R., Amerson, E. W., Myers, M. W., Kepler, J. A., Taylor, G. F., and Christensen, H. D. (1976): Caffeine in plasma and saliva by a radioimmunoassay procedure. *J. Pharmacol. Exp. Ther.*, 199:679–686.
34. Daly, J. W., Bruns, R. F., and Snyder, S. H. (1981): Adenosine receptors in the central nervous system: Relationship to the central actions of methylxanthines. *Life Sci.*, 28:2083–2097.
35. de Gubareff, T., and Sleator, W. (1965): Effects of caffeine on mammalian atrial muscle, and its interaction with adenosine and calcium. *J. Pharmacol. Exp. Ther.*, 148:202–214.
36. Desmond, P. V., Patwardhan, R., Parker, R., Schenker, S., and Speeg, K. V., Jr. (1980): Effect of cimetidine and other antihistamines on the elimination of aminopyrine, phenacetin and caffeine. *Life Sci.*, 26:1261–1268.
37. Dews, P. B. (1982): Caffeine. *Annu. Rev. Nutr.*, 2:323–341.
38. Diamond, I., and Goldberg, A. L. (1970): Uptake and release of ⁴⁵Ca by brain microsomes, synaptosomes and synaptic vesicles. *J. Neurochem.*, 18:1419–1431.
39. Drouillard, D. D., Vesell, E. S., and Dvorchik, B. H. (1978): Studies on theobromine disposition in normal subjects: Alterations induced by dietary abstention from or exposure to methylxanthines. *Clin. Pharmacol. Ther.*, 23:296–302.
40. Drury, A. N. (1936): The physiological activity of nucleic acid and its derivatives. *Physiol. Rev.*, 16:292.
41. Dunwiddie, T. V., and Worth, T. (1982): Sedative and anticonvulsant effects of adenosine analogs in mouse and rat. *J. Pharmacol. Exp. Ther.*, 220:70–76.
42. Eddy, N. B., and Downs, A. W. (1928): Tolerance and cross tolerance to the diuretic effect of caffeine, theobromine, and theophylline. *J. Pharmacol. Exp. Ther.*, 33:167–174.
43. Eichler, O. (1976): In: *Kaffee and Coffein*, edited by H. P. T. Ammon, C. J. Estler, G. Fulgraff, P. Mitznegg, E. Schmid, O. Strubelt, and O. B. Vitzhum, pp. 491. Springer-Verlag, Berlin.
44. Ekas, R. D., Steenberg, M. L., Eikenberg, D. C., and Lokhandwala, M. F. (1981): Presynaptic inhibition of sympathetic neurotransmission by adenosine in the rat kidney. *Eur. J. Pharmacol.*, 76:301–307.
45. Eldridge, F. L., Millhorn, D. E., and Waldrop, T. G. (1982): Adenosine receptors and the methylxanthines: Involvement in the neural control of respiration. *Fed. Proc.*, 41:1960 (Abstr.).
46. Farmer, J. B., and Farrar, D. G. (1976): Pharmacological studies with adenine, adenosine and some phosphorylated derivatives on guinea pig tracheal muscle. *J. Pharm. Pharmacol.*, 28:748–752.
47. FASEB (1978): Select Committee on GRAS Substances. Evaluation of the health aspects of caffeine as a food ingredient. SCOGS-89, *Federation of the American Society for Experimental Biology*, Bethesda, Maryland. SCOGS-89.
48. Feldberg, W., and Sherwood, S. L. (1954): Injections of drugs into the lateral ventricle of the cat. *J. Physiol. (Lond.)*, 123:148–167.
49. Finke, A., and Czok, G. (1980): Metabolisierung von coffein durch leberschnitte der maus und deren beeinflussing durch athanol und aminophenazon sowie phenobarbital-vorbehandlung der versuchstiere. *Z. Ernahrungswiss*, 19:179–190.
50. Foote, W. E., Holmes, P., Pritchard, A., Hatcher, C., and Mordes, J. (1978): Neurophysiological

and pharmacodynamic studies on caffeine and on interactions between caffeine and nicotinic acid in the rat. *Neuropharmacology*, 17:7–12.

51. Fox, I. H., and Kelley, W. N. (1978): The role of adenosine and 2'deoxyadenosine in mammalian cells. *Annu. Rev. Biochem.*, 47:655–686.

52. Fredholm, B. B. (1980): Are the actions of methylxanthines due to antagonism of adenosine? *Trends Pharmacol. Sci.*, 1:129–132.

53. Fredholm, B. B., Brodin, K., and Strandberg, K. (1979): On the mechanism of relaxation of tracheal muscle by theophylline and other cyclic nucleotide phosphodiesterase inhibitors. *Acta Pharmacol. Toxicol.*, 45:336–344.

54. Fredholm, B. B., and Hedqvist, P. (1980): Modulation of neurotransmission by purine nucleotides and nucleosides. *Biochem. Pharmacol.*, 29:1635–1643.

55. Fredholm, B. B., and Vernet, L. (1978): Morphine increases depolarization-induced purine release from rat cortical slices. *Acta Physiol. Scand.*, 104:502.

56. Friedman, L. (1980): Biochemical effects of methylxanthines. *FDA By-lines*, No. 2, April, pp. 78–103.

57. Garattini, S. (1980): Selected comparative data on metabolic and kinetic differences between human and other species. Report submitted to the FDA.

58. Gorodischer, R., Warzawski, D., and Karplus, M. (1977): Caffeine pharmacokinetics and toxicity in the neonate: Human and animal studies. In: *Proceedings of the 15th International Congress of Pediatrics*, pp. 1209–1210.

59. Gourley, D. R. H., and Beckner, S. K. (1973): Antagonism of morphine analgesia by adenine, adenosine, and adenine nucleotides. *Proc. Soc. Exp. Biol. Med.*, 144:774–778.

60. Haulica, I., Ababei, L., Branisteano, D., and Topoliceahu, F. (1973): Preliminary data on the possible hypnogenic role of adenosine. *J. Neurochem.*, 21:1019–1020.

61. Haylor, J., and Towers, J. (1982): Renal vasodilator activity of prostaglandin E_2 in the rat anesthetized with pentobarbitone. *Br. J. Pharmacol.*, 26:131–137.

62. Hedqvist, P., Fredholm, B. B., and Dakskog, M. (1980): Theophylline-induced release of renin from the rabbit kidney, and its inhibition by adenosine. *Acta Physiol. Scand.*, 108:A35.

63. Hedqvist, P., Fredholm, B. B., and Olundh, S. (1978): Antagonistic effect of theophylline and adenosine on adrenergic neuroeffector transmission in the rabbit kidney. *Circ. Res.*, 43:592–598.

64. Henon, B. K., Turner, D. K., and McAfee, D. A. (1980): Adenosine receptors: Electrophysio-logical actions at pre- and postsynaptic sites. In: *Society for Neuroscience Meeting*, Cincinnati, Ohio. (Abstr.).

65. Ho, I. K., Loh, H. H., and Way, E. L. (1973): Cyclic adenosine monophosphate antagonism of morphine analgesia. *J. Pharmacol. Exp. Ther.*, 185:336–346.

66. Hopkins, S. V. (1973): The potentiation of the action of adenosine on the guinea pig heart. *Biochem. Pharmacol.*, 22:341–348.

67. Horning, M. G., Haegele, K. D., Sommer, K. R., Nowlin, J., Stafford, M., and Thenot, J. P. (1975): Metabolic switching of drug pathways as a consequence of deuterium substitution. In: *Proceedings of the Second International Conference on Stable Isotopes*, pp. 41–54.

68. Huang, M., and Drummond, G. I. (1976): Effect of adenosine on cyclic AMP accumulation in ventricular myocardium. *Biochem. Pharmacol.*, 25:2713–2719.

69. Jhamandas, K., and Sawynok, J. (1976): Methylxanthine antagonism of opiate and purine effects on the release of acetylcholine. In: *Opiates and Endogenous Opiate Peptides*, edited by H. W. Kosterlitz, p. 161. Elsevier, Amsterdam.

70. Jhamandas, K., Sawynok, J., and Sutak, M. (1978): Antagonism of morphine action on brain acetylcholine release by methylxanthines and calcium. *Eur. J. Pharmacol.*, 49:309–312.

71. Jones, T. R., Lefcoe, N. M., and Hamilton, J. T. (1980): Pharmacological study of adenosine and related compounds on isolated guinea pig trachea: Evidence for more than one type of purine receptor. *Can. J. Physiol. Pharmacol.*, 58:1356–1365.

72. Kolbeck, R. C., Speir, W. A., Jr., Carrier, G. O., and Bransome, E. D. C., Jr. (1979): Apparent irrelevance of cyclic nucleotides to the relaxation of tracheal smooth muscle induced by theo-phylline. *Lung*, 156:173–183.

73. Kraynack, B. J., Gintautas, J., and Hinshaw, J. (1981): Adenosine triphosphate increases survival time in hypoxia. *Neuropharmacology*, 20:887–890.

74. Kuroda, Y., Saito, M., and Kobayashi, K. (1976): High concentrations of calcium prevent the inhibition of postsynaptic potentials and the accumulation of cyclic AMP induced by adenosine in brain slices. *Proc. Jpn. Acad.*, 52:86–89.

75. Latini, R., Bonati, M., Castelli, D., and Garattini, S. (1978): Dose-dependent kinetics of caffeine in rats. *Toxicol. Lett.*, 2:267–270.
76. Lokhandwala, M. F. (1979): Inhibition of cardiac sympathetic neurotransmission by adenosine. *Eur. J. Pharmacol.*, 60:353–357.
77. Maitre, M., Ciesielski, L., Leeman, A., Kempf, E., and Mandel, P. (1974): Protective effect of adenosine and nicotinamide against audiogenic seizure. *Biochem. Pharmacol.*, 23:2897–2816.
78. Major, P. P., Agarwal, R. P., and Kufe, D. W. (1981): Clinical pharmacology of deoxycoformycin. *Blood*, 58:91–96.
79. Marais, O. A. S., and McMichael, J. (1937): Theophylline-ethylenediamine in Cheyne-Stokes respiration. *Lancet*, 2:437–440.
80. Marley, E., and Nistico, G. (1972): Effects of catecholamines and adenosine derivatives given into the brain of fowls. *Br. J. Pharmacol.*, 46:619–636.
81. Marone, G., Findlay, S. R., and Lichtenstein, L. M. (1979): Adenosine receptor on human basophils: Modulation of histamine release. *J. Immunol.*, 123:1473–1477.
81a. McCall, A. L., Millington, W. R., and Wurtman, R. J. (1982): Blood-brain barrier transport of caffeine: dose-related restriction of adenine transport. *Life Sci.*, 31:2709–2715.
82. Mitoma, C., Lombrozo, L., Lavalley, S. E., and Dehn, F. (1969): Nature of the effect of caffeine on the drug-metabolizing-enzymes. *Arch. Biochem. Biophys.*, 134:434–441.
83. Mosher, B. A. (1981): The health effects of caffeine. A position paper of the American Council of Science and Health.
84. Mueller, R. A., Lundberg, D. B., and Breese, G. R. (1981): Alteration of aminophylline-induced respiratory stimulation by perturbation of biogenic amine systems. *J. Pharmacol. Exp. Ther.*, 218:593–599.
85. Mueller, R. A., Widerlov, E., and Breese, G. R. (1982): Effect of 2-chloroadenosine on respiratory activity. *Fed. Proc.*, 41:1725 (Abstr.).
86. Ogilvie, R. I., Fernandez, P. G., and Winsberg, F. (1977): Cardiovascular responses to increasing theophylline concentrations. *Eur. J. Clin. Pharmacol.*, 17:409–414.
87. Oliw, E., Auggard, E., and Fredholm, B. B. (1977): Effect of indomethacin on the renal actions of theophylline. *Eur. J. Pharmacol.*, 43:9–16.
88. Osswald, H. (1979): Renal effects of adenosine and their inhibition by theophylline in dogs. *Naunyn Schmiedebergs Arch. Pharmacol.*, 288:79–86.
89. Osswald, H. (1982): Adenosine and renal function. In: *International Symposium on Adenosine*, Charlottesville, Virginia.
90. Osswald, H., Schmitz, H.-J., and Heidenreich, O. (1975): Adenosine response of the rat kidney after saline loading, sodium restriction and hemorrhagia. *Pfluegers Arch.*, 357:323–333.
91. Parsons, W. D., and Neims, A. H. (1978): Effect of smoking on caffeine clearance. *Clin. Pharmacol. Ther.*, 24:40–45.
92. Parsons, W. D., and Neims, A. H. (1981): Prolonged half-life of caffeine in healthy term newborn infants. *J. Pediatr.*, 98:640–641.
93. Patwardhan, R. V., Desmond, P. V., Johnson, R. F., and Schenker, S. (1980): Impaired elimination of caffeine by oral contraceptive steroids. *J. Lab. Clin. Med.*, 95:602–608.
94. Persson, C. G. A., Erjefalt, I., and Karlsson, J.-A. (1981): Adenosine antagonism, a less desirable characteristic of xanthine asthma drugs? *Acta Pharmacol. Toxicol.*, 49:317–320.
95. Persson, C. G. A., Karlsson, J.-A., and Erjefalt, I. (1982): Differentiation between bronchodilation and universal adenosine agitation antagonism among xanthine derivatives. *Life Sci.*, 30:2181–2189.
96. Phillis, J. W. (1982): Evidence for an A_2-like receptor on cerebral cortical neurons. *J. Pharm. Pharmacol.*, 34:453–454.
97. Phillis, J. W., Edstrom, J. P., Kostopoulos, G. K., and Kirkpatrick, J. R. (1979): Effects of adenosine and adenine nucleotides on synaptic transmission in the cerebral cortex. *Can. J. Physiol. Pharmacol.*, 57:1289–1312.
98. Phillis, J. W., Jiang, Z. G., Chelack, B. J., and Wu, P. H. (1979): Morphine enhances adenosine release from the *in vivo* rat cerebral cortex. *Eur. J. Pharmacol.*, 65:97–100.
99. Pitts, R. F. (1959): *The Physiological Basis of Diuretic Therapy*, pp. 204–211. Charles C Thomas, Springfield, Illinois.
100. Poisner, A. M. (1973): Direct stimulant effect of aminophylline on catecholamine release from the adrenal medulla. *Biochem. Pharmacol.*, 22:469–476.
101. Polson, J. B., Krzahowski, J. J., Anderson, W. H., Fitzpatrick. D. F., Hwang, D. C., and Szen-

tivanyi, A. (1978): Analysis of the relationship between pharmacological inhibition of cyclic nucleotide phosphodiesterase and relaxation of canine tracheal smooth muscle. *Biochem. Pharmacol.*, 28:1391–1395.

102. Rall, T. W. (1980): In: *The Pharmacological Basis of Therapeutics*, 6th edition, edited by A. G. Gilman, L. S. Goodman, and A. Gilman, pp. 592–607. Macmillan, New York.

103. Rall, T. W., and West, T. C. (1963): The potentiation of cardiac inotropic responses to norepinephrine by theophylline. *J. Pharmacol. Exp. Ther.*, 139:269–274.

104. Rapoport, J. L., Jensvold, M., Elkins, R., Buchsbaum, M. S., Weingartner, H., Ludlow, C., Zahn, T. P., Berg, C. J., and Neims, A. H. (1981): Behavioral and cognitive effects of caffeine in boys and adult males. *J. Nerv. Ment. Dis.*, 169:726–732.

105. Robertson, D., Frolich, J. C., Carr, R. K., Watson, J. T., Hollifield, J. W., Shand, D. G., and Oates, J. A. (1978): Effects of caffeine on plasma renin activity, catecholamines and blood pressure. *N. Engl. J. Med.*, 298:181–186.

106. Robertson, D., Wade, D., Workman, R., Wooslet, R. L., and Oates, J. A. (1981): Tolerance to the humoral and hemodynamic effects of caffeine in man. *J. Clin. Invest.*, 67:1111–1117.

107. Ross, D. H., Medina, M. A., and Cardenas, H. L. (1974): Morphine and ethanol: Selective depletion of regional brain calcium. *Science*, 186:63–65.

108. Satchell, D. G. (1982): ATP and adenosine cause excitatory or inhibitory responses in the guinea pig trachealis muscle: Studies on mechanism of action (poster abstract #58). *International Symposium on Adenosine*, Charlottesville, VA.

109. Sattin, A. (1971): Increase in the content of adenosine 3′, 5′-monophosphate in mouse forebrain during seizures and prevention of the increase by methylxanthines. *J. Neurochem.*, 18:1087–1096.

110. Sattin, A., and Rall, T. W. (1970): The effect of adenosine and adenine nucleotides on the cyclic adenosine 3′,5′-phosphate content of guinea pig cerebral cortex slices. *Mol. Pharmacol.*, 6:13–23.

111. Schallek, W., and Kuehn, A. (1959): Effects of drugs on spontaneous and activated EEG of the cat. *Arch. Int. Pharmacodyn. Ther.*, 120:319–333.

112. Snider, S. R., and Waldeck, B. (1974): Increased synthesis of catecholamines induced by caffeine and theophylline. *Naunyn Schmiedebergs Arch. Pharmacol.*, 281:257–260.

113. Snyder, S. H. (1981): Adenosine receptors and the actions of methylxanthines. *Trends Neurosci.*, 4:242–244.

114. Snyder, S. H., Katims, J. J., Annau, Z., Bruns, R. F., and Daly, J. W. (1981): Adenosine receptors and behavioral actions of methylxanthines. *Proc. Natl. Acad. Sci. USA*, 78:3260–3264.

115. Statland, B. E., and Demas, T. J. (1980): Serum caffeine half-lives: healthy subjects vs. patients having alcoholic hepatic disease. *Am. J. Clin. Pathol.*, 73:390–393.

116. Strubelt, O. (1969): Uber indirekt-sympathikomimetische wirkungen der methylxanthine. In: *Coffein und andere Methylxanthine*, edited by F. Heim and H. P. T. Ammon. F. K. Schattauer Verlag, Stuttgart.

117. Sved, S., and Wilson, D. L. (1977): Simultaneous assay of the methylxanthine metabolites of caffeine in plasma by high performance liquid chromatography. *Res. Commun. Chem. Pathol. Pharmacol.*, 17:319–331.

118. Sydbom, A., and Fredholm, B. B. (1982): On the mechanism by which theophylline inhibits histamine release from rat mast cells. *Acta Physiol. Scand.*, 114:243–251.

119. Syndbom, A., Fredholm, B. B., and Uvnas, B. (1981): Evidence against a role of cyclic nucleotides in the regulation of anaphylactic histamine release in isolated rat mast cells. *Acta Physiol. Scand.*, 112:47–56.

120. Takeuchi, K., Kogo, H., and Aizawa, Y. (1980): Effect of methylxanthines on urinary prostaglandin E secretion in rats. *Jpn. J. Pharmacol.*, 31:253–259.

121. Takeuchi, K., Kogo, H., and Aizawa, Y. (1981): Effect of theophylline on the release and contents of prostaglandins E and F in rat renal medulla. *Jpn. J. Pharmacol.*, 31:477–479.

122. Thurston, J. H., Hauhart, R. F., and Dirgo, J. A. (1978): Aminophylline increases cerebral metabolic rate and decreases anoxic survival in young mice. *Science*, 201:649–651.

123. Tithapandha, A., Maling, H. M., and Gillette, J. R. (1972): Effects of caffeine and theophylline on activity of rats in relation to brain xanthine concentrations. *Proc. Soc. Exp. Biol. Med.*, 139:582–586.

124. Trang, J. M., Blanchard, J., Conrad, K. A., and Harrison, G. G. (1982): The effect of vitamin C on the pharmacokinetics of caffeine in elderly men. *Am. J. Clin. Nutr.*, 35:487–494.

125. Triner, L., Vulliemoz, Y., and Verosky, M. (1977): Cyclic 3',5'-adenosine monophosphate and bronchial tone. *Eur. J. Pharmacol.*, 41:37–46.
126. Twente, J. W., Twente, J., and Giorgio, N. A. (1970): Arousing effects of adenosine and adenine nucleotides in liberating *Citellus lateralis*. *Comp. Gen. Pharmacol.*, 1:485–497.
127. Van Calker, D., Muller, M., and Hamprecht, B. (1978): Adenosine inhibits the accumulation of cyclic AMP in cultured brain cells. *Nature*, 276:839–841.
128. Vogl, A. (1953): *Diuretic Therapy*, pp. 42–45. Williams & Wilkins, Baltimore.
129. von Borstel, R. W., Wurtman, R. J., and Conlay, L. A. (1983): Chronic caffeine consumption potentiates the hypotensive action of circulating adenosine. *Life Sci.*, 32:1151–1158.
130. Wakade, A. R. (1981): Studies on secretion of catecholamines evoked by acetylcholine or transmural stimulation of the rat adrenal gland. *J. Physiol. (Lond.)*, 313:463–480.
131. Wakade, A. R., and Wakade, T. D. (1978): Inhibition of noradrenaline release by adenosine. *J. Physiol. (Lond.)*, 282:35–49.
132. Warszawski, D., Ben-Zvi, B., and Gorodischer, R. (1981): Caffeine metabolism in liver slices during postnatal development in the rat. *Biochem. Pharmacol.*, 30:3145–3150.
133. Warszawski, D., Gorodischer, R., Moses, S. W., and Bark, H. (1977): Caffeine pharmacokinetics in young and adult dogs. *Biol. Neonate*, 32:138–142.
134. Welch, R. M., Hsu, S. Y., and DeAngelis, R. L. (1977): The effect of Arochlor 1254, phenobarbital and polycyclic aromatic hydrocarbons on the plasma clearance of caffeine in the rat. *Clin. Pharmacol. Pharm.*, 22:791–798.
135. Welton, A. F., and Simko, B. A. (1980): Regulatory role of adenosine in antigen-induced histamine release from the lung tissue of actively sensitized guinea pigs. *Biochem. Pharmacol.*, 29:1085–1092.
136. Winn, H. R., Morii, S., Ngai, A. C., Weaver, D. D., and Berne, R. M. (1982): Effects of theophylline on cerebral blood flow in the rat (poster abstract #27). *International Symposium on Adenosine*, Charlottesville, Virginia.
137. Winn, H. R., Rubio, R., and Berne, R. M. (1981): The role of adenosine in the regulation of cerebral blood flow. *J. Cerebr. Blood Flow Metab.*, 1:239–244.
138. Yarbrough, G. G., and McGuffin-Clineschmidt, J. C. (1980): Neuropharmacological characterization of CNS purinergic receptors (abstract #270.16). *Society for Neuroscience meeting*, Cincinnati, Ohio.

Nutrition and the Brain, Vol. 6 edited by
R. J. Wurtman and J. J. Wurtman.
Raven Press, New York © 1983.

Role of the Food and Drug Administration in Regulation of Neuroeffective Food Additives

*David G. Hattan, *Sara H. Henry, *Stephen B. Montgomery,
*Marvin J. Bleiberg, **Alan M. Rulis, and *P. Michael Bolger

*Division of Toxicology and **Division of Food and Color Additives, Bureau of Foods,
Food and Drug Administration, Washington, D.C. 20204*

I. INTRODUCTION

A number of substances that exhibit neurotoxic potential have been associated, either directly or indirectly, with the food supply. The purpose of this chapter is to analyze some prime examples of this type of toxicity and to acquaint the reader with the role of the Food and Drug Administration (FDA) in the regulation of such substances.

We address first the relationship between the requirements of the law, on the one hand, and scientific knowledge about these substances, on the other. Next we consider at some length several specific chemical substances with known neurotoxic potential, examining both the scientific and the public policy issues that make these examples notable. Finally, we conclude this chapter with a summary of regulatory processes and events utilized in control of substances with neurotoxic potential, and a brief assessment of the present usefulness of routine neurotoxicological testing of food additives.

II. INTERACTION OF LAW AND SCIENCE

The manner in which the FDA handles neuroeffective substances in food, as it does any other chemical substance of concern, must be studied against the backdrop of the Federal Food, Drug, and Cosmetic Act (the Act) (22). The concern of the FDA with regard to such substances originates in this law, and it is often only within the context of the law that the agency's different means of handling such substances, even when they may exhibit similar toxicological properties, may be perceived as consistent. The present food law provides, among other things, statements about (a) the types of food-related substances and associated health effects that are of societal concern and thus subject to FDA authority; (b) the scientific standards of safety that are to be brought to bear on such substances (including assignment of the burden of proof and the degree of uncertainty to be tolerated with such proof); and (c) the administrative and legal procedures that are to be used by the FDA to ensure compliance with these standards.

By its very nature, therefore, FDA's enabling legislation invites interaction with science, may influence the direction of scientific research, and, in turn, must itself respond to the challenges often posed by new scientific knowledge. A prime historical example of such reciprocal influence is the famed Delaney Clause that forbids the purposeful addition to food of food additives or color additives that have been shown to cause cancer. Incorporation of this clause into the Act in 1958 reflected new scientific knowledge and societal concerns about the carcinogenic potential of chemicals (29,192). The Act as presently written makes no such specific mention of neurotoxic substances. Therefore, FDA's treatment of chemical compounds that exhibit a capacity to affect human neurological functions derives from generic, legal, and scientific standards that could as well apply to any other "classic" toxic phenomenon.

There are two important characteristics of the law–science interaction that will assist readers of this chapter to understand FDA's treatment of specific neurotoxic substances in food. First, because of the way the sections of the Act have been structured and amended over the years, food-related substances subject to the Act may fall into one or more separate regulatory "categories." These categories include food, food additives, color additives, naturally occurring environmental contaminants, inherent constituents of raw agricultural commodities, pesticide residues, and animal drug residues. Table 1 contains a more complete listing of these regulatory categories along with references to sections of the Act that pertain to them. The existence of such categories in the law means that the scientific and legal standards applied to substances may differ from one category to another. Therefore, the standards that FDA may apply in controlling risk from a neurotoxic substance will be partly determined by the category(ies) into which the substance falls.

Second, the agency may choose from a range of regulatory options and administrative procedures in handling different problems. This flexibility allows the agency to act appropriately, depending on the degree of risk or potential risk to the public, and to continue to apply the static language of the present law to different situations that are part of an ever-changing scientific and technological landscape.

TABLE 1. *Food-related regulatory categories derived from the Food, Drug, and Cosmetic Act*

Category	Generic example(s)	Specific example(s)	Safety standard	Section of the Act
Food	Raw agricultural commodities; traditional food—raw, unprocessed, processed	Apples, potatoes, bread, meat	"May render injurious"[a] "Ordinarily render injurious"	201(f), 402(a)(1), 201(r)
"GRAS" ingredients	Antioxidants, emulsifiers, texturizers	Salt, dextrose, caramel, benzoic acid, caffeine	"May render injurious" "Ordinarily render injurious"	201(s), 402
Prior sanctioned ingredients[b]	Directly added ingredients, packing materials	Lead solder seams in cans, nitrite (for certain uses)	"May render injurious" "Ordinarily render injurious"	402
Nutrients (added essential)	Vitamins, minerals, amino acids, proteins	Vitamin A, zinc, tryptophan	"May render injurious" "Ordinarily render injurious"	402, 411
Food additives				
Direct	Antioxidants, emulsifiers, flavors, sweeteners	Sodium nitrite, aspartame	Reasonable certainty of no harm	201(s), 409, 402
Indirect	Packaging materials and components	Acrylamide, polyvinyl chloride, vinyl chloride monomer	Reasonable certainty of no harm	
Secondary direct	Ion-exchange resins		Reasonable certainty of no harm	
Color additives	Natural colors	Carotene, grape skin extract, turmeric	Reasonable certainty of no harm	201(t), 706, 402
	Synthetic colors	FD & C Red 40, FD & C Red 3		
Animal drugs	Growth promotants coccidiostats, therapeutics			201(w), 402, 512
Pesticides (residues)	Insecticides herbicides	Organophosphates, chlorinated hydrocarbons	Standard of section 402 residues set by EPA	201(q), 402, 408
Unavoidable contaminants	Ubiquitous—poisonous and deleterious substances, both industrial and naturally occurring (environmental)	MeHg, polychlorinated biphenyls, lead, saxitoxin, aflatoxin	Standard of section 402 tolerance levels	402, 406

[a]Section 402(a) states, "A food shall be deemed to be adulterated if it bears or contains any poisonous or deleterious substances which may render it injurious to health."
[b]"Prior sanctioned" food ingredients are substances permitted for specific uses prior to 1958 on the basis of an explicit written agency opinion.

A. Categories

The Act, as written at present, is the product of numerous amendments that have been made over the span of time since passage of the first United States food law, the Food and Drugs Act of 1906. It is, however, the 1938 version that forms a substantial foundation for the present law. At that time, Congress added provisions (the present Section 402) for determining whether food was adulterated because of the presence of poisonous or deleterious substances (including inherent constituents of raw agricultural products). More recently, in 1958 and in 1960, Congress again amended the Act to require the premarket safety testing of new food additives (Section 409) and color additives (Section 706), respectively. There is also a section that addresses the question of pesticides on raw agricultural commodities (Section 408) and one (Section 406) that deals with environmentally added contaminants in food.

Individual sections of the present law, therefore, address different *categories* of food-related substances, any one of which conceivably could comprise a material with neurotoxic potential. The category into which a food or food-related substance may fall is a result of factors such as the chemical nature, the intended use, and the origin or intrinsic toxicological character of the substance. The safe use of a given substance in food may even be governed simultaneously by the standards of more than one category.

This concept of food-related regulatory categories is perhaps the greatest source of misunderstanding of FDA's actions, because many believe that the law strictly forbids *any* amount of any "toxic" substance to be present in food and that the agency ensures complete safety in this way.

In spite of popular misconceptions, no standard of absolute safety is demanded (except for a food or color additive that is a carcinogen); FDA may apply a variety of safety standards to substances depending on the regulatory categories in which they are placed. These differing standards reflect Congress' implicit intent over the years both to provide for the safety of food (including substances added to food) and to maintain an economically affordable and abundant food supply.

Table 1 lists the food-related regulatory categories that the present law prescribes. Listed also are some examples of substances likely to comprise such categories, the various sections of the law that address these categories, and the relative standards of safety that apply in each case. The requirements for proof of safety under these standards are not always fixed absolutely either by law or by regulation. They have always been subject to interpretation by both the FDA and the courts. Each standard designates who bears the burden of proof of safety. But the actual level of uncertainty tolerated in the scientific data and the level of possible risk to public health that is tolerated from category to category can best be seen by comparing several specific examples. The examples were chosen because they contain at least one substance discussed in detail later in this chapter.

1. Food and General Food Safety (Section 402)

In determining whether food itself is adulterated (and hence unsafe), the law prescribes two related standards of safety depending on whether the substance of concern is "naturally occurring" in food or is an "added" substance.[1] For convenience we refer to them as the "may render" standard (for added substances) and the "ordinarily render" standard (for naturally occurring substances). These standards originate in the 1938 version of the Act, and remain unchanged to the present day in Section 402.

These safety standards are sometimes referred to as the "general adulteration provisions," and leave the burden on the FDA to produce a proper level of evidence of actual harm or possible harm to consumers before the agency may seize or take other legal action against a food that appears to violate these standards.

For a large number of possible substances present in food, such as the so-called GRAS (Generally Recognized As Safe) substances (18–20,146), as well as traditional food items, the choice of safety standard (whether "may render," or the more lenient "ordinarily render") depends on whether the substance is present in food naturally or is determined to be an added substance. Substances with a history of use in food (such as salt, for example) can be used as long as they remain Generally Recognized as Safe. If a concern arises about a particular food to which such a substance is added, the agency then concludes whether the addition of such a substance "may render" the food injurious to health. In the case of nonadded substances, the determination of whether the substance is indeed subject to the more lenient "ordinarily injurious" standard may depend on the intended use or the processing conditions of the final food product. Aflatoxin, discussed below, though found naturally in many common food crops, has been considered by the FDA to be an "environmentally added" substance. However, some agricultural products that are meant to be consumed as harvested and that contain a naturally occurring poisonous or deleterious component, such as the solanine present in potatoes (49,103,113,297), will usually be subject to the "ordinarily injurious" standard. The agency would consider such foods not adulterated if the substance of concern does not "ordinarily render" the food injurious to health. An example of a neuroeffective food component present as a nonadded substance in food is the caffeine occurring naturally in coffee beans.

Certain types of food-related substances are either exempt from these Section 402 standards or are addressed specifically elsewhere in the Act. Examples of these are approved food additives (Section 409), approved color additives (Section 706), approved pesticide residues (Section 408), environmentally added contaminants (Section 406), and certain drugs used in food-producing animals (Section 512). In

---

[1] Section 402(a)(1) of the Food, Drug, and Cosmetic Act states: "A food shall be deemed to be adulterated—if it bears or contains any poisonous or deleterious substance which *may render* it injurious to health; but in case the substance is not an added substance such food shall not be considered adulterated under this clause if the quantity of such substance in such food does not *ordinarily render* it injurious to health . . .".

the case of environmental contaminants and pesticides, the safety standard applied is the same as in Section 402, although the legal procedures for determining safety may differ.

2. *Environmental Contaminants (Section 406)*

Certain "poisonous or deleterious" substances including possible neurotoxins are environmental contaminants that may be present in food, but also may be unavoidable by good manufacturing practice. These substances are not legally food additives but may be allowed under Section 406 to be present in food, and if used in accordance with a Section 406 tolerance do not cause the food to be adulterated according to the safety standards of Section 402 (above).

Examples of unavoidable contaminants are the following: (a) mycotoxins (232) such as aflatoxin, produced by mold and present in raw agricultural products such as wheat, corn, peanuts, or even milk, or saxitoxin, a naturally occurring neurotoxin responsible for paralytic shellfish poisoning and discussed later in this chapter; (b) ubiquitous industrial pollutants such as polychlorinated biphenyls and methylmercury; or (c) ubiquitous naturally occurring heavy metals such as lead or mercury. To avoid removing from the food supply large amounts of valuable agricultural produce, Section 406 allows the FDA, in some cases, to set either "tolerances" or the less formal so-called "action levels" for such contaminants (13) so that food containing these chemicals can be safely consumed. When a tolerance or action level is set for a specific substance, the food containing it at or below the announced level is not considered "adulterated" according to the safety standard of Section 402 *(see above)*. Action levels and tolerances represent limits at or above which FDA may take legal action to remove adulterated products from the market. Where no established action levels or tolerances exist, the FDA may take action against the product at the minimal detectable level of the contaminant.

Legally, the setting of a formal tolerance under Section 406 requires the FDA to use a very time-consuming formal rulemaking process. Therefore, to date, only one formal tolerance has been set (for polycholorinated biphenyls in foods and food packaging) (52). On the other hand, the agency has set "action levels" for the presence of substances such as methylmercury and aflatoxin in foods (13). At present, the action level for mercury in fish is 1.0 parts per million (ppm) (mg/kg of product) and for aflatoxin in peanuts it is 20.0 parts per billion (ppb) (μg/kg of product).

The FDA may establish these action levels and tolerances on the basis of unavoidability of poisonous or deleterious substances and on the basis of the actual health risks associated with ingestion of such materials at the levels of occurrence.

Action levels and tolerances do not represent permissible levels of contamination where it is avoidable (13). The blending of a food containing a substance in excess of an action level or tolerance with another food with a contamination that is below the action level is not normally permitted, and the final product resulting from blending is unlawful, regardless of the level of the contaminant in the blended product.

3. Food Additives (Section 409)

In 1958, Congress amended the Act by adding Section 409. This provision requires that manufacturers assume the burden of adequately testing new food additives[2] to ensure their safety before they may be added to any food. The manufacturer is required by law to file with FDA a written petition that contains the scientific data adequate to support safety. The agency reviews the petition and if the data are adequate, publishes a regulation in the *Federal Register* permitting the safe use of the additive.

This provision ensures that the intended use of the substance in food (when both the toxic potential and consumer exposure is taken into account) meets the safety standard of "reasonable certainty of no harm."[3] This standard is more stringent than the general food safety provisions of Section 402.

The "reasonable certainty of no harm" safety standard, sometimes referred to as the general safety provision for food additives, requires that the petition submitted in support of any new food additive contain detailed data from adequately performed toxicological feeding studies and an adequate evaluation of the probable exposure of consumers to the new substance (23,24). However, the additive need not be shown to be absolutely safe.[4] The boundaries of this "reasonable certainty" have never been formalized rigidly by the FDA. In the past, the agency has taken the position that even though the wording of the law is indeed static, the diverse results of many scientifically valid types of data may properly support a finding that the proposed use of a food additive will cause "no harm" to consumers. Section 170.20 of the Code of Federal Regulations (21 CFR 170.20) at present explains the general scientific criteria that FDA uses in evaluating a food additive petition. That regulation cites the "principles and procedures ... stated in 'current' publications of the National Academy of Sciences, National Research Council" as a guide for agency

---

[2]The term "food additive" refers only to a specific set of substances defined by Section 201(s) as follows: "The term 'food additive' means any substance the intended use of which results or may reasonably be expected to result, directly or indirectly, in its becoming a component or otherwise affecting the characteristics of any food (including any substance intended for use in producing, manufacturing, packing, processing, preparing, treating, packaging, transporting, or holding food; and including any source of radiation intended for any such use), if such substance is not generally recognized, among experts qualified by scientific training and experience to evaluate its safety, as having been adequately shown through scientific procedures (or, in the case of a substance used in food prior to January 1, 1958, through either scientific procedures or experience based on common use in food) to be safe under the conditions of its intended use; except that such term does not include

(1) a pesticide chemical in or on a raw agricultural commodity; or
(2) a pesticide chemical to the extent that it is intended for use or is used in the production, storage, or transportation of any raw agricultural commodity; or
(3) a color additive; or
(4) any substance used in accordance with a sanction or approval granted prior to the enactment of this paragraph pursuant to this Act, the Poultry Products Inspection Act or the Meat Inspection Act; or
(5) a new animal drug."

[3]The Act uses only the word "safe." The term "reasonable certainty of no harm" derives from the legislative history of the bill and has been incorporated into FDA regulations (23).

[4]The exceptions, of course, are carcinogens, which are not permitted as food additives at any level.

use in safety evaluation of food additives. NAS has written testing standards from time to time in separate publications for both public and agency use, but these testing requirements have been stated in relatively general terms (35,36,44,47,48). In practice FDA has, through the years, applied the current toxicological criteria and exposure information in assessing the safety of each food additive. The agency has, in effect, continuously adjusted food additive safety requirements as necessary to reflect both the steady progress of science and the most current information about population exposure to additives.

The FDA has recently published a document entitled "Toxicological Principles for the Safety Assessment of Direct Food Additives" (51). This document comprises the most up-to-date articulation of the toxicological safety testing required by the "reasonable certainty of no harm" safety standard.

None of the routinely required tests has protocols solely designed for investigating neurotoxic phenomena. Nevertheless, during the review of any required test, the appearance of any neurotoxic effects is noted and is relevant to the outcome of the final safety evaluation of the food additive.

The evaluation of the toxicological studies performed on any food additive results in knowledge about the potential adverse effects that may arise from ingestion of the substance, the levels of exposure likely to cause such effects, and the "no-adverse-effect" level. On the basis of this no-adverse-effect level, an appropriate safety factor (often a value of about 1:100, when the data are derived from lifetime feeding studies in rodents) is applied to arrive at an estimate of maximum "acceptable daily intake" (ADI) of the additive for humans. This ADI is then compared with the estimated daily intake (EDI) of the substance for use in food. If the EDI is less than the ADI, the use of the substance as a food additive is considered safe by FDA.

Aspartame, discussed at length below, is one example of a potentially neuroeffective substance that falls under the strict legal definition of "food additive." As in the case of other potential food additives, aspartame was subjected to a premarket

TABLE 2. *Certified color additives permitted for food use*

Color additive	Approved listing		
	Provisional	Permanent	Restricted use
FD & C Red No. 3 (Erythrosine)		*	
FD & C Red No. 40		*	
FD & C Yellow No. 5 (Tartrazine)		*	
FD & C Yellow No. 6 (Sunset Yellow FCF)	*		
FD & C Blue No. 1 (Brilliant Blue FCF)		*	
FD & C Blue No. 2 (Indigotene)	*		
FD & C Green No. 3 (Fast Green FCF)	*		
Citrus Red No. 2			*
Orange B			*

safety evaluation, with the burden of proving safety placed squarely upon the company sponsoring the compound.

In addition to the so-called "direct" food additives, there are also "indirect" additives. These are substances that satisfy the legal definition of food additives (see footnote 2), usually because of their use in packaging materials that come into contact with food. Acrylamide, a known neurotoxic agent, is a possible low-level constituent of some common food packaging materials and is discussed below.

4. Color Additives (Section 706)

Color additives[5] for use in food, like the food additives considered in Section 409, require premarket safety evaluation by the FDA. The toxicological testing criteria essentially are the same, as is the prohibition against carcinogens.[6] These requirements were added to the law in 1960 as the "Color Additive Amendments." The amendments, now in Section 706, (a) provide the FDA with the authority to set forth conditions for the safe use of color additives in foods, drugs, and cosmetics; (b) require premarketing clearance from the FDA by establishing the safe conditions of use of the color additive; (c) include the anticancer Delaney Clause; and (d) provide for a temporary (provisional) listing of color additives already in use as of July 12, 1960 as well as a permanent listing for color additives. The temporary listing (initially for $2\frac{1}{2}$ years) was established to allow the time necessary to complete safety testing of the colors then in use and evaluation of analytical methods.

There are two categories of color additives used in food: those that are derived through synthetic chemical manufacturing (artificial) and those that are derived from natural products (natural pigments). Table 2 lists those artificial color additives currently approved for use in foods and Table 3 lists those natural color additives currently approved for use in foods (21 CFR Part 73).

A color additive intended for food use is regulated by two procedures. One is through premarketing approval to ensure human safety; the other is through postmarketing surveillance to assure good manufacturing practices (GMP). Premarketing approval procedures establish the safety of a compound, using appropriate animal models as in the case of food additives, while postmarketing surveillance entails certification of the dye to ensure that it meets predetermined chemical specifications.

Scientists have speculated for some time about the potential of certain color additives to effect changes in neuronal activity, especially with respect to possible behavioral disturbances. The example chosen for detailed discussion later in this chapter, erythrosine, although studied more thoroughly than some color additives, is still the source of much disagreement concerning its neuroeffective potential.

---

[5] Section 201(t) of the Act defines "Color additive" as . . . material which

(A) is a dye, pigment, or other substance made by a process of synthesis or similar artifice, or extracted, isolated, or otherwise derived, with or without intermediate or final change of identity, from a vegetable, animal, mineral, or other source, and

(B) when added or applied to a food, drug, or cosmetic, or to the human body or any part thereof, is capable (alone or through reaction with other substance) of imparting color thereto."

[6] Section 706 has its own version of the Delaney Clause, namely Section 706(b)(5)(B).

TABLE 3. *"Natural" food color additives permitted for food use*

	Earliest reported use
β-APO-8′-carotenal	1960
Caramel	1900
β-Carotene	1950
Annatto extract	1878
Paprika[a]	1877
Paprika oleoresin[a]	1927
Turmeric	1877
Turmeric oleoresin[a]	1948
Saffron	1930
Titanium dioxide	1959
Cochineal extract (Carmine)	1940
Grape skin extract (Enocianina)[a]	1950
Ferrous gluconate	1932
Dehydrated beet extract[a]	1952
Riboflavin[a]	1940
Canthaxanthin	1964
Carrot oil	—
Fruit juice	—
Vegetable juice	—
Toasted partially defatted cooked cottonseed flour	—

[a]May be used as either a flavoring or a coloring additive.

B. Options for Regulatory Control

The wording of the law is static (and demands that definitive judgments be made). But science, on the other hand, by its very nature, is constantly evolving and improving and not always amenable to pat answers. The discontinuity between these two aspects (i.e., law and science) of the work of the FDA may mean that, over time, one aspect can get out of step with the other. For example, scientific developments such as the increased capacity to detect and identify toxic trace contaminants, including potentially neurotoxic ones in certain foods, may require the agency to adopt policies not anticipated when the law was drafted. On the other hand, the law may demand a judgment or require a finding of fact that scientific knowledge is at present unable to deliver.

Fortunately, the law is worded generally enough to allow some interpretation by both the agency and the courts. In addition, the law mandates that FDA write interpreting regulations to implement the law's various provisions, and that the agency publish these regulations in the *Federal Register*, thus amending Title 21 of the *Code of Federal Regulations*. By means of such regulations, the agency interprets and administers the law in specific situations.

Of course, more than just the science may change over the years. As a result of lifestyle as well as technological changes, public exposure to different food-related substances may change over time as well (34). Because the exposure of people to various substances in the food supply may change with time, the agency develops data and writes guidelines for estimating the levels of exposure of consumers to food substances (21,53). It then may use these exposure estimates to arrive at and continually update the EDI of given substances. In this way, the agency may continually survey the food supply to determine that exposure of the public to substances remains within acceptable limits.

The law and FDA regulations provide for a number of alternative procedures for the agency to address public health concerns that relate to consumer exposure to toxic substances in food. The enforcement tools that are used depend on the category in which the substance has been placed, as well as the degree to which the substance in question might violate a particular safety standard for that category.

The FDA has several alternatives for protecting the public from unsafe food itself. When food has been shown to be unsafe because an added substance present *may render* the food injurious to health, the FDA on reasonable grounds may simply warn a manufacturer by letter, may order a product recall, may impound the suspect food, or may actually seize food products if the threat to public health is great enough. Methods such as these may also be used in the case of food containing a nonadded, naturally occurring substance that renders the food *ordinarily injurious* to health.

In the case of food additives that are already approved, the agency, on finding new information that questions the safety of an additive, may ban the substance or place the additive on an "interim list" as long as new studies to answer safety questions are performed on the substance within an acceptable time.

Many agency actions, such as bans, proposals of tolerances, or interim listing, proceed by "notice and comment" rulemaking, a process during which all interested parties, including scientists, may comment or file objections. For food additives, color additives, or the setting of Section 406 tolerances, persons adversely affected by a final regulation may have recourse to a hearing before an administrative law judge, or as an alternative, a scientific board of inquiry. After a final agency decision on any action, persons have recourse to the courts of law (14,23,28,37–40).

III. FDA ACTIVITY IN THE ASSESSMENT OF THE NEUROTOXIC POTENTIAL OF SUBSTANCES OCCURRING IN FOODS

A. Food Additives

1. Direct: Aspartame

a. Aspartame regulation history

With respect to the safety assessment of direct food additives, a consideration of the history of aspartame regulation is quite useful from two important perspectives. First, this substance was subjected to a greater number of administrative regulatory procedures than most substances and will serve to illustrate those procedures discussed in Section II, A, 3 above. Second, the safety assessment for this compound involved the resolution of several complex neurotoxicological issues, including analyses of the *potential* of aspartame to exacerbate preexisting capacity for mental retardation, and to cause brain lesioning and central nervous system neoplasms in animals.

In February, 1973, the sponsor submitted a food additive petition to the FDA, Bureau of Foods, requesting the approval of aspartame as a sweetener and flavor enhancer (33). Since there were a number of toxicological questions to be answered, it was more than 1 year later before the Bureau of Foods published the regulation for aspartame (25). Shortly thereafter, interested parties requested a hearing on possible safety hazards inherent to consumption of aspartame (211).

The usual procedure for evaluation of these types of objections to a food additive has been to hold a formal evidentiary public hearing before an administrative law judge. In the instance of aspartame, however, the FDA's General Counsel sent a letter in January, 1975 suggesting that a Public (Scientific) Board of Inquiry (PBOI) be held (31,149). The PBOI was to consist of presentations of the scientific data used to assess the compound's safety and the data would be presented to a panel or "Board" of three experts appointed by the FDA commissioner. After presentations and time for analysis of these scientific data, the board of experts would present its decision on the safety of the subject compound to the FDA Commissioner. The FDA Commissioner would then make the final decision on the regulatory status of the compound, i.e., whether the FDA would approve or reject the sponsor's application for the use of aspartame (31).

There was agreement by the concerned parties to discuss the following issues at the PBOI:

(a) Does aspartame pose a risk of contributing to mental retardation or other brain damage when ingested alone or in combination with glutamate?

(b) If approval of aspartame marketing is not withdrawn, what label warnings, if any, are appropriate?

At the same time, April, 1975, the sponsor agreed to a voluntary postponement of the marketing of aspartame until the toxicological significance of uterine polyps in aged female rats in the chronic study with the aspartame breakdown product, diketopiperazine (DKP), could be determined (191). Later that same year, three outside independent pathology groups had been consulted and the consensual interpretation of the uterine polyp data was that there was no evidence of damage to rat uterine tissue (polyps) that could be specifically associated with DKP administration in the chronic rat feeding study (242).

At about the same time, however, the FDA Commissioner had testified before a Senate subcommittee that questions concerning the authenticity of certain of the sponsor's data that had been used to establish the safety of aspartame had been discovered (46). A few months later the FDA Commissioner stayed the effectiveness of the aspartame regulation until the sponsor's safety data on aspartame could be reviewed and authenticated (190).

There followed a protracted dialogue between the FDA and the sponsor about how the safety data for aspartame could be authenticated; i.e., who would do the authentication, and who would pay for the procedure. Finally, in September, 1976, the sponsor agreed to pay an independent pathology group, Universities Associated for Research and Education in Pathology (UAREP), for the authentication of selected studies that served as the basis for the safety assessment of aspartame (285). Near the end of this same year, after invitation by the FDA Chief Counsel, interested parties proposed four additional studies to be authenticated by UAREP. Following the acceptance of three of these four studies for review and authentication, the FDA clarified UAREP's role in the authentication procedures. UAREP was to ascertain whether the reports of the critical aspartame studies accurately, completely, and reliably reflected the primary data collected. UAREP did not consider the technical competence demonstrated in the planning and execution of the studies or the correctness or meaning of the conclusions to be drawn from the studies. This latter role was undertaken by the FDA (160).

The authentication report on three of the studies was performed by FDA personnel and the FDA Commissioner informed Searle that the data from studies examined by the FDA were basically consistent with the raw data in the firm's possession (164). More than 1 year later, in December, 1978, UAREP's authentication report on the 12 pivotal Searle studies was received by the FDA. A few months later the FDA Bureau of Foods released a document that reported the UAREP report's conclusions that there were no discrepancies in any of the sponsor's reports that were of sufficient magnitude or of a nature that would compromise the data as originally submitted (249).

With the authenticity of the sponsor's safety data on aspartame affirmed, the FDA proceeded to prepare for a PBOI on the potential hazards that might accompany the ingestion of aspartame. During April, 1979, the Bureau of Foods published a letter that outlined the scientific issues to be discussed at the PBOI (196). These issues were agreed to by the objectors to aspartame approval and the Bureau of Foods:

(a) Whether ingestion of aspartame, alone or together with glutamate, poses a risk of contributing to mental retardation, brain damage, or undesirable effects on the neuroendocrine system.

(b) Whether ingestion of aspartame may induce brain neoplasms in the rat.

(c) On the basis of answers to the above questions, should aspartame be allowed for use in foods or should approval be withdrawn? If allowed for use in foods, what conditions of use and labeling (if any) should be required?

The Public Board of Inquiry on aspartame was held early in 1980 and during a 3-day period factual testimony and expert opinion were supplied by a number of participants: representatives of the sponsor, the FDA Bureau of Foods, and other interested scientists. This survey of aspartame data and presentation of expert opinion were heard by a panel of three scientists who subsequently will be referred to as the "Board." The following section will review and discuss a number of the more significant scientific questions and interpretations that the Bureau of Foods and other scientists considered during the safety assessment of aspartame.

b. Major scientific issues

The regulation of aspartame is based on one of the most complete series of toxicological tests ever compiled for a single food additive. Not only was there a complete series of toxicological tests in animals, but an ambitious program of clinical testing was conducted as well. G.D. Searle and Company submitted to the FDA Bureau of Foods the results of more than 100 studies on the safety of aspartame. As indicated in the previous section, the regulation of aspartame involved the resolution of a number of complex scientific issues; however, in this discussion only the most important and comprehensively deliberated issues relating to neurotoxicity will be considered.

For the purpose of food additive safety determinations, the types of toxic response or risk potentially present in substance use are of two classes: first, food additives that have demonstrated reasonable probability of no harm (are safe) at or below a certain level of consumption as evidenced by safety data and that have demonstrated reasonable probability of being harmful or potentially unsafe at higher levels, and second, food additives that may not be safe at any level of consumption, for instance, substances that have been proven to be carcinogens in animals or man. Among the general issues discussed at the PBOI, the issues of phenylalanine and aspartic acid toxicity are of the first general class of toxic response. The question of whether aspartame ingestion increased brain tumor incidence in animals that were part of chronic rat feeding studies is an example of the second general class of toxic response; i.e., those without an apparently discernible safe level of consumption.

The discussion of these issues will be placed in appropriate context by first considering estimates of probable levels of aspartame ingestion. Next, the level of probable aspartame exposure will be compared with the level that might result in brain damage in susceptible individuals. Finally, the evidence concerning the incidence of spontaneous brain tumors in rats and the incidence in the aspartame animal studies will be presented.

(1) Levels of aspartame ingestion.   The safe use of aspartame is ensured if the concentrations of phenylalanine and aspartic acid remain below certain levels. The concentrations that these substances reach in the blood are dependent on the dose of aspartame given and the route by which it enters the body. For these reasons, it was important to use estimations of aspartame consumption that were in fact exaggerations of what was actually expected. Thus, all three methods of estimated consumption listed below were designed to provide conservative (greater than anticipated) predictions of use.

The consumption estimate utilized by the Bureau of Foods assumed that *all* the sucrose in the diet of a 60-kg man was replaced by aspartame. Under this set of conditions, about 9.3 mg/kg/day would be ingested (137). This does not consider the heavy user of aspartame, but the fact that all sucrose is assumed to be replaced should more than compensate for this shortcoming of this estimate. As an additional conservatism, the Bureau of Foods calculated that about 25 mg/kg/day might be ingested if *all carbohydrates* in the diet of a 60-kg man were replaced by aspartame. This appears to be a definite exaggeration of projected usage levels.

A second means of projecting aspartame consumption was based on data supplied by the Market Research Corporation of America (MRCA). This company receives information of levels of food ingestion by actual dietary records kept by 4,000 households. These estimates are based on what food is actually eaten by people of various age brackets and include data for both average and heavy users (262). MRCA surveyed food use in category "A," products that would contain aspartame as presently intended, and category "B," products that encompassed seven additional kinds of food products (including soft drinks). The MRCA estimate of daily aspartame intake at mean exposures was 11.1 mg/kg and the intake based on maximum exposure on 9 out of 10 days (90th percentile) was 25 mg/kg/day. For all age groups, the 99th percentile was 34 mg/kg/day (262).

One of the sponsor's witnesses used a 10-kg infant, to optimize exposure level, and based an estimate for it of 19 mg/kg/day on the replacement of all sucrose normally ingested each day (262). However, to be sure to use a cautious approach the decision of the PBOI (196) and the final decision of the FDA Commissioner (140) both adopted the 99th percentile level from the MRCA survey of 34 mg/kg/day as the level of daily aspartame exposure.

(2) Phenylalanine toxicity. It is a well known fact that a certain small proportion of the babies delivered each year (about 1 in 15,000) (196) are born with an autosomal recessive genetic disorder. In these infants, homozygous for this particular gene, the hepatic phenylalanine hydroxylase enzyme does not mediate the usual effect of changing phenylalanine to tyrosine. Thus, in these phenylketonuric (PKU) infants, phenylalanine and other normally minor metabolites, such as phenylpyruvic, phenylacetic, and phenyllactic acids accumulate to toxic concentrations in body tissues (233). These children have plasma phenylalanine levels in the range of 120 to 600 μmoles/dl rather than the normal range of 6 to 12 μmoles/dl (162). The Bureau of Foods was aware of this particular genetic disorder and also recognized that these individuals and/or their parents were accustomed to carefully checking food for phenylalanine content. Therefore, the Bureau of Foods recommended labeling of all aspartame-containing foods with the statement "Phenylketonurics: Contains Phenylalanine." Treatment of these individuals consists of limiting their intake of phenylalanine-containing foods so that their blood levels of phenylalanine are at or below 70 to 80 μmoles/dl.

The board of experts from the PBOI considered the phenylalanine hazard assessment in the following manner: What conditions of aspartame ingestion would result in plasma levels of phenylalanine of 100 μmoles/dl or higher, the levels associated with impaired brain development (162,196)? In addition, because there is a maternal-to-fetal concentration gradient with phenylalanine of 1:2 maintained by the placenta, what conditions of aspartame ingestion would result in greater than 50 μmoles/dl of phenylalanine to accumulate in the circulation of women of child-bearing age (196)?

When normal human adults are given a single, loading dose of aspartame of 34 mg/kg body weight (the 99th percentile of expected aspartame consumption for the entire day), dissolved in orange juice, the plasma phenylalanine concentration rises from a fasting level of 6 to 11 μmoles/dl. This latter concentration is found in both adults and children following ingestion of a protein-rich meal (196).[7] Following a 100 mg/kg loading dose (the same as drinking 12 liters of aspartame-sweetened beverage at a single sitting), the plasma phenylalanine rises to 20 μmoles/dl. Thirty-four milligrams of aspartame/kg of body weight was given to a number of 1-year-old infants and their plasma phenylalanine concentrations rose from a resting level of 6 to 10 μmoles/dl. This latter finding demonstrates that a 1-year-old infant metabolizes phenylalanine just as effectively as an adult (196).

Another group of individuals have a hepatic phenylalanine hydroxylase enzyme that is less effective than that of normal individuals in converting phenylalanine to tyrosine. They are referred to as individuals heterozygous for PKU. If a 34 mg/kg loading dose is given to these individuals, the peak plasma phenylalanine reaches 16 μmoles/dl, and this concentration of phenylalanine decreases somewhat more slowly than in a normal individual (265). Even following an enormous dose of 100 mg/kg (about 3 times the 99th percentile level, the plasma phenylalanine concentration, 42 μmoles/dl, is less than the level that would place the fetus of a pregnant woman at risk (196). It should be emphasized that in normal circumstances, even this abusive dose would be taken at several different sittings and throughout the day, not all at one time as in this experimental study. For this reason, the concentration of plasma phenylalanine would be expected to stay well below 50 μmoles/dl if this very large dose were consumed in a normal mealtime environment (196).

The issue has been raised by certain objectors that a risk might occur in unidentified PKU children as a result of the presence of aspartame in the food supply. Although most states (47) require that newborns be screened for PKU, 10 to 30% of the 200 PKU children born annually may go undiagnosed. It is important to note that expert testimony at the PBOI (203) indicates that the infant, if not diagnosed at birth, will be diagnosed by 8 to 10 months of age because of abnormal development. The mean projected intake of aspartame for children under 2 years of age is 3 mg/kg/day, while this same infant would be consuming 80 mg/kg/day of phenylalanine from breast milk or infant formula (196). The undiagnosed PKU child is certainly and primarily at risk from consumption of normal meals; one expert concluded that the undiagnosed PKU infant will not be at additional risk by the marketing of aspartame (203).

In a somewhat related group of people, diagnosed PKU children not on phenylalanine-restricted diets, a similar question may be asked: What risk is present for them because of the presence of aspartame in the food supply? A 99th percentile dose of aspartame of 34/mg/kg contains 17 mg of phenylalanine/kg. This is less than 10% of the 200 mg of phenylalanine/kg, which the PKU child would receive from normal food protein. When one considers that daily variation in protein ingestion can easily exceed 10%, it is apparent that the ingestion of aspartame by these children does not provide a significant additional risk (196).

---

[7] See *Editor's note* on page 99.

A final group of people to be considered are the offspring of women who suffer from elevated blood concentrations of phenylalanine, so-called hyperphenylalaninemics. These women have plasma phenylalanine levels between 25 and 120 μmoles/dl. Most of these individuals are of normal intelligence and lack any of the other physical signs of PKU. Since they do not have physical signs of PKU, neither they nor their doctors are aware of their anomolous state (196). Approximately 50% of 1750 women hyperphenylalaninemics have blood concentrations of phenylalanine in the range of 60 to 120 μmoles/dl, which place their offspring at risk for mental retardation. The only effective means of ensuring normal offspring is to reduce systematically their dietary intake of phenylalanine. However, this treatment is contingent on an awareness of the condition. Thus prevention of brain damage caused by maternal hyperphenylalaninemia cannot be achieved until screening tests have identified these women. The PBOI decision concluded that a hyperphenylalaninemic woman is at much higher risk from the consumption of normal foods than she would be from the use of aspartame (196).

The overall conclusion of the PBOI was that aspartame ingestion by normal humans cannot be expected to increase the severity of mental retardation that is contingent on sustained plasma phenylalanine concentrations up to or beyond 120 μmoles/dl during immature stages of brain development (196). In individuals on phenylalanine-restricted diets, the package label specifically informing that aspartame is a source of phenylalanine should prevent liberal use of the sweetener by these patients. With respect to the undiagnosed hyperphenylalaninemic pregnant woman, the risk to the mother (or the unborn child) from food-derived sources of phenylalanine is much greater than any risk associated with aspartame use. The only effective management of the risk to the offspring is knowledge of the disorder and limitation of phenylalanine intake from all dietary sources (196).

(3) Neurotoxic potential of aspartic acid. It has been known since 1969 that under appropriate experimental conditions in test animals, both glutamic acid (GLU) and aspartic acid (ASP), one of the amino acid constituents of aspartame, are capable of inducing lesions in the arcuate nucleus of the hypothalamus (214). In this same report, it was demonstrated that GLU and ASP can act similarly, are about equal in potency, and in combination can be additive in this brain-lesioning effect (214). At higher doses, other portions of the brain and the retina of the eye may be permanently damaged (210).

Many scientists have agreed that when ASP is given in proper dosage and route of administration, it can cause lesioning in the brain of certain animals. Thus, the real safety question to be answered is: At what plasma concentration is there a reasonable probability that humans are at potential risk to these toxic effects of ASP, and are these plasma concentrations attainable in humans under the proposed conditions of aspartame use? Actually, it is the combined level of GLU and ASP in the plasma that must be monitored because a significant proportion of ingested ASP is metabolized to GLU by enzymatic transamination once it is absorbed into cells lining the gastrointestinal tract, and then released into the systemic circulation (196). For the purposes of ascertaining toxic potential, monosodium glutamate

(MSG), GLU, monosodium aspartate, and ASP may be considered to be nearly equipotent, in that the neurotoxic dose for each of these substances appears to be virtually equivalent (196).

Scientific evidence indicates that the age of the animal is an important consideration in the development of brain lesions resulting from exposure to the excitotoxic amino acids, GLU and ASP (142,205,208,276). When MSG is given by gavage, the lowest effective dose inducing hypothalamic lesions in mice is approximately 0.5 g/kg body weight in the newborn, 0.7 g/kg body weight in 10-day-old infant animals, and about 2 g/kg body weight in weanlings or adult mice (142,205,208,276). In terms of plasma levels of GLU required to produce hypothalamic lesioning, neonatal or infant mice require 100 μmoles/dl (276).

A second factor that has been demonstrated to affect the lesioning potency of these excitotoxic amino acids, GLU and ASP, is the route of administration utilized. In the weanling mouse, for example, the lowest effective dose for hypothalamic lesioning by GLU was 0.7 g/kg when given subcutaneously or 2 g/kg body weight when given by oral intubation (277). This control of the extent of lesioning by route of administration is also observed in the neonatal and infant rodent (5,121,204,267). In addition, one study has reported that GLU fed with meals (doses ranging from 10 to 35 g/kg body weight) does not produce neuronal damage (277).

A third factor that has been shown to control the appearance and extent of hypothalamic lesioning is the species of animal used for experimentation. The most sensitive animal species appears to be the mouse, with rats and guinea pigs somewhat less sensitive. GLU-mediated brain lesions have not been demonstrated in dogs (142). The data concerning the sensitivity of primates to the hypothalamic lesioning effect of GLU are the subject of some controversy. Although one study reported lesions in infant monkeys with plasma GLU concentrations of about 120 μmoles/ dl (215), data from four other laboratories failed to confirm this effect (3,4, 199,228,229,300). These latter authors, utilizing oral, dietary, or subcutaneous administration of MSG in doses ranging from 0.25 to 4.0 g/kg body weight, failed to find any evidence of neuronal damage to the hypothalamus (3,4,199,228,229,300). The plasma level of GLU and ASP combined was 445 μmoles/dl in one of these studies in which the monkeys exhibited no hypothalamic lesioning (268). Because neither the aspartame PBOI experts nor the FDA Commissioner could resolve these conflicts in the reported experimental findings, both the Board and the Commissioner chose to adopt a conservative plasma level of GLU and ASP combined of 100 μmoles/dl as the potential neurotoxic concentration in humans (140,196).

The next step in the safety assessment of aspartame was to review how various doses of aspartame, when given alone or in combination with GLU (an approved additive) to human subjects, affected the combined plasma levels of GLU and ASP. Aspartame was administered to adults in doses of 100, 150, and 200 mg/kg body weight as a single dose in 500 ml of orange juice. These doses are equivalent to 3, 4.5, and 6 times the projected 99th percentile level of intake for an entire day; i.e., 34 mg/kg body weight. The 200 mg/kg dose is the level that a 3-year-old child would be exposed to if he or she accidentally ingested the entire contents of a container of aspartame coffee sweetener (100 tablets of 20 mg each). In this study, both the plasma GLU and ASP concentrations were within or well below, respectively, the normal postprandial plasma levels for these two amino acids (264).

In addition to studies on normal adults, Searle also conducted studies to ascertain any risk of aspartame ingestion in special population groups, such as the effect on breast milk composition in lactating women, the degree of placental transfer of aspartate in pregnant primates, and the metabolism of aspartame by 1-year-old infants. In lactating women, 50 mg of aspartame/kg body weight (more than 1.5 times the 99th percentile level of projected consumption) was given dissolved in orange juice. The concentrations of GLU and ASP in the milk of the lactating women rose from 109 to 120 μmoles/dl and 2.3 to 4.8 μmoles/dl, respectively. While these increases are just statistically significant acutely, they are not statistically increased for the 24-hr period following this single large dose (32). This increase in ASP concentrations would result in the infant increasing the amount of its overall intake of ASP by less than 1%, an amount that is not biologically significant (32). It is important to know what amounts of the ASP portion of the aspartame molecule may be expected to be transferred across the placental membranes to the fetus. If the levels of ASP were concentrated from maternal to fetal circulation, as in the case of certain neutral amino acids (190,285), there would be concern that high maternal levels of ASP might damage the hypothalamus of the fetal brain. However, data available on ASP demonstrate that the placenta actually provides a substantial barrier to ASP transfer to the fetus. It was only after an enormous elevation of the maternal plasma level of ASP was achieved (237 μmoles/dl) that placental transfer of ASP occurred. With this maternal plasma level, the fetal concentration rose from 0.6 to 4.5 μmoles/dl (266). These data suggest that it would be almost impossible for humans to ingest enough aspartame under all expected conditions of use to cause an increase in maternal plasma of ASP that would result in the transfer of significant quantities of ASP to the fetal circulation.

One final special population, 1-year-old infants, was tested for its response to ingested aspartame. These infants and control adult subjects received aspartame in a flavored beverage mix, at levels of 34, 50, and 100 mg/kg body weight. Plasma GLU and ASP concentrations did not increase significantly in either infants or adults (265).

Another concern addressed during the safety assessment of aspartame was whether the combined intake of aspartame and MSG could result in unsafe plasma concentrations of GLU and ASP in humans. When aspartame at the projected 99th percentile level of ingestion, 34 mg/kg body weight, and MSG at the 90th percentile level of ingestion, 34 mg/kg body weight, were given with a hamburger and milkshake meal, there were no significant differences in plasma GLU and ASP concentrations among the individuals fed the meal alone, those fed the meal plus MSG, and those fed the meal plus MSG and aspartame (263). Another study was conducted utilizing the same experimental design except that 150 mg of GLU/kg body weight and 23 mg of aspartame/kg body weight were ingested. The combined plasma

GLU–ASP concentration was 13.9 μmoles/dl after the meal alone and 23.5 μmoles/dl after the meal plus MSG and aspartame (263).

An example of food ingestion where one would expect the highest plasma levels of GLU and ASP to result is when a high concentration of MSG(GLU) in a consommé-type soup is coadministered with aspartame in a beverage. A study was performed with human subjects using three treatment regimens: (a) soup and beverage with no addition; (b) soup with 50 mg of MSG/kg body weight and unsweetened beverage; and (c) soup with 50 mg of MSG/kg body weight and beverage sweetened with 34 mg of aspartame/kg. With the MSG-in-soup meal, the combined plasma GLU–ASP levels were 21.0 ± 7 μmoles/dl. With the meal plus added MSG and aspartame, the same plasma levels were 25.7 ± 10.5 μmoles/dl (263). Thus, there was a slight but not statistically significant increase in the elevation of GLU and ASP plasma levels produced when aspartame plus MSG were added compared with these same values determined for the GLU–ASP plasma levels resulting from MSG in soup alone. Each of these studies, in an increasingly more sensitive manner, tests the hypothesis that combined ingestion of MSG and aspartame will result in unacceptable plasma levels of GLU and ASP in human subjects. On the basis of the available data, one concludes that this hypothesis is not supported and that there is reasonable certainty of no harm resulting from the combined consumption of aspartame and MSG.

The final argument in this general area concerning the safety of aspartame was whether ASP from aspartame ingestion could mediate changes in neuroendocrine function, ostensibly by stimulating cells in the hypothalamus, which could, in turn, cause alterations in pituitary and subsequent endocrine gland function. It has been established that if very high doses of MSG (2.2 to 5.8 g/kg body weight) are administered repeatedly on successive days postnatally, mice show marked adiposity, skeletal stunting, and female infertility (209). A markedly undersized pituitary has been observed in adult rats and hamsters after repeated subcutaneous injection of about 4 g of MSG/kg body weight in these animals as neonates (56,168,198,226). In these treated rodents, the pituitary contents of growth hormone, luteinizing hormone, follicle-stimulating hormone, thyroid-stimulating hormone, and prolactin are depressed (145,168,194,198,226,277). Indeed, there are reduced plasma levels of these hormones (90,198,277,280) and reduced weight of reproductive organs and diminished reproductive capacity (90,197,209,222, 226,271,282). Further, this same obesity, stunting, and decreased weights of ovaries, testes, and anterior pituitary are also observed in ASP-treated mice that as neonates received subcutaneous doses of 4 g/kg body weight on days 1 through 4 postnatally (238). Certain investigators have reported that sublesioning doses of MSG (1 g/kg) produced acute changes in plasma levels of gonadotropins in adult male rats following subcutaneous injection (210,213). These authors propose that the doses used in this study are sublesioning (although no histopathologic studies were performed to confirm this assumption), yet acute changes in hormones were effected. One of these investigators speculates that high but nonlesioning doses of GLU may cause endocrine peturbations in man. In the aspartame PBOI decision, the Board concluded that the hormone level changes observed in these and other studies (308) were within the range of normal hormonal fluctuations and may have resulted from normal circadian or ultradian periodicity of hormone release (196).

(4) Tumorigenic potential of aspartame. The final major scientific issue considered during the safety assessment of aspartame was whether ingestion of this food additive resulted in the induction of brain tumors in rats. The discussion below considers many of the most critical elements of the scientific dialogue concerning this important topic. The Bureau of Foods requires chronic feeding studies in two rodent species, normally the rat and mouse, to evaluate the carcinogenic potential of food additives (165). In fulfillment of this requirement, the sponsor conducted chronic feeding studies with aspartame added to the diet of both rats (sponsor's data submission, Vols. 43–44 or E-33, 34 and Vol. 81 or E-70) and mice (Vol. 85 or E-75). A second series of chronic feeding studies was performed with a degradation product of aspartame, its diketopiperazine (DKP), in rats (Vols. 89–90 or E-77, 78) and in mice (Vol. 88 or E-76). All parties at the PBOI on aspartame agreed that the mouse data were negative (140); therefore, only the interpretation of the brain tumor incidence data from the rat studies was controversial. The three rat studies consisted of the following experimental design:

(a) E-33, 34 was a 104-week study with exposure to dietary aspartame beginning after weaning. Doses were 0, 1, 2, 4, and 6 to 8 g/kg body weight.

(b) E-70 was a two-generation study with aspartame exposure beginning *in utero*, during lactation and for 104 weeks thereafter. Doses were 0, 2, and 4 g/kg body weight.

(c) E-77, 78 was a 115-week study with dietary exposure to DKP beginning after weaning. Doses used were 0, 0.75, 1.5, and 3.0 g/kg body weight.

The FDA Commissioner has found that on the basis of general principles of statistical and biological significance, carcinogenicity studies may be categorized as (a) positive; (b) inconclusive but suggestive of a carcinogenic effect; (c) negative; or (d) deficient (17). Utilizing this system of classifying results, one scientist would place E-33, 34 in the suggestive category and E-70 in the deficient category. The main scientific objection brought forth by one objector to aspartame approval was that the spontaneous rate of brain tumors in Sprague-Dawley rats (similar to the strains used in the three rat studies by the sponsor) indicated by scientific literature is well below the incidence of brain tumors found in both the control animals in E-70 and the treated animals in E-33, 34 (212). The objector claimed that if one rejects the results of certain "unreliable" or "irrelevant" studies, the spontaneous incidence of brain tumors in rats is 0.15% (212).

Testimony by the Bureau of Foods at the PBOI on aspartame suggests that there is a wide variation in the spontaneous incidence of brain neoplasms in rat studies reported in the literature. The incidence of spontaneous brain neoplasms in rats varies from 0.09 to 5.8% (138). In several of the studies that indicate low spontaneous brain tumor rates, a number of unresolved methodological questions exist, such as (a) whether the rats were of the same age, sex, and strain; (b) whether rats were treated or control animals; (c) whether tissue sectioning was routine or done only after observation of clinical symptoms; (d) how many areas of each brain were sectioned; and (e) whether examination of the slides was macroscopic or microscopic (95,110,123,128,138,186,200,224,240,281). Because of the methodological short-comings or uncertainties of almost all these studies, the Bureau of Foods concluded that the most appropriate indicators of the spontaneous brain tumor rates in these studies were those demonstrated by the control animals in Searle studies E-33, 34; E-70; and E-77, 78 (15). Ultimately, the FDA Commissioner agreed with this conclusion and used a comparison of brain neoplasm incidences between the control and treated groups in the Searle studies to ascertain the carcinogenicity potential of aspartame (140).

The conclusion of the panel of scientists selected for the aspartame PBOI was that the evidence from the Searle studies ". . . do not rule out an oncogenic effect of aspartame, and that, to the contrary, they appear to suggest the possibility that aspartame, at least when administered in the huge quantities employed in the studies, may contribute to the development of brain tumors" (196). Thus, the Board agreed with one of the objectors that the chronic rat feeding study with E-33, 34 is suggestive of carcinogenic potential and that the chronic *in utero* feeding study with aspartame is deficient.

The Bureau of Foods and the sponsor disagreed with these conclusions; discussed below are several of the more important topics that were the focus of their disagreement with the Board. The Bureau of Foods is convinced that for a carcinogenicity analysis to implicate a compound as a carcinogen, a study must show one of the following: a statistically significant increase in the number of tumors when the treated animals are compared with controls, an earlier occurrence of tumors in the treated animals, a compound-related increase in rare tumor occurrence, or a dose-related relationship in conjunction with a statistically significant increase in the number of tumors (26, 30, 41–43).

In the aspartame PBOI decision, there was no statistical analysis of the brain tumor incidence data. This is unfortunate because in carcinogenicity testing the mere occurrence of tumors is not conclusive. The increase in tumor incidence must be analyzed statistically to assess to a stated level of probability, for instance, 95%, whether an observed increase in tumor incidence between treated animals and controls is higher than can be expected by random biological variation alone (and is, therefore, a result of treatment) (15,122). The Bureau of Foods utilized a number of statistical analyses to test whether there had been a statistically significant increase in brain tumor incidence between treated and control groups in study E-33, 34. After adjusting for multiple comparisons of treatment groups with control group, no significant increase was indicated by the Fisher's exact test (one-tailed), and without adjustments for multiple comparisons, no statistically significant results were observed with a second chronic rat feeding study, E-70 (45). The Bureau of Foods also applied three separate trend tests (Exact, Cox-Tarone, Breslow) to these same data. These statistical tests enable one to test for a decreased time-to-tumor appearance and to determine whether any dose–tumor response relationship exists

(45). When one very early occurring tumor, a medulloblastoma, is eliminated from the brain tumor incidences, none of these tests when applied to the data from E-33, 34 or E-70 demonstrated a decreased time-to-tumor appearance nor a dose–tumor response relationship (45).

The Bureau of Foods excluded the single medulloblastoma from their data analysis for the following reasons: The animal with the medulloblastoma died from tumor-related pathology at 12 weeks of age and after aspartame treatment for only 8 weeks. For the rat to have died of tumor-related pathology at 12 weeks of age, the medulloblastoma must have originated in embryonic tissue (45). However, embryonic brain tissue would not be expected to be present at 4 weeks after birth, the time when aspartame administration was begun (230,231,304).

The Bureau of Foods also disagreed with the manner in which the Board demonstrated a relationship between the dose of aspartame ingested and brain tumor incidences in study E-33, 34. The Board combined the brain tumor incidences found in the two lowest and two highest dose groups together. With the data combined in this way, the respective tumor incidences are: control 0.8%; 1 and 2 g/kg, 3.1%; and 4 and 6 to 8 g/kg, 4.3% (45). The Bureau of Foods concluded that this *ad hoc*, postexperimental combining of dosage groups is not scientifically tenable. Unless adequate justification is provided, one must analyze the data resulting from a particular study as it was originally designed. Thus, when the data were analyzed as stipulated in the original protocol, the incidences were: 0.8% (one tumor) in the control group; 3.9% (three tumors) in the 1 g/kg dose group; 1.25% (one tumor) in the 2 g/kg dose group; 6.2% (five tumors) in the 4 g/kg dose group; and 2.5% (two tumors) in the 6 to 8 g/kg dose group. These results do not demonstrate the type of increasing effect one normally associates with a dose–response relationship (15).

In addition to the lack of concurrence on the topics described above, the Bureau of Foods accepted the histopathological findings of an independent group of pathologists regarding the number of brain tumors in study E-33, 34. A panel of pathologists appointed by UAREP diagnosed 12 tumors in study E-33, 34, while the Board accepted that 13 tumors were found in this same study. The difference of one tumor was in the 1 g/kg treatment group, where the Board accepted the number of brain tumors as four rather than three as described by UAREP (15,45,122). Further, the Board reported that two rats died of brain tumor-related pathology early in the E-33, 34 study, one rat at 8 weeks and another at 16 weeks (196); however, these early tumor-related deaths were not confirmed when the Bureau of Foods reexamined the record for study E-33, 34 (15).

Finally, the Board concluded that the second chronic rat feeding study was "bizarre" in that the incidence of control tumors was 3.5% (196). This rate of brain tumors, which seemed too high to the Board, is within the range of brain tumors incidences, 0.5 to 5.0%, that have been reported recently in Sprague-Dawley Caesarean-derived albino rats from Charles River Breeding Laboratories when a comprehensive, systematic search for brain tumors was conducted (140).

Following the conclusion of the aspartame PBOI, the sponsor submitted evidence of a new chronic rat feeding study. In this very large study, there was no statistically significant increase in the incidence of brain tumors in Wistar rats fed 1, 2, or 4 g/kg of aspartame when compared with that in the concurrent control group (151). Thus, in the Commissioner's decision on aspartame he states, "For all the reasons stated above, I conclude that the available data, taken as a whole, establish that there is a reasonable certainty that aspartame and DKP do not cause brain tumors in laboratory rats (140)."

(5) Regulatory resolution of scientific issues. Eight months following the Aspartame Board of Inquiry, after study and evaluation of testimony by the PBOI participants and consultants and safety data submitted by the sponsor, and review of conclusions and rebuttals of participants, the Board released its conclusions and recommendations regarding aspartame. The Board concluded that the ingestion of aspartame, in even high but conceivable doses, could not be expected to increase the incidence of mental retardation associated with sustained elevations of phenylalanine, nor could aspartame ingestion be expected to result in focal brain damage or dysfunction of the neuroendocrine regulatory systems. However, with regard to the issue of whether aspartame ingestion results in brain neoplasms in rats, the Board concluded that the available evidence on laboratory rats did not rule out the possibility that aspartame might induce brain tumors. Thus, the Board recommended that aspartame should not be approved for marketing until further animal testing was conducted to resolve the brain tumor issue (196).

The various PBOI participants provided further discussion and comment on the conclusions published in the Board's decision. Following an analysis and interpretation of the data and arguments of all parties, the FDA Commissioner published his final decision on aspartame on July 24, 1981. Commissioner Hayes found that the sponsor had met its responsibility of proving that aspartame is safe for its proposed use. In coming to this decision, the Commissioner agreed with the Board on the issue of aspartame providing no risk of contributing to mental retardation or causing brain damage or dysfunction of the neuroendocrine system; however, he decided in favor of the data interpretations by the Bureau of Foods and the sponsor with regard to the brain tumor issue (140). In ruling that there was reasonable certainty that aspartame does not cause an increased occurrence of brain tumors in rats, the FDA Commissioner relied on results, from an additional chronic rat study, that were not available at the time of the aspartame PBOI (151). Thus, after protracted scientific debate, the marketing of aspartame as a sweetener in selected foods was approved 90 days after the publication (July 24, 1981) of the Commissioner's final decision on aspartame.

2. Indirect: Acrylamide and Polyacrylamides

a. Regulatory history

The polyacrylamides are examples of polymers with potential neurotoxicity that are regulated by Bureau of Foods as indirect or secondary direct food additives (see

Table 1 and Section II, A, 3). Acrylamide monomer ($CH_2=CHCONH_2$) is a three-carbon compound, molecules of which polymerize easily in the presence of a catalyst to form long-chain compounds (144). These reaction products are water-soluble polymers, the polyacrylamides. If humans are exposed to excessive and cumulative amounts of acrylamide monomer, they develop a disturbance in walking gait, with ataxia and postural tremor (107).

Since acrylamide monomer is neurotoxic under certain conditions, it is not permitted as an intentional direct food additive. It is, however, an unavoidable "migrant," i.e., a substance retained as a contaminant and released in minute, nontoxic concentrations from the polymeric substances (polyacrylamides) on contact with food. Dilute concentrations of various polyacrylamide polymers in aqueous solution are permitted in manufacture of paper for food packaging (12), as flocculating agents in filtration of sugar juice and liquors that are intermediates in the processing of beet and cane sugar, and as water filtration aids (16). The safe use of the polyacrylamide resins is based on the extremely limited migration of the acrylamide monomer to foods. The resulting concentrations in food from this migration is manifold less than the levels mediating neurotoxicity. In addition, it has been demonstrated that the polymers are chemically stable and are not absorbed or metabolized.

A petition requesting a clearance for a regulation permitting the use of a specific polyacrylamide resin in the manufacture of paper intended for contact with food was submitted in 1961 (101). Earlier, the Bureau of Foods had received a petition that requested approval of an anionic polyacrylamide for improving the wet strength of paper and paperboard used in food containers (7). Both of these petitions were submitted following the congressional passage of the Food Additives Amendment of 1958 which required that scientific data be supplied to the FDA to establish the safety of food additives before these substances could be approved for addition to the food supply. Later, petitions were received requesting approval of other polyacrylamide resins that differed chemically in regard to molecular weight, monomer content, and proportions of acrylamide and acrylic acid used as reactants in synthesis. These copolymers were designed to meet specialized requirements for other uses (279).

Some polymers consist in part of polyacrylic acid, in which free carboxyl groups (COOH) substitute for the amide ($CONH_2$) side chain. The acrylic acid monomer is not neurotoxic. Such polymers were designed for clarifying sugar solutions during processing (102). An additional approved use of a polyacrylamide resin is for the washing of fruits and vegetables. For this purpose, polyacrylamide resin is permitted to contain 0.2% (2,000 ppm) residual acrylamide (16). By a series of specifications controlling residual acrylamide monomer content in the polymer and the concentration in the washwater, the detectable concentration of acrylamide monomer left on unwashed foods was at levels well below 20 ppb. As additional uses for polyacrylamide polymers were proposed, concern over possible exposure to toxic levels of these chemicals was being expressed by consumers (1,130,189,236). As a result, the latter petitioners were requested to submit more detailed chemical and toxicity data to establish that their products could be safely used.

b. *Scientific data*

Studies were conducted to investigate the fate of [^{14}C]polyacrylamide in the rat. In one study three rats received 10 to 75 mg of material orally; urine and feces were collected in a metabolic chamber. After 24 hr the rats were sacrificed and tissues assayed. More than 97% of the administered radioactivity was recovered in feces or from the gastrointestinal tract (101). It may be concluded that polyacrylamide is not systemically absorbed after oral administration (101).

In the investigations of toxic potential, the safety of polyacrylamide resins used in paper manufacture was established in pharmacokinetic, acute, subchronic (90-day), and chronic (2-year) feeding studies of polymer to rats and dogs and of acrylamide monomer to rats, cats, and monkeys (7,101). Studies were conducted with various polyacrylamides containing several different residual levels of acrylamide monomer to determine the quantity of monomer necessary to demonstrate neurotoxicity as revealed by changes in posture and walking gait. In these subchronic studies, rats received a diet containing 10% polyacrylamide that resulted in a final concentration of acrylamide monomer in the powdered feed of 300 ppm. Several of these rats showed hindquarters paralysis with a loss of proprioception (position sense). When rats were maintained on a diet containing 3% polyacrylamide or 90 ppm of acrylamide monomer, one of 10 rats showed a loss of proprioceptive control after 56 days on experiment (101).

A number of additional short-term tests were conducted in rats using diets containing variable amounts of acrylamide monomer. Samples of four resins with acrylamide content ranging from 0.07 to 0.81% were synthesized. Dietary levels of 3, 9, 30, 70, 90, 110, 300, or 400 ppm of acrylamide monomer were administered with resin to rats for 90 days. The resins with the higher acrylamide content were achieved by adding monomer to polymer. It was concluded that dramatic and severe neurotoxic signs (ataxia and inability to stand) could be produced in rats with polymer containing small amounts of residual acrylamide. With respect to these neurotoxic symptoms, the no-effect dietary level for acrylamide monomer was 70 ppm. Those rats receiving 300 to 400 ppm monomer developed other signs such as failure to grow at a normal rate; pathological changes in kidney, liver, and testis; urinary retention; and penile erection. The rats showed recovery if the administration of the test substance was stopped before 3 months and the usual chow diet was then resumed (101).

Another study to determine the neurotoxicity of acrylamide monomer was conducted with six groups of 10 rats each. Each group received diets of polyacrylamide with monomer content ranging from 10 to 320 ppm. The no-effect level of monomer in the presence of polymer from this 1-year study was determined to be 80 ppm (7).

Studies were also conducted in cats and monkeys to establish the neurotoxic dose of acrylamide. Two cats each (12 cats) received oral doses of acrylamide at levels of 0.03, 0.1, 1, 3, or 10 mg/kg, respectively, for 5 days/week (101). At the highest dose level (10 mg/kg), the treated cats showed definite limb weakness at 26 days, leading to loss of control at 40 days, at which time dosing was stopped. At 85 days, there were definite signs of recovery. "No-effect" was noted at dose levels of 0.03 to 0.1 mg/kg, and one cat at 0.3 mg/kg showed no grossly observable effects during 1 year of acrylamide dosing. A similar study was also conducted in rhesus monkeys. The "no-effect" level was determined as 1.0 to 3.0 mg of acrylamide/kg/day for neurotoxicity (101).

The following additional studies were done to establish the safety of the polyacrylamide approved for use as a processing aid in manufacture of paper. In rats, dietary levels of 1, 3, and 10% polymer (0.5 to 5 g/kg) per day were fed (101); in dogs, levels of 0, 2.5, and 5% were fed (7). The 2-year rat study established a no-effect level of 2 mg/kg/day for the polymer, using as criteria no change in organ weights at necropsy and no observable compound-induced gross or histopathological changes in body organs. On the basis of a 100-fold safety factor to the "no-effect level" of 3%, a safe daily dose of polyacrylamide was calculated to be 0.02 mg/kg body weight or 1.4 mg polymer for a 70-kg adult. On the basis of this study, the safe daily exposure to monomer would be 1.12 μg of acrylamide. When this no-effect level is compared with actual levels of acrylamide migrants in food, a safety factor of greater than 1 million-fold is present. It should be understood that no neurological effects were reported at any dose level of polymer that was fed and that the criteria of no observable effects were based on growth effects and absence of tissue changes.

To reduce the residual acrylamide monomer content of polyacrylamides, the company treated polymer with sodium bisulfite (101). As a reaction product of acrylamide with sodium bisulfite, sodium sulfopropionamide is formed. This reaction product was subjected to toxicology protocols consisting of acute oral toxicity determination (LD_{50}), irritation, absorption, effects of intraperitoneal injection, and 90-day and 2-year dietary feeding to rats and 1-year dietary feeding to cats. A no-effect level of 3% was observed in rats; as much as 1.5 g/kg/day had no adverse effects (101). The absence of neurotoxicity of the reaction product was established in these studies.

In addition to laboratory data, a summary of the medical histories of workmen involved in research, development, and production of polyacrylamide was furnished (101). These records were said to show no adverse effects on the workmen involved. Because of the multiple possible routes of exposure industrially and possible multiple exposures to other chemicals, the records of industrial experience were of limited value.

Another petition was submitted for approval of polyacrylamide for use in sugar processing. For this use the polymer is regulated as a Secondary Direct Food Additive Permitted in Food for Human Consumption (71). The polymer was modified by greater hydrolysis of polymer amide linkages (30% hydrolysis of the amide side branches). Two-year feeding studies in dogs and rats were conducted at feeding levels of 0, 1, 2, 5, 10, and 15%. While no neurotoxic effects were noted in the rat, toxic effects such as increased liver weight were observed at the 15% dietary level and increased kidney weights were detected at the 5 to 10% dietary level. The no-observed effect level was considered to be 1% in the rat and 2% in the dog. Absorption of the compound was considered to be less than 1% of the dietary level. The use level of this polymer during sugar manufacture is 10 ppm for cane sugar at an early step in the process, giving residues of less than 1 ppb of acrylamide monomer in the final product.

c. Mechanism of action

The mechanism of action of acrylamide was unknown at the time these studies were conducted. Early studies which were conducted by Hazleton Laboratories showed that addition of alanine or thiamine to diets of dosed rats was without effect in protecting against neurotoxicity; cholinesterase activity of plasma, red cell, or brain was not affected. It was noted that acrylamide-dosed dogs had hypotension, which did not respond to epinephrine but was supersensitive to acetylcholine (7). Kuperman (166) noted the similarity of the neurological syndrome produced by acrylamide to that exhibited by animals with a cerebellar deficit. He administered acrylamide, both orally and parenterally, to cats that had been subjected to surgical decortication or decerebration. Posture, gait, and EEG changes were studied. In intact cats he noted no differences in the neurotoxic syndrome attributable to route of administration, either in degree of effect or latency for appearance of ataxia or changes in EEG pattern. When single large doses of acrylamide were given, central excitability and convulsions and accompanying EEG changes occurred. With continued daily dosing, blood pressure was decreased until shock was produced. If administration of acrylamide was terminated before hypotension developed, animals recovered from the postural and gait deficits. On the basis of these studies, Kuperman concluded that the postural tremor and ataxia originated from an impairment of subcortical function and proposed that the mesencephalic tegmentum was the site of action (166).

McCollister and co-workers (187) reported in the open literature on their laboratory studies of acrylamide. They did not comment on the mechanism of action. Many of these studies had been submitted to the FDA and reviewed in the safety determination of polyacrylamide as a food additive (101).

In intact rats, Fullerton and Barnes (114) found that acrylamide depressed peripheral nerve conduction velocity in motor fibers to small muscles of the hind paw. Histologically, they noted that a form of axonal degeneration of the nerve fiber was produced. Thus, they ascribed acrylamide effects to a peripheral neuropathy.

Spencer and Schaumberg (259,260) recently reviewed aspects of acrylamide toxicity. They and Edwards (104) concluded that the histologic structural changes it produces are similar to those seen following local application of drugs known to inhibit axonal flow in nerves. Over the last several years reports have been published indicating that a neuron-specific enolase, glyceraldehyde-3-phosphate dehydrogenase, and phosphofructokinase, enzymes involved with the glycolytic cycle of nerve tissue, are inhibited by acrylamide both *in vitro* (in studies conducted on rat and cat tissues) and *in vivo* (in the cat) (147).

d. Conclusions

The safety of the approved indirect or secondary direct food additive uses of the polyacrylamides rests on the small concentrations used in a particular application and on strict limitations on the content of residual monomers present in the polymeric product, as well as on their chemical stability. Short- and long-term toxicity tests conducted in mice, rats, cats, dogs, and monkeys established the "no-observed effect" levels, and the application of 100-fold safety factors was used to set an upper permissable limit of ingestion. No cases of human neurotoxicity have been reported to FDA as resulting from ingestion of polyacrylamides with limitations on acrylamide monomer content as set forth in the regulations.

B. Food Color Additive: Toxicity Assessment of FD & C Red No. 3 (Erythrosine)

1. Historical Perspective of Erythrosine

As in the case of other industrial dyes used in foods, the history of erythrosine began in the late 1800s. With the Food and Drug Act of 1906, erythrosine and six other dyes were permitted for use in foods because they "had been examined physiologically, with no unfavorable results" (201). The FD & C Act of 1938 also permitted the use of erythrosine in foods, since additional pharmacology studies had not indicated any adverse effects from the dye. Following the 1960 Amendments to the Act (see Section II, A, 4, Table 1) and the completion of several toxicity studies, in March, 1968 a formal petition was filed on behalf of the Certified Color Industry Committee to list permanently FD & C Red No. 3 for use in the coloring of foods, dietary supplements, and ingested drugs (Federal Register Notice of July 2, 1968). By October, 1968 the toxicological evaluation of the color additive had been completed with the establishment of an estimated maximum acceptable daily intake level (ADI) for humans of 2.5 mg/kg/day. A notice of proposed rulemaking to list permanently FD & C Red No. 3 for the petitioned uses appeared in the Federal Register in April 8, 1969, and 90 days later the regulation was promulgated (Federal Register July 12, 1969). In the early 1970s, new reports on the toxicity and carcinogenicity of several of the color additives brought attention to the need for more extensive toxicity testing according to more recent protocols. In addition, reports surfaced that suggested involvement of artificial food colors in the clinical syndrome of hyperkinesis. Erythrosine acutely administered at high dose levels has been specifically implicated in this regard. In September 1976, an in-house review of the toxicity data on erythrosine revealed that the study protocols previously used to assess its safety had not been designed according to contemporary standards and that additional testing would be needed to support a more extensive use of the dye (i.e., in cosmetics and lipsticks). Hence, a new series of studies was designed and initiated in 1977 to assess the potential chronic toxicity or carcinogenicity effects of oral administration of erythrosine to rats and mice. These studies are to be complete by October, 1982.

2. Chemical and Physical Characteristics

Erythrosine is the disodium salt of 2,4,5,7-tetraiodofluorescein ($C_{20}H_6O_5I_4Na_2$) and belongs to the class of xanthene compounds (Table 1). It is produced by the condensation of resorcinol and phthalic anhydride to form fluorescein, which is then iodinated to yield the tetraiodo compound (201).

Erythrosine is an anionic water-soluble dye that is slightly soluble in alcohols and alkaline solutions. It is fairly stable both in acidic and basic solutions compared with the lower halogenated fluoresceins, which can be subjected to chemical deiodination (296). However, deiodination of erythrosine to lower iodinated fluoresceins may occur in some foods held under acid storage conditions (100).

3. Exposure Information

In the 1981 National Academy of Sciences Phase III Survey of Food Additives, the annual poundage for FD & C Red No. 3 used in foods was reported to be 81,000. The use of the color additive spans the entire spectrum of food categories from baked goods and dairy products to beverages and reconstituted vegetable protein (27,182). Mean levels of the color additive used in foods ranged from 0.00001% for gravies/sauces to 0.1% for bubble gum.

On the basis of reports submitted to the FDA in support of the safety of the color additive, the average daily intake allowed for human ingestion (ADI) is 2.5 mg/kg body weight or 100 ppm of total diet (utilizing a 100-fold safety factor). The estimated per capita daily intake (EDI) of erythrosine for humans from food and dietary supplement sources is expected to be no greater than 7.88 mg/day (34.07 mg/day for all reported ingested uses, i.e., food, drugs, and cosmetics).

4. Pharmacokinetics

In vitro studies with erythrosine have shown the dye to be highly lipid-soluble in cholesterol-lecithin mixed micelles (119). Erythrosine also complexes with the phospholipid fraction of plasma (68), and binds readily and spectrally alters both rodent and human serum proteins (albumin and β-globulins) (119,176). This binding to rodent serum proteins, however, greatly reduces its lipid solubility.

For erythrosine, only limited information exists on the disposition of the dye *in vivo*. Erythrosine is not extensively absorbed across the gastrointestinal tract. Studies using [^{14}C]erythrosine have indicated that less than 20% of the dye is absorbed across the gastrointestinal lumen with no apparent tissue accumulation (68). In addition, erythrosine does not undergo metabolic degradation in the intestine, which is a major pathway for the disposition of the azo dyes (125,225). Erythrosine may, however, be subject to deiodination in the gastrointestinal tract. Recent studies have shown a decoloration of the color additive following its incubation with intestinal extracts from rodents (139). Whether this is actually the result of intestinal degradation or the result of a leuco dye formation (intact but immobilized chromophore) has not been determined.

Erythrosine is bound to plasma proteins (mainly the β_1 fraction) and circulates in the animal as such (68). Initial studies with rodents indicated that erythrosine was not subject to either systemic deiodination, such as occurs for the lower halogenated fluoresceins, or to type II conjugation, such as occurs for fluorescein (296). Paper chromatographic techniques, for instance, depicted only one urinary metabolite that was identical to that of erythrosine following oral intubation of doses up to 1% in rats (296). However, more recent studies in rats indicate that from 25 to 33% of an absorbed dose of erythrosine can be metabolized (deiodinated) (97,293). Failure to observe metabolic changes in earlier studies may have occurred because of the acute nature of the administration and observation times as well as the insensitivity of the analytical methods.

Erythrosine is excreted primarily via the biliary route, with less than 10% of the unchanged compound appearing in the urine after 24 hr (150,176,293,296). Pink coloration of the urine has been observed following high-dose administration (75,307) and at least one study has shown evidence of accumulated staining of the renal tubules (75). *In vitro* inhibition of organic acid transport in the kidney also occurs with erythrosine (77). Whether this plays a role in determining its excretion pattern or its propensity for staining renal tissues has not been examined.

5. Neurobehavioral and Systemic Toxicity Aspects

In 1975, Feingold published his thesis on behavioral disorders (hyperkinesis) in children in whom he claimed dramatic success in alleviating behavioral symptoms after placing patients on a predefined diet (Kaiser-Permanente, K-P) devoid of artificial food and color additives (108). It had been Feingold's premise that many children diagnosed as hyperkinetic were genetically predisposed (sensitive) to artificial food additives. This sensitivity could be manifested by neurobehavioral changes. Thus, altering the diet to eliminate these food components was reported to ameliorate the dysfunction. In attempts to validate this hypothesis scientifically, several investigators tested the utility of the K-P diet in crossover and challenge designs in children identified as hyperkinetic (135,136,286,299). An analysis of these results has been presented elsewhere (173,254,255). Needless to say, the undertaking of such clinical trials has posed a number of problems in the interpretation of the results: defining the hyperkinetic group, compliance with the program, appropriate crossover designs, nutritional balance, choice of challenge material, and the subjective nature of the behavioral ratings among others (93,109,173, 254,255,298). From the available evidence, it appears that within the heterogenous population of hyperkinetic children, there may exist a subgroup of individuals who respond favorably to the K-P diet.

Since exposure to food colors has been implicated in mediating this hyperkinetic response pattern, a number of clinical studies have attempted to examine the behavioral effects of giving hyperkinetic children, on the K-P diet, a challenge with a food dye mixture (containing among other dyes FD & C Red No. 3) masked in a particular food item (109,135,273,299,303). Again, the results from at least one study are suggestive of a subgroup of the hyperkinetic children that may be sensitive to the color additive. Swanson and Kinsbourne (273) recently reported that a group of hyperactive children exhibited impaired performance in paired-associated learning tests when administered a mixture of artificial food color additives of which 6% was FD & C Red No. 3. Because of the acute nature of the response pattern, these results and others (303) have been indicative of a pharmacologic rather than an allergic or immunologic action to the color additives. It has been suggested that FD & C Red No. 3 may be involved in a direct neurotoxic reaction since this color additive has been shown experimentally to affect neurochemical processes. However, the evidence to date utilizing various *in vivo* animal model systems has not supported this contention.

As a preliminary index of toxicity in animal test systems, the acute lethal dose (LD_{50}) for erythrosine was found to range from 0.70 mg/kg (intravenous administration) to 1.84 to 6.80 mg/kg (oral administration) in rodents (75,133,176,294,307). Clinical signs of toxicity have included depression, diarrhea, distension of the abdomen, intestine and cecum, ataxia, decreased spontaneous motor activity, irritability, and a loss of righting reflex. Hindlimb paralysis has been observed in both rats and mice following intravenously administered erythrosine (68,294). Variations in the actute oral LD_{50} values reported probably reflect differences in the purity of the dye used in these studies.

More definitive means of assessing the potential toxicity and neurotoxicity of erythrosine have been performed in several animal species over varying dosing periods. Initial reports on the subchronic bioassay testing of erythrosine indicated that anemia, hypocholesterolemia, and elevations in protein-bound iodine (PBI) were present in rats receiving the dye by stomach intubation (69). In subsequent studies by other investigators, only diarrhea and dose-related increases in PBI were observed in rats receiving up to 4% erythrosine in the diet for 90 days (75,132). No signs of neurotoxicity were present. The changes in PBI were later attributed to the interference by erythrosine in the assay technique (248). However, dose-related thyroid effects (including changes in T_3, T_4, and PBI) from erythrosine ingestion (167 to 1500 mg/kg/day) were apparent in another study using minipigs (76). Whether these effects were in fact attributable to erythrosine or to dye impurities was not ascertained. Recent studies in minipigs have shown that as much as 50% of an ingested dose of erythrosine may be absorbed, and can effect T_4 levels, thyroid uptake, and thyroid iodine retention (143). Interestingly, in this latter study, the distribution of "radioactivity" of labeled erythrosine appeared first in the liver and later in the thyroid, with maximum levels reached by 2 weeks. Again, in neither minipig study were there reports of neurotoxicity.

In the chronic bioassay testing of erythrosine, neither rats (up to 5% in the diet) nor mice (up to 2% in the diet) gave substantial evidence of either thyroid gland dysfunction or neurotoxicity from ingestion of the dye (133,287,295,302). Similarly, beagle dogs receiving the color additive at levels of 0.5% to 2.0% in the diet for 2 years did not exhibit any specific toxic manifestations (although subclinical thyroiditis was present in two of ten animals at the high-dose level) (133). Prolonged administration of erythrosine in a less common animal model, the mongolian gerbil, has been associated only with dose-related changes in thyroid function (92). What relationship these latter findings have to man is not known at present. Other studies have examined erythrosine for reproductive and teratogenic effects in several animal species (73,220). In neither case were neurotoxic changes elicited following *in utero* exposure with the color additive.

In further attempts to identify the neurotoxic potential of erythrosine, several animal model systems have been used. Goldenring et al. (127) observed increases in locomotor activity and disruptions of avoidance performance in both control and 6-hydroxydopamine-treated rats receiving a mixture of food dyes of which 6% was FD & C Red No. 3. In further studies by these authors, however, erythrosine (1 mg/kg/day) administered to neonatal pups for 30 days did not affect locomotor activity nor cognitive performance (126). Analysis of whole brain homogenates for catecholamines (norepinephrine and epinephrine) did not reveal any differences between dye-treated animals and their corresponding controls.

Similar findings in developing rats administered erythrosine in the diet have been reported by Vorhees et al. (289,290). In investigations of the potential psychotoxicity of erythrosine (up to 1%) in rats exposed *in utero* and through 90 days postweaning, the results were suggestive of an increase in locomotor activity in some of the treated groups (290). In a repeat study using the same neurobehavioral testing paradigms (such as reflex development, open-field activity, rotorod coordination, and active avoidance) as well as physical milestones, Butcher et al. (74) and Vorhees et al. (289) failed to confirm any consistent adverse or delayed developmental responses when the dye was administered chronically. In neither study was gross or histochemical evidence of brain lesions found. Increased pup mortality (decreased viability) was apparent at the high-dose level and was attributed to stressful handling of the animals at testing (74). Mailman et al. (180) have observed an attenuated response pattern in an avoidance-approach paradigm when erythrosine was acutely administered intraperitoneally to rats. There is some question regarding the interpretation of this study, since the dye is relatively unabsorbed by this route of administration (119). Although the above studies have not provided sufficient evidence of a neurotoxic potential for the color additive, they have posed the question of whether erythrosine can alter neuronal processes in certain situations.

Both clinical and experimental studies have suggested that abnormalities in monoaminergic neurons at specific loci in the CNS may underlie the hyperkinetic syndrome (131,169,253). Utilizing *in vitro* techniques to focus on specific neurochemical events in the brain, several investigators have attempted to ascertain whether erythrosine has the potential to modify neuronal function. Levitan and coworkers addressed this question using lower-order biological systems. They observed that erythrosine could bind nonspecifically to lipophilic regions of plasma membranes and thus promote alterations in ion permeability and conductance

(78,79,110,170,171). Its interaction with membrane lipoproteins was apparently responsible for its inhibitory effects on membrane activity and/or surface charges. Presynaptically, erythrosine was shown to affect miniature end-plate potentials (MEPP) and postsynaptically to alter potassium conductance in the frog neuromuscular junction preparation (54). In subsequent studies employing rat brain synaptosomes as a model system, erythrosine inhibited dopamine uptake, decreased nonsaturable binding of dopamine, and displaced [^{3}H]oubain binding (an inhibitor of the Na$^+$/K$^+$-ATPase system) (167,174,180,245,246,247). Because of the inhibitory actions by erythrosine on dopamine- and other neurotransmitter-uptake systems (such as those of choline, γ-aminobutyric acid (GABA), glycine, glutamate, and norepinephrine], it was proposed that the color additive may alter membrane fluidity, thereby decreasing the stability of membrane coupling complexes (174). Spin-labeling techniques have further supported this thesis, since erythrosine has been shown to migrate into the membrane lipid bilayer and interfere with oxidation–reduction events (111). However, the use of the certified color (which by definition is only 87% pure) in these investigations has raised questions about the influence of dye impurities, especially the free iodine molecule, on the uptake processes. Fluorescein, for example, has not been shown to affect ATP-dependent norepinephrine uptake into chromaffin granule cell membranes (a neuronal storage model system), as opposed to other neuroleptic agents known to be psychopharmacologically active (223). Although Lafferman and Silbergeld (167) have reported that NaI does not inhibit the neuronal uptake processes, there may be other factors involved that could best be resolved by using purer dye preparations.

Mailman et al. (180) concluded from their experiments that the neurochemical changes observed with erythrosine were tissue-dependent (i.e., protein) and arose from its nonspecific interactions with brain membranes. Hence, alterations in synaptosomal uptake by erythrosine were caused by a "pseudoirreversible inhibition" of either dopamine or other neurotransmitters. Inability of erythrosine to displace [^{3}H]spiperone, a dopamine antagonist, from the dopamine receptor binding sites and its failure to inhibit dopamine-stimulated adenylate cyclase activity in synaptosomal preparations gave further evidence that erythrosine does not participate in specific binding to alter functional neuronal processes (180). However, it should be recognized that other types of receptor interaction, such as serotoninergic, GABAergic, and α- or β-adrenergic, may be more specific for the erythrosine moiety. Functional changes in these receptors (e.g., number or affinity) may alter molecular events at the synapse level either directly or indirectly through interruptions in receptor interactions. The use of ligand-binding techniques in these types of *in vitro* systems to identify the affected receptors has not been fully examined.

In vivo studies designed to assess the effects of dietary administration on specific neuronal receptor areas, using these binding assays (65), may also help to resolve the question of whether erythrosine can modify brain activity. These studies should include an examination of its systemic pharmacokinetics, especially tissue distribution and accumulation in the suggested target areas such as the brain. Recent studies, for example, suggest that erythrosine does not cross the blood–brain barrier in significant amounts (172). If this evidence is borne out, then erythrosine should be examined to determine if it may act to modulate molecular events at the barrier itself such as influx or efflux of organic acids, ions, or neurochemical precursors. Other possible studies include unit recording (electrophysiological events) to identify potential ionic conduction disturbances.

From the previous discussions it appears as though there may be two potential target organ sites for erythrosine in mammals: the thyroid and the central nervous system (CNS). Ample evidence exists in both animals and humans that thyroid dysfunction may evoke neurological manifestations. Hyperthyroidism, for example, can present symptoms of hyperactivity, emotional lability, and irritability (272). It has been suspected that in some instances hyperthyoidism may be responsible for the hyperactivity syndrome in children (173). Whether thyroid function is compromised in these individuals (either as a group or as a subpopulation) has not been adequately tested. For example, it is not known how sensitive these individuals may be to subtle changes in T_4, T_3, or iodine itself. It is known that alterations in thyroid hormone levels can lead to CNS changes in (a) energy-dependent transport mechanisms in the synthesis and release of neurotransmitters; (b) nerve conduction; and (c) pre- and postsynaptic adrenergic receptor sites (169,183,272). However, evidence that acute or chronic exposure to erythrosine can alter thyroid function in humans has not been verified. Although large doses of erythrosine have been associated with increases in iodine uptake by the thyroid (181), erythrosine ingested by humans either in foods or in drug capsules has been associated only with serum elevations in PBI, and these may be caused by interference in the assay technique (305). Other thyroid parameters such as T_3, T_4, or ^{131}I-thyroid uptake do not change significantly with acute dye exposure (11,50,62,66,129,305). Increases in PBI from organic iodine intake, however, may occur without appreciable evidence of thyroid toxicity in humans (98,273). Apparently, functional changes in the thyroid are evident only after more prolonged periods of iodide intake at high dose levels (306). A number of cases of iodine-induced hyperthyroidism (Jod-Basedow phenomenon) have been reported (57). With smaller doses of iodine, uptake of iodine into the thyroid may be enhanced (237), possibly because of the absolute clearance of iodine by this organ (306). In animal models, both acute and chronic administration of iodine at high dose levels has been preceded by increases in PBI and decreases in ^{131}I-thyroid uptake (94,118,293). In these instances, histological evaluation of the thyroid revealed slight increases in follicular size but no indication of hypothyroidism.

It is possible, therefore, that minor alterations in thyroid function may be manifested as behavioral changes, especially in settings of environmental challenges. Thus, a delicate neurological balance in susceptible individuals may be altered by factors that influence the fine tuning of thyroid hormone homeostasis (169). Although no evidence exists at present that would indicate that erythrosine can act in this capacity, it is possible to hypothesize that, because of its structural similarity to T_4, erythrosine might act in a manner analogous to that of thyroxine. Indeed, erythrosine has been shown to bind and to migrate in the same protein fraction as

T_4 (68). Whether these changes could occur from erythrosine displacement of T_4 from binding protein sites, from interference with T_4 activity (feedback or metabolism), or from alterations in T_4-dependent neuronal receptor populations has not been experimentally evaluated. Studies along this line could provide important information on the biological activity of the color additive and its potential for inducing neurological consequences.

6. Discussion

There are a number of factors to be considered in determining the neurotoxic potential of erythrosine and the taking of regulatory actions. Although erythrosine appears to be somewhat membrane-soluble and may undergo at least some metabolism, evidence of a direct CNS involvement has not been established. Studies conducted *in utero* to demonstrate potential teratogenic responses have not identified any neurobehavioral effects from erythrosine administration. Similarly, other bioassay testing models used to assess the safety of FD & C Red No. 3 have not revealed any clinically overt signs of neurotoxicity or neurobehavioral changes associated with the ingestion of the color additive. This may be the result of the relative inertness of the dye or to the unusual sensitivity of animal model systems needed to elicit an observable response. The attention paid in the past to recording behavioral changes during prolonged administration of the color additive may have been less than adequate. Moreover, subtle changes may not be evident in unchallenged testing paradigms. The extent of observations in most chronic and subchronic testing schemes centers about the quantitative rather than the qualitative changes in animals receiving the additive.

As indicated in Table 4, the fluorescein compounds in general appear to be nontoxic. Overt clinical signs of neurotoxicity from acute administration of these compounds are similar to those previously reported for erythrosine. It has been noted that the acute toxicity (LD_{50}) of the xanthene compounds increases with the addition of a halogen to the fluorescein molecule (307), an effect that may be attributable to its altered excretion pattern (296) and/or its increased lipid solubility (partition coefficient). For example, fluorescein, in contrast with erythrosine, has a lower partition coefficient and is almost exclusively excreted by the kidney (as a glucuronide conjugate) with little biliary elimination (296).

Indications of neurological effects have not been associated with ingestion of the other fluorescein-related compounds (Table 5). Although some studies suggest that erythrosine may produce operant behavior changes when examinations are made under a selective testing paradigm, they have not provided definitive evidence of neurotoxicity. Similarly, the lack of convincing clinical evidence showing that erythrosine is involved in the hyperkinetic syndrome further increases the uncertainty that any regulatory actions could be upheld. The problem in taking such actions to reduce or eliminate human exposure to erythrosine lies in the question of appropriateness of the scientific evidence implicating erythrosine as a neuroactive agent. Studies using dye mixtures containing erythrosine, for instance, are unsuitable for

TABLE 4. *Fluorescein compounds used as color additives*

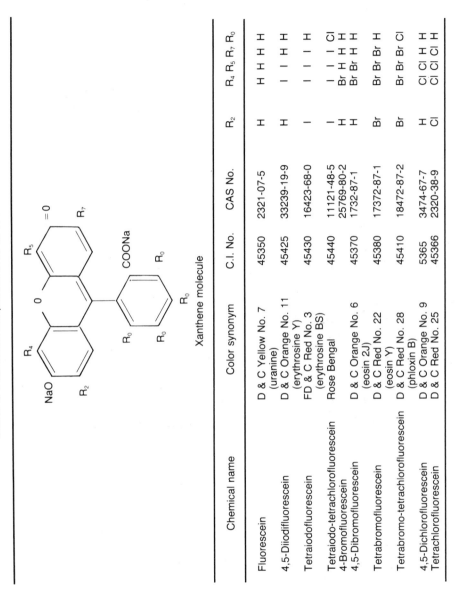

Xanthene molecule

Chemical name	Color synonym	C.I. No.	CAS No.	R_2	R_4	R_5	R_7	R_0
Fluorescein	D & C Yellow No. 7 (uranine)	45350	2321-07-5	H	H	H	H	H
4,5-Diiodifluorescein	D & C Orange No. 11 (erythrosine Y)	45425	33239-19-9	H	I	I	H	H
Tetraiodofluorescein	FD & C Red No. 3 (erythrosine BS)	45430	16423-68-0	I	I	I	I	H
Tetraiodo-tetrachlorofluorescein	Rose Bengal	45440	11121-48-5 25769-80-2	I	I	I	I	Cl
4-Bromofluorescein			1732-87-1	H	Br	H	H	H
4,5-Dibromofluorescein	D & C Orange No. 6 (eosin 2J)	45370		H	Br	Br	H	H
Tetrabromofluorescein	D & C Red No. 22 (eosin Y)	45380	17372-87-1	Br	Br	Br	Br	H
Tetrabromo-tetrachlorofluorescein	D & C Red No. 28 (phloxin B)	45410	18472-87-2	Br	Br	Br	Br	Cl
4,5-Dichlorofluorescein	D & C Orange No. 9	5365	3474-67-7	H	Cl	Cl	H	H
Tetrachlorofluorescein	D & C Red No. 25	45366	2320-38-9	Cl	Cl	Cl	Cl	H

TABLE 5. *Structure–activity relationship of fluorescein dyes*

Chemical name	M.W.	Partition coefficient[a]	LD_{50}	Animal model systemic toxicity	Animal model neurotoxicity	Human neurotoxicity
Fluorescein	352.31	−4.77	6.7[b]	Kidney; granulation	Nontoxic	None reported
4,5-Diiodofluorescein	589.12	−2.46	15.4	Nontoxic	Nontoxic	None reported
Tetraiodofluorescein	835.88	−0.15	2.9[b]	Kidney tubular pigmentation; thyroid(?)	Questionable	Hyperactivity (suspected)
Tetraiodo-tetrachlorofluorescein	973.67	+3.14			Nontoxic	None reported
4,5-Dibromofluorescein	490.07	−3.02	11.3	Kidney; glomerularnephritis	Nontoxic	None reported
Tetrabromofluorescein	647.89	−1.27	13.9	Nontoxic	Nontoxic	None reported
Tetrabromo-tetrachlorofluorescein	785.67	2.02	8.4	Kidney tubule pigmentation; testes and brain mineralization	Nontoxic	None reported

[a]From Levitan et al., ref. 110.
[b]From Yankell and Loux, ref. 307.

extrapolating an effect to a single dye component. On the other hand, the lack of a neurotoxic effect from high dose levels of erythrosine in the chronic toxicity studies provides some assurance of the safety at the low dose level of dietary exposure in humans. As such, current regulations regarding the use of erythrosine in foods are based on quantitative findings from previous chronic toxicity tests that did not suggest any untoward effects. In addition, current ongoing chronic toxicity studies in rodents with *in utero* exposure to erythrosine have not as yet been suggestive of any adverse neurological effects from oral ingestion (up to 4%) of the color additive. It is anticipated that the results from these studies will provide the agency and the consumer with a better definition of the potential toxicity of FD & C Red No. 3.

C. Contaminants

1. Industrial: Methylmercury

a. Historical overview of the methylmercury problem

The contamination of fish and shellfish by methylmercury (MeHg) serves as an appropriate example of how the FDA has approached the problem of contamination of the food supply by ubiquitous industrial compounds. In this particular instance, neurotoxicity induced by MeHg had a significant impact on the regulatory action taken by the agency with regard to this public health problem (see Section II, A,2 and Table 1). Indeed, the establishment of the action level for MeHg was based in large part on its demonstrated human neurotoxicity. Other industrial contaminants, such as lead and polychlorinated biphenyls, also have adverse effects on the structure and function of the nervous system; however, for these compounds this is but one of several toxic endpoints produced by each. In the case of MeHg, its neurotoxicity formed almost the entire basis for the toxicological assessment that was used as part of the regulatory procedures undertaken by the FDA.

The concern surrounding mercury contamination of the food supply was greatly accentuated by the episodes of MeHg poisoning that occurred in Minimata Bay and Niigata, Japan in the 1950s and 1960s. In these particular instances, severe neurological damage occurred in individuals (several hundred cases reported) who had consumed fish taken from local estuarine waters. It was determined that the fish were contaminated with MeHg that originated from industrial (plastics) sources located in these areas (163,278,283). In the Niigata incident, six deaths were reported in addition to the neurotoxic aberrations. There were also other episodes of MeHg-induced neurotoxicity that occurred in Iraq in 1960 and 1972 (55). In these incidents, seed wheat treated with an MeHg antifungal compound was processed as flour for baking bread. In the earlier incident, approximately 1,000 persons were affected and the mortality rate was 30 to 40%, whereas in the 1972 incident over 6,000 individuals demonstrated symptoms and 459 eventually succumbed. These occurrences, along with others in Guatemala (134), Ghana (217), Pakistan

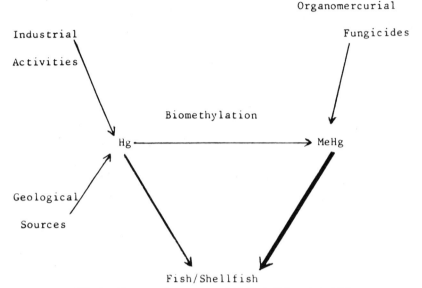

FIG. 1.   Sources of mercury and MeHg in fish and shellfish.

(99), and the United States (221), brought attention to the potential problem of contamination of the food chain, particularly fish and shellfish, by MeHg.

Mercury, as derived from geological sources, is normally found in the aquatic environment. However, normal environmental levels can be elevated by man's activities. Therefore, mercury contamination of water and, as a result, contamination of fish can result from geological, industrial, and/or agricultural sources. The geological contamination results from the leaching or volatilization of natural geological sources. Agricultural use of organomercurial fungicides is a source of the direct release of MeHg into the environment. Mercury also enters the environment as a result of its use in a number of products including cosmetics, paint, paper, pulp, pharmaceutics, electrical equipment, and chloralkali materials. Other sources of mercury contamination are from the burning of fossil fuels and the refining of mercury-contaminated ores. As a result of these activities the contamination of drinking water and the food supply, especially fish and shellfish, can occur from either inorganic or organic mercury (89,163).

The most prevalent and biologically active form of mercury in the edible portions of fish is the methylated form (163). As previously stated, the most obvious source of this form of mercury is from agricultural sources, but this alone cannot account for all of the MeHg found in fish. Apparently, inorganic mercury in the aquatic environment can be converted by microorganisms found in bottom sediments to the more toxic MeHg (154,163). MeHg, in turn, can be taken up by shellfish and bottom-feeding fish and from there can move up the food chain to man, as depicted in Fig. 1 (89).

The FDA surveyed 10 basic food items and found that fish and shellfish contaminated with MeHg were the only commodities that would pose a potential human health risk (241,247). What is particularly distressing about these food items is that the mercury is present, almost entirely, in its methylated form in the edible portions of these species. MeHg has been shown to be quite persistent with a biological half-life of over 2 years. The disappearance of MeHg from fish occurs in two stages. The first phase is rapid and coincides with the distribution of the compound to various tissues throughout the fish. The second phase involves the removal of the compound from the tissue where it is bound, and it is this process that is extremely slow and accounts for the long biological half-life of MeHg (241).

b. Toxicological overview

(1) *Pharmacokinetics.* Once ingested, MeHg is bound to proteins in the gastrointestinal tract and from there it is efficiently absorbed and distributed systemically. This absorption is more efficient and much greater than that occurring with inorganic mercury. Studies using both test animals and humans have shown that nearly 90% of orally administered MeHg is absorbed, whereas only 2 to 15% of ingested inorganic mercury will be absorbed (2,59,89). Studies in germ-free animals have shown that intestinal microflora metabolize orally administered MeHg in such a way as to reduce the tissue content of mercury (234).

Once absorbed, MeHg binds to sulfhydryl and disulfide groups of large molecules, particularly those of proteins. In the plasma, MeHg is primarily bound to plasma proteins, while in the erythrocytes it is bound in a reversible fashion to hemoglobin (59). The mechanism by which MeHg enters cells is unknown, but it appears that the primary reservoir of MeHg in the blood is the erythrocyte (59,115). Once bound, whether in the plasma or erythrocytes, MeHg is slowly disseminated to the rest of the body by intracellular distribution (58,61,193). Although uptake in the nervous system is slow, it appears that both fetal and adult brain have an affinity for this heavy metal (59,61,301). Indeed, although the overall distribution in the fetus is similar to that found in the adult, it appears that fetal brain levels are relatively higher than those found in the adult (63). In the human male, MeHg was shown to accumulate in the liver and brain and to have a biological half-life of 70 to 74 days. The removal of the heavy metal from the nervous system occurred more slowly than that from the other tissues (2).

It is apparent that because of the neurophilicity of MeHg, the nervous system is the primary target organ. Although the initial uptake by nervous tissue of orally administered MeHg is slow, undoubtedly because of the blood–brain barrier, the compound is eventually distributed to most segments of the nervous system (81). In rodents it accumulates in the hippocampus, subcortical portion of the forebrain, cerebellum, cerebral cortex, and spinal dorsal root ganglia, and perturbations in these areas appear to correspond somewhat with the clinical symptomatology (81,82,83,105,115,258,309). In monkeys, there is a linear correlation between the concentrations of MeHg in the blood and brain up to a blood concentration of 1 $\mu g/g$; however, once this blood level is exceeded, the ratio increases (59). On the cellular level, MeHg is bound to protein (most probably sulfhydryl groups) in the mitochondria, endoplasmic reticulum, Golgi complex, and nuclear envelope, whereas little is found in the nucleus and nucleolus. In nerve cells, MeHg is localized in the mitochondria, myelin, cytoplasm, and axoplasm (81,82,83,219,310).

Other *in vitro* work has demonstrated that MeHg can be degraded to inorganic mercury by the action of ascorbate and soluble proteins (116). The release of inorganic mercury from MeHg is also thought to occur by enzymatic cleavage, and it has been suggested that this catabolic reaction is one mechanism by which this heavy metal elicits its toxicity (115,152). However, it must be stressed that this is not the sole mechanism responsible for its toxic effects (58,81,117). While this transformation of MeHg is considered to be a minor pathway of metabolism and has been shown to be almost nonexistent in the rat kidney and liver, it is present to a small degree in the CNS of the rat (275). In contrast, another study demonstrated significant hepatic and renal levels of inorganic mercury after administration of the methylated form to primates, which suggests species differences in the metabolism of MeHg (59). The exact mechanism by which the demethylation of MeHg takes place and its role in MeHg toxicity remain to be resolved.

MeHg is removed from the body via two routes, renal and biliary (88). The latter is the major route of excretion, where the initial step involves the conjugation of MeHg primarily to glutathione, with a minor fraction conjugated to cysteine (2,227). This complex is formed in the liver and is introduced into the intestine via the bile (207). A major portion of this metabolite is reabsorbed in the intestine, resulting in the establishment of an enterohepatic circulation (88,202). MeHg can also be removed via the bile in its inorganic form. The latter is derived by a demethylation process and undergoes less absorption in the intestine, and as a result is readily excreted via the feces (58,59). In humans, the fecal mode of elimination accounts for approximately 90% of the MeHg excreted (2,55,250). The kidney constitutes a minor route of elimination of MeHg, and, although the exact mechanism(s) has not been determined, it has been suggested that glomerular filtration, tubular transport, exocytosis, and exfoliation may be involved. In the neonate these excretory systems are not fully developed, and therefore it is very likely that the newborn will not be able to remove MeHg as efficiently as the adult. In women, MeHg is passed via lactation to infants, with concentrations in the breast milk reflecting the dose and the magnitude of maternal blood levels (8,184). MeHg also reaches the fetus in animals and humans by crossing the placenta, on exposure of the pregnant female. It readily traverses the placenta as evidenced by the observation that MeHg concentrations in cord blood are equivalent to or exceed concentrations in maternal blood (55,158,185,252).

(2) Animal toxicology. Work with laboratory animals has shown MeHg-induced neurotoxicity to be complex, multifaceted, and dependent on a variety of variables including sex, age, and species (177,178,193).

Studies in rats have shown that the initial toxic event in the nervous system, prior to any neurological signs, is a disruption of protein metabolism (80,141,155,310). When the adverse clinical effects are eventually seen, then a decrease in oxygen consumption, a slight diminution of lactic acid formation, a decrease in neuronal RNA levels, and a breakdown in polyribosomes occur (310). MeHg has pronounced and complex effects on nervous tissue enzymatic systems, particularly those involved in glycolysis, which is of central importance in mammalian nervous tissue metabolism (72,161,218). In cerebral and cerebellar synaptosomes, MeHg elicited a reduction in glutamate-, succinate-, or pyruvate-supported respiration during the initial phase of toxicity (288). It was postulated that the disturbance in glycolysis is due to a decrease in State 3 respiration (ADP-stimulated) with a resulting increase in State 4 respiration (seen as glutamate-supported respiration) (288). The reoxidation of nicotinamide-adenine dinucleotides elicited by electrical stimulation of rat cerebral cortical slices is significantly inhibited by MeHg (72). Histochemical studies in the rat have demonstrated an accumulation of lysosomes in the nervous system, as evidenced by a decrease in the activity of acid phosphatase with chronic MeHg intoxication (86). The activities of neurotransmitter enzymes, such as tryptophan hydroxylase, monoamine oxidase, catechol-*O*-methyltransferase, choline acetyltransferase, and acetylcholinesterase, are also reduced by MeHg in the rat (284). These studies indicate that MeHg brings about complex changes in the metabolic activity of nervous tissue, possibly through mercury-sulfur interactions, which result in the impaired coordination of energy metabolism to functional activity.

One of the initial toxic lesions seen with MeHg is an impairment of the blood–brain barrier (81). This occurs soon after the organic metal is absorbed from the intestine and is evidenced by trauma to the endothelial and glial plasmalemma, which results in increased permeability and dysfunction of the barrier. This dysfunction is responsible for the reduction in the uptake of amino acids and metabolites by the CNS and the extravasation of plasma seen with MeHg intoxication (80,309). The primary neuropathology observed in a variety of animal studies closely resembles that seen with human exposure to MeHg. In the CNS, there is a marked loss of granule cells and, as a result, atrophy of the granule cell layer and proliferation of Bergmann's glial fibers occur in the areas of granule cell loss (153).

In the peripheral nervous system, the primary target tissue is the cell body of the sensory ganglion cell, which results in axonal degeneration beginning at the nodes of Ranvier (84,85,141,153,258). In addition, demyelination of the dorsal nerve roots and peripheral nerves has been noted (193). In the dorsal root ganglion the larger myelinated fibers are affected to a greater extent than the small-diameter fibers (258). These changes are characterized by focal degranulation of the cytoplasm, disintegration of the rough endoplasmic reticulum and ribosomes, and formation of hyloid inclusion material in the cytoplasm, resulting in intracellular vacuolation (82,83,84,85,141). Electrophysiological studies showed retardation of conduction velocity, elevation of threshold, and reduction of amplitude and "area" of the evoked action potential in dorsal roots, as well as minor weakening of skeletal muscle (257).

A number of effects that have been seen in various tissue culture systems with MeHg include degeneration of the axon, myelin sheath, and cytoplasmic organelles (58,124). Tissue culture systems have also been used to demonstrate that MeHg profoundly inhibits neuronal migration in the developing human fetal cerebrum.

This is thought to be the result of cytotoxic effects. Indeed, injury to the plasma membranes and neurotubules in neurons and astrocytes was shown to be prominent and to result in irreversible cell degeneration (87).

The prenatal exposure of rodents to MeHg results in histopathological abnormalities in the CNS, such as degeneration and loss of Purkinje cells (185), transitory inhibition of cerebellar migration from the external granule layer, ultrastructural alteration of cerebellum (81), and depressed reaction of oxidative enzymes (161). In the infant monkey, the histopathological assessment of the CNS revealed extensive neuronal degeneration of the cerebrum, particularly the occipital cortex, with minimal damage to the cerebellum and cerebellar nuclei (301). Behavioral and learning deficits have also been noted in rats and mice that were exposed during gestation and lactation (67,216,261). In the infant monkey, the first signs of MeHg toxicity were losses in dexterity and locomotor ability that were followed by ataxia, blindness, coma, and death. The latter effects developed even after dosing with MeHg was discontinued. In addition to these effects, a reduction in growth and deficits in touch sensation, motor coordination, and/or visual impairment were noted (301). These neurological aberrations are similar to those seen with MeHg intoxication of adult monkeys (60,105,175,193,243).

(3) Human toxicology. The toxicity of inorganic and organic mercury to humans has been known for centuries, especially that associated with occupational settings. The neurological disorders associated with exposure to MeHg were first documented by Hunter and co-workers in 1940 (148). These included observations of paresthesia of the tongue, fingers, and toes, astereognosis, loss of peripheral vision, dysphasia, diminished hearing, impaired speech, ataxia, and incoordination. The clinical symptoms demonstrated by affected individuals varied depending on the degree and length of exposure.

Beginning in 1953, Japanese fishermen and their families in the Minimata Bay area began demonstrating symptomatology similar to that found by Hunter et al. (148), and it was concluded that fish contaminated with MeHg were responsible (163). The illness began with numbness around the mouth and in the extremities, slurred speech, awkward gait, and deafness. The primary neurological symptoms eventually demonstrated by these individuals were the absence of superficial and deep sensation of the extremities, concentric constriction of the visual field, and later, cerebellar ataxia and dysarthria, tremor, and slight mental disturbance (see Table 6). Fifteen years after these individuals first demonstrated the disease, some of the neurological disturbances still persisted, and generally included visual field constriction, deafness, ataxia, and numbness of extremities (163). Other symptomology that occurred in this poisoning incident and others (Niigata, Japan, and Iraq) included exaggerated or reduced muscle tone and tendon reflexes, positive Romberg sign, bilateral motor weakness, ocular convergence paresis, nystagmus on pursuit, tinnitus, dysarthria, and astereognosis (55,163,221,235,283).

Although it must be stressed that not all of these symptoms appeared in every instance, there was a similar pattern of disease response in all of them. These acute neurological disorders constituted the entire toxic response seen in humans. They

TABLE 6. *Primary neurological symptoms resulting from major human exposures*

Minimata Bay	Niigata	Iraq
Paresthesia (100%)[a]	Paresthesia (95%)	Paresthesia (100%)
Concentric constriction of vision (100%)	Concentric constriction of vision (58%)	Concentric constriction of vision (100%)
Slurred speech	Deafness (76%)	Ataxia (100%)
Tremor (75.8%)	Incoordination (87%)	Dysarthria (85%)
Mental disturbance (70.5%)	Positive Romberg's sign (63%)	Deafness (66%)
Tendon reflexes increased (38.2%)	Bilateral motor weakness (60%)	
Tendon reflexes decreased (8.8%)	Convergence paresis (41%)	
	Nystagmus on pursuit (33%)	
	Tinnitus (33%)	

[a]Numbers in parentheses indicate percentage of afflicted individuals demonstrating symptoms.

generally demonstrated a latent period of from several weeks to months before paresthesia became evident as the first clinical symptom. These neurological defects were generally persistent, but did not progress once exposure ceased (163).

As was noted in the animal studies, chronic intoxication with high doses of MeHg in the adult produced atrophy of the brain. This was evidenced by atrophy of the cerebellar folia with extensive thinning of the cerebellar gray matter. In the cerebellar cortex, there was a marked disintegration of the granule cells and, to a lesser extent, the Purkinje cells. Other common findings were involvement of basket climbing and parallel fibers, proliferation of Bergmann's glia, astrocytes, and glial fibers, and development of axonal torpedoes of the Purkinje cells. In the calcarine regions of the occipital lobes there was marked atrophy with degeneration of nerve cells and myelin sheaths. Other findings that did not occur as frequently included astrocytosis, glial fiber proliferation, tissue disruption, proliferation of capillary networks, and mobilization of fat granule cells (81).

MeHg-induced fetal and/or neonatal toxicity has occurred in infants of mothers who were asymptomatic or mildly affected on exposure to the heavy metal (184). The effects in the infants were noted early, and included delays in motor and psychological development, blindness, incoordination, ataxia, deafness, exaggerated muscle tone and reflexes, persistence of primitive reflexes, involuntary movements, and sialorrhea. Although not all of these defects were seen in every child, many were noted to be persistent in follow-up examinations years later (163,252). Indeed, in the Iraqi incident the damage to the fetal nervous system was permanent, with varying degrees of developmental retardation in addition to exaggerated tendon reflexes and pathological extensor plantar reflex (9,10,184). There was a definite relationship between the maximum maternal hair mercury concentration during pregnancy and the frequency of neurological effects in the infants. The frequency of abnormal findings was significantly greater in the infants whose mothers had maximum hair mercury concentrations in the range of 99 to 384 ppm than in infants whose mothers had hair mercury concentrations between 0 and 85 ppm (184).

The distribution of lesions within the CNS of the adult tends to be preferentially localized in the areas of the cerebrum and cerebellum cited above. However, the distribution in the fetus and neonate differs in that it is more generalized. Indeed, it was apparent in the cases detected in Japan that the earlier the involvement the more widespread was the pathology in the CNS (81,278).

The neurotoxicity of MeHg in both animals and humans appears to be the total of the adverse effects on the blood-brain barrier, metabolism, and cellular membranes of the nervous system that lead to sensory, motor, and behavioral disturbances.

c. Derivation of action level

As it became evident that contamination of fish and shellfish with MeHg posed a potential human health problem, the presence of this contaminant was determined to be unavoidable. This conclusion was reached because, even though certain sources of mercury contamination could be controlled, the levels of MeHg that were found in water and fish resulting from man's activities (e.g., industrial and agricultural) could not be reduced. Further, it was impossible to reduce the concentrations found in fish and shellfish, since the technology to do so was not available at the time. Thus, the only available means of controlling human consumption of mercury-adulterated fish was to establish a maximum permissible limit on the mercury content of commercially marketed fish and shellfish.

The data base that was used to establish the proposed action level consisted of the following:

(a) metabolic/pharmacodynamic studies of MeHg in man;

(b) clinical studies of patients from Minamata Bay and Niigata, Japan, and Iraq;

(c) correlation of blood, hair, and occasionally brain levels of MeHg with adverse health effects;

(d) estimates of contaminated fish intake levels in the poisoning incidents;

(e) determination of the relationship between blood and hair levels with the ingestion of MeHg-contaminated fish; and

(f) data on relationship of intake of MeHg to body burdens of MeHg (242).

Since no suitable analytical test for MeHg existed at the time of the proposed action level and, as a result, the ratio between inorganic mercury and MeHg could not be determined, it was assumed that all mercury present in fish and shellfish was in the methylated form.

The analysis of the Japanese incident established that the lowest estimated blood mercury concentration at which toxicity occurred was 0.2 μg/g or 200 ppb (total body burden 20–40 mg). This was later confirmed by preliminary analysis of data from the Iraqi episode and studies by Birke and co-workers (63) of Swedish fisherman with a high daily intake of MeHg. This lowest effect dose was based on a theoretical extrapolation of the data from these incidents of high exposure to an estimate of the potential body burden of mercury that could be expected from the long-term ingestion of low levels of MeHg. This low-dose exposure was determined to be proportional to the daily intake of MeHg and attained a steady state after approximately 1 year of exposure. Intake data indicated that a blood level of 200 ppb could be attained from a daily intake of 0.3 mg MeHg by an average adult male (70 kg). By applying a safety factor of 10 to the estimated blood level of 200 ppb, a maximum tolerable level for whole blood was set at 20 ppb, which would correspond to a daily intake of 0.4 μg/kg of body weight. It was next determined that if fish were consumed at a daily rate of 60 g and contained 0.5 ppm, then the maximum daily intake of 0.4 μg/kg of body weight would be attained.

Although a 10-fold safety factor was applied in this instance, it must be stressed that an additional safety margin exists because the actual levels of MeHg found in fish surveyed were normally well below the proposed action level. The safety margin is increased further by the use of 60 g/person/day as an intake figure for fish and shellfish, but only 1.8% of the population consumes this quantity and the average consumption of fish in this country is actually much less. To protect the individual with the highest intake of fish would have required an action level of 0.18 ppm. However, this would have placed an inordinately heavy economic burden on the fishing industry, since a major portion of the fish catch would have exceeded such an action level, and therefore, would have been excluded from the market place. Under these circumstances the question of avoidability becomes relevant and it was determined that it was not appropriate to exclude or ban a major portion of the fish catch so as to protect the fish consumer with the highest rate of consumption (241).

Other issues that were considered in the development of the action level were the presence of MeHg in other foods and the toxic interaction of MeHg with other compounds, particularly heavy metals such as selenium (6,64,120,157,179,206,269). The former was disregarded because the levels detected in other foods were shown to be extremely low (247), whereas the latter could not be analyzed at the time because of the lack of definitive information to suggest such an interaction (241). This proposed action level of 0.5 ppm was subject to the following limitations:

First, information on individual sensitivity was not available;

Second, the action level was based on the lowest effect level, rather than the no effect level in man;

Third, the dose/response relationship in the fetus and neonate could not be assessed; and

Fourth, the likelihood that long-term exposure to low levels of MeHg could result in subclinical effects is unknown (241).

The original proposal for an action level of 0.5 ppm for MeHg was later modified to 1 ppm. This resulted from a consideration of newer data on fish consumption in the United States, particularly of those species known to be contaminated with mercury. These data, which were developed by the National Marine Fisheries, indicated that the average intake of fish in this country was much less than the 60 g/person/day that was the intake figure used to develop the 0.5 ppm action level, and therefore the action level was adjusted upward to 1 ppm (159).

In addition to the review of intake data for fish, further analysis of the association between blood mercury concentrations and toxicity in the Iraqi incident and in other fish-eating populations showed that many of these individuals were asymptomatic but had blood mercury concentrations that clearly exceeded those that would be attained with an action level of 0.5 ppm. Indeed, this analysis showed that the lowest blood concentration in these individuals that was associated with toxic responses varied between 400 and 600 ppb, and that this amount clearly exceeded the lowest effect level of 200 ppb determined in studies on Japanese patients (251). This new information suggested that the lowest effect level used to derive the proposed action level of 0.5 ppm in the original proposal was too low. However, other data indicated that there was a marked variability in the individual response to MeHg and that late-onset or subclinical effects could result from the exposure to MeHg. Because of these uncertainties concerning the newer data on the health effects of MeHg, it was concluded that the data could not be used to support an adjustment of the proposed action level. Therefore, the decision to raise the action level for MeHg in fish and shellfish was based primarily on the new fish consumption data that had been generated since the original proposal of 0.5 ppm (159).

The development of this action level for MeHg is a clear example of how the FDA has dealt with a food-borne industrial contaminant which has pronounced neurotoxicity in humans. It was developed using data derived from human studies available at the time, and is intended to provide a safety margin for the average consumer from MeHg-contaminated seafoods.

2. Natural: Paralytic Shellfish Poison

a. Cause, origin, and symptoms

Sporadic outbreaks of intoxication from the consumption of fresh, unspoiled mussels and clams have long been known and have served to provide the reason for the FDA interest in this area of commerce (see Section II, A, 2 and Table 1). Since the 1920s, these outbreaks of paralytic shellfish poisoning (PSP) have come to be associated with the occurrence of "red tides." To the oceanographer, "red tide" means concentrations or blooms of planktonic organisms that discolor the ocean. In United States coastal waters, shellfish become toxic after ingesting the dinoflagellates *Gonyaulax tamarensis (excavata)* and *G. catenella.* In Alaska the dinoflagellate still has not been unequivocally identified, but is a *protogonyaulax* spp. Unfortunately, the shellfish may be toxic to humans without the presence of a sufficient growth of dinoflagellates to color the water (96).

The causes of the dinoflagellate blooms are not well understood; their explosive growth may be triggered by a combination of temperature, nutrient concentration, salinity, and other factors, including, perhaps, pollution. The frequency of occurrence of PSP is increasing, and it is occurring in new areas. South of the coast of Maine, for example, there had never been a reported serious incident until the fall of 1972; since that time, blooms due to *G. tamarensis (excavata)* and resulting toxicity of shellfish have become routine incidents along the coasts of Maine, New Hampshire, and Massachusetts (244).

The toxin responsible for PSP was first isolated from the Alaska butter clam *Saxidomus giganteus* and named saxitoxin. At least 10 related toxins have been isolated from *G. tamarenis (excavata)*, *G. catenella*, *protogonyaulax*, and *Gymnodinium breve*. Saxitoxin is stable under acidic conditions (pH 4 to 5), but quickly loses toxicity at higher pH values. For many years the structure of saxitoxin was elusive, but in 1976 X-ray crystallographic studies indicated the structure to be that shown in Fig. 2.

Prior to 1937 there were no analytical methods for detection of PSP. In 1937, Sommer and Meyer (256) developed the mouse bioassay to detect PSP in shellfish tissue and in the "red tide" organism itself. They established the mean death time of an LD_{50} dose injected intraperitoneally into mice and constructed a dose:death-time titration curve. As modified by Schantz et al. (239), this method has been adopted as official by the United States and Canadian governments. One mouse unit[8] is the amount of toxin needed to kill a 20-g mouse in 15 minutes or the asymptote of the dose-to-death curve. Mouse units differ depending on the strain of mouse used, and are usually corrected using a standard saxitoxin solution. Currently there are no proven rapid chemical assay methods for saxitoxin and its analogs in shellfish (244), although there is an intense effort underway to develop such a method.

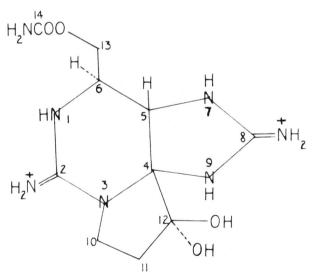

FIG. 2. Structure of saxitoxin. (From Shimizu, ref. 244.)

---

[8]0.18 μg of saxitoxin = 1 mouse unit.

PSP is a type of food poisoning known to occur worldwide with at least 300 cases on record in 1978 (96). The symptoms are summarized in Table 7. The speed of onset is related to the severity of intoxication, but the first symptom—the tingling sensation described in Table 7—occurs within 5 to 30 min after ingestion of the toxic shellfish.

A study of clinicians' reports has failed to reveal any essential difference between the neurological manifestations of PSP occurring on the U.S. Pacific coast and those on the U.S. Atlantic coast. However, one nonneurological symptom seems to be consistently different; during Pacific coastal outbreaks, nausea, vomiting, and other gastrointestinal disturbances are rarely reported, whereas this is a common symptom in Atlantic coastal outbreaks of PSP (106).

The human lethal dose has been suggested to be 1 to 2 mg of saxitoxin, although individual sensitivity is highly variable. Some workers have reported, but not definitively established, that individuals who habitually eat contaminated shellfish can build up a limited immunity; the mechanism is unknown. The toxin accentuates the symptoms of drunkenness, and thus detection of cases may be neglected without vigorous public health education. Cooking slightly reduces the toxin, but is not an adequate method of protection (96). A comparative characterization of toxicity from oral administration of saxitoxin to various species is provided in Table 8.

Prevention of intoxication by avoidance of toxic shellfish is the best way to cope with this public health problem. There is no antidote to the poison. A patient with severe symptoms has his stomach pumped and is given artificial respiration in an iron lung. Otherwise, death due to respiratory paralysis may occur within 24 hr after ingestion, depending on the dose ingested. In survivors, saxitoxin leaves no lasting symptoms once the toxin has been eliminated (96).

b. Pharmacological action

Saxitoxin is a potent neuropoison whose mechanism of action on nerve membranes has been studied by means of various advanced electrophysiological tech-

TABLE 7. *Symptoms of PSP, classified according to degree of severity of intoxication*

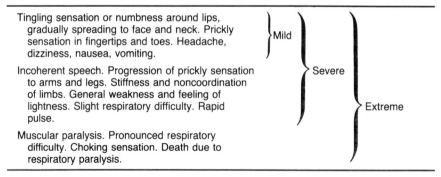

Tingling sensation or numbness around lips, gradually spreading to face and neck. Prickly sensation in fingertips and toes. Headache, dizziness, nausea, vomiting.	Mild		
Incoherent speech. Progression of prickly sensation to arms and legs. Stiffness and noncoordination of limbs. General weakness and feeling of lightness. Slight respiratory difficulty. Rapid pulse.		Severe	
Muscular paralysis. Pronounced respiratory difficulty. Choking sensation. Death due to respiratory paralysis.			Extreme

From Dale and Yentsch, ref. 96.

TABLE 8. *Acute oral toxicities of*
saxitoxin dihydrochloride in
different animals

Animals	LD_{50} (μg/kg)
Pigeon	91
Guinea pig	135
Rabbit	181
Dog	181
Rat	192
Cat	254
Mouse	382
Monkey	264–727

From Shimizu, ref. 244.

niques. Saxitoxin inhibits membrane action potentials by preventing the permeability increase to sodium or by blocking sodium channels.

The membrane resting potential is not affected by the toxin, but the action potential is drastically reduced. Saxitoxin appears to inhibit the sodium conductance increase responsible for the rising phase of the potential. Saxitoxin is totally ineffective when applied internally; for example, a squid giant axon squeezed out with a roller and perfused internally with a saxitoxin solution shows no impairment of excitability, yet saxitoxin is extremely potent when applied externally at nanomolar concentrations. Saxitoxin is poorly soluble in organic solvents, and thus presumably penetrates lipid membranes very poorly. The site of action of the toxin is presumably on or near the external surface of the nerve membrane (195).

Saxitoxin has been demonstrated to bind to the receptor in the nerve membrane on a one-to-one stoichiometric basis. Thus, the toxin is a useful probe to characterize and identify the sodium channel in the nerve membrane (195).

Strichartz (270) has studied the binding of purified radiolabeled saxitoxin to nerve membranes and to receptors from these membranes solubilized by detergents. Binding of tritium-labeled saxitoxin was studied with intact nerves from rabbits, lobsters, and garfish and with solubilized receptors from garfish olfactory nerve. Saxitoxin binds to nerves in two modes. One is a first-order binding and is inhibited by 100-fold concentrations of saxitoxin. This is saturable or specific binding activity. The second mode of binding is an uptake by the nerve that is never saturated, even at concentrations of 10^{-6}M. Solubilized receptors bind saxitoxin only in the saturable mode.

In competition studies, agents that block action potentials by binding in the sodium channels near the outside of the nerve membrane had the capacity to block saxitoxin uptake; examples are lithium, thallium, calcium, and trivalent metal cations. Local anesthetics and veratridine, which affect sodium conductance at the inside of the nerve membrane, do not depress saxitoxin binding. Inhibitory reactions, like the toxin binding action itself, are reversible. Preliminary experiments have indicated that thiamine and its antimetabolites modulate saxitoxin binding; this suggests the use of thiamine as a saxitoxin antidote (270).

Saxitoxin has a direct effect on skeletal muscle. In studies with intact animals (106), saxitoxin, when administered by a low intravenous infusion, did not affect the spinal cord reflexes until the dose became sufficient to start blocking conduction in nerve fibers. In an anesthetized animal, the toxin caused a progressive hypotension and diminishing respiratory movements. When the animal was given a lethal dose, the peripheral action of the poison on nerve conduction and muscle contraction cause respiratory paralysis, with death following. There is no central failure of respiration, since the medullary respiratory centers continue to function for a time after tidal volume has fallen to zero. If the animal is artificially ventilated before the terminal collapse, the heart continues to beat and the animal may eliminate sufficient poison after an hour or longer to resume respiration. Only when saxitoxin is directly injected into the cerebrospinal fluid in the lateral cerebral ventricles does it cause a direct failure of the respiratory center (106).

Saxitoxin has important actions on the cardiovascular system in whole animals (156). Saxitoxin causes a marked fall in arterial blood pressure followed by a moderate compensatory pressor response. The hypotensive action is not due to any selective action of saxitoxin on the central vasomotor system or the heart, but rather to a combination of a direct relaxant effect on vascular smooth muscle at low doses, and to a release of vasomotor tone (which blocks the adrenergic vasoconstrictor nerves) at higher doses. Released catecholamines are responsible for the latter compensatory pressure phase. In clinical cases of PSP, the initial hypotensive phase is rarely seen, but the late pressor phase may be a presenting sign.

c. Regulation of PSP

PSP is a costly problem to public health officials as well as to the shellfish industry. Either shellfish toxicity must be monitored or coastal areas must be closed to shellfishing altogether. Parts of the coastline of Alaska have been closed to fishing of clams and mussels since 1947, following a severe PSP outbreak; this is clearly a great economic loss to the state (96).

In North America, the earliest reported control program designed to protect persons from PSP was established by certain West Coast Indian tribes before the arrival of Russian or European trappers. Sentries posted on high points along the beaches searched for bioluminescence on the water, which was believed to presage a toxic red tide; shellfish harvesting in toxic areas could then be prohibited.

Modern public health control efforts for PSP began in California in the 1920s. Federal attempts to develop guidelines for the control of toxic shellfish also began in the 1920s with the establishment of the National Shellfish Sanitation Program (NSSP) administered by the FDA. A series of conferences in 1955, 1957, and 1958 sponsored by the U.S. Public Health Service established a standard bioassay procedure (the mouse test) for PSP and resulted in the setting of a quarantine limit based on Canadian epidemiological investigations (188) (See Table 9).

Current PSP management programs involve the following actions:

TABLE 9. *Typical toxicity levels, based on mouse test results*

	Toxin level expressed as $\mu g/100$ g tissue
Lower limits of mouse test sensitivity	58
Closure level in United States for shellfish	80
Moderate symptoms in human adult	1,000
Usual lethal level in human adult	10,000
Highest level found in mussels at Mohegan, Maine, in the 1975 outbreak	22,000

From Dale and Yentsch, ref. 96.

1. Key shellfish sampling stations are located.

2. Seasonal sampling plans are developed.

3. Most sensitive species are used as indicators, usually mussels.

4. As PSP levels rise at key stations, satellite stations are established and monitored.

5. Areas exceeding quarantine levels are closed to harvesting, posted, and patrolled.

6. Sampling may be conducted as warranted, and affected shellfish are embargoed.

7. Public education measures are taken to alert recreational and commercial harvesters.

8. Areas are reopened to harvesting when PSP levels in shellfish meats fall consistently below quarantine levels.

California, Maine, and Washington have routine PSP surveillance programs. Since the 1972 PSP outbreak, Massachusetts has conducted an extensive sampling program. The FDA, through the NSSP, evaluates the effectiveness of the state shellfish sanitary control programs. This responsibility also includes foreign countries that have signed bilateral agreements on terms that they will only export shellfish to the U.S. in accordance with NSSP provisions (currently Canada, Japan and Korea). There is a great need for a simple field test to detect the presence in shellfish of PSP (91).

IV. SUMMARY OF FDA ACTIVITIES TO CONTROL EXPOSURE TO NEUROEFFECTIVE FOOD ADDITIVES

The preceding discussions exemplify how the FDA has regulated potentially neurotoxic substances that have inadvertently or intentionally been added to the food supply. These examples serve to emphasize several important points concerning the relationship between regulatory law and science in the protection of public health. First, it is important to note the diverse nature of the sources of these compounds. Aspartame and erythrosine, for example, are intentionally added to food. Acrylamide, on the other hand, migrates into food from plastic packaging materials used to contain and protect food. MeHg is ingested from seafood through a combination of environmental and industrial contamination. Finally, exposure to the natural toxicant PSP or saxitoxin in seafood occurs episodically from poorly understood changes in marine food chain conditions.

Second, it is important to be aware of the various means utilized to uncover the neurotoxic properties of these substances. For both MeHg and saxitoxin, human epidemiology as well as extensive animal tests confirmed the neurotoxicity of these substances. Acrylamide was observed to elicit a neurotoxic effect (paralysis) in animal feeding studies. Indication of a neurotoxic effect from aspartame arose from clinical studies that demonstrated that ingestion of phenylanine has adverse consequences in individuals with PKU and from separate studies conducted on animal models with glutamic and aspartic acids. Implication of a neurobehavioral effect from erythrosine was suggested from clinical observations on a small group of individuals who appeared to be unusually and adversely responsive to the presence of certain food and color additives in their diet.

Third, it should be noted how the agency has utilized various regulatory procedures to maximize public health protection by assuring that the public is not exposed to these substances at neurotoxic concentrations. The first example of these regulatory procedures is the extensive development and analysis of supporting biological data to establish safe conditions of use, followed by the opportunity, provided by the FDA, for the public to comment on the agency's approval of a new food additive. For the purpose of establishing a safe level for food additive intake or action levels for contaminants, it is particularly important to have extensive scientific data and careful evaluation of these agents prior to their final approval or other action by the FDA. Certain of these substances, for example, aspartame and FD & C Red No. 3, may be consumed by large populations of varying age groups in appreciable amounts on a daily basis.

A second example of opportunity for public comment provided in the regulatory process is the Public Board of Inquiry, in which facts of science are deliberated in the context of public health protection. This process was utilized during the approval process for aspartame. A third example of regulatory procedures is the process by which the FDA has established "action levels" for contaminants such as MeHg. When this substance is detected in seafoods above a certain concentration, the seafood can be withheld from interstate commerce as being potentially toxic. Other examples of these regulatory procedures are discussed in the section of this chapter dealing with application of the Food, Drug, and Cosmetic act in controlling exposure to substances which are incorporated into food (see especially section II,B above).

Although most scientific information on the potential toxicity of a foodborne substance is useful, there are a number of other questions that must be answered to place that potential neurotoxic effect in the proper regulatory context. For instance, is more than one animal species affected similarly? If certain species are not similarly affected, are there pharmacokinetic differences that might explain the species difference in toxic response? What are the doses and routes of administration which cause the toxic effect? Are they appropriate when compared with the human exposure route? Thus, one must carefully evaluate the merit and significance of toxic effects demonstrated with doses that may be many times higher than the levels present in foods or toxic effects observed following administration of the substance by other than the oral route. One must also be cautious when attempting to extrapolate the results of *in vitro* test systems to *in vivo* circumstances. To what extent is the implicated substance absorbed from the gastrointestinal tract? Does the substance, when ingested, reach the proposed site of toxic effect within the CNS? Or is it rapidly metabolized, sequestered, or excreted and therefore not available for distribution to the nervous system? The FDA must weigh all of these kinds of evidence concerning each individual compound before it can make an informed decision concerning the presence or lack of neurotoxicity by a putative food additive substance or rationally determine whether there is a risk to public health from an environmental contaminant.

At present the Bureau of Foods is conducting a retrospective analysis of the toxicological data on 1571 food additive compounds. This extensive project, referred to as the priority based assessment of food additives, involves, along with a large number of other toxicological objectives, a correlation of the chemical structure of each compound and its projected or determined neurotoxicological characteristics. It is hoped that a careful review of the structural characteristics of compounds mediating neurotoxic effects may provide a valuable data base for the prediction of comparable untoward responses in untested or poorly tested compounds. This systematic and comparative neurotoxicological analysis may allow the Bureau of Foods to determine the testing priorities among compounds with unresolved questions concerning their neurotoxic potential.

In the past, the Bureau of Foods has relied upon the results from an extensive series of classic toxicological tests, including long-term feeding studies in rodents and nonrodents, to provide evidence, along with many other toxicological end points, of neurotoxic effects by potential food additive substances.

However, the Bureau of Foods recognizes the desirability of developing methodologies to test for neurotoxicity in a more specific manner. As a means of encouraging this development of methodologies designed to detect food additives with neurotoxicologic potential, the FDA Bureau of Foods has for several years supported the development of neurobehavioral testing methods which it hopes will be sensitive, reliable, and comprehensive (292). The discipline of neurotoxicological testing has developed along with the related discipline of behavioral teratology. Behavioral teratology has as its goal the understanding of causes of abnormal behavioral development and the creation of methods for detecting substances that may be potentially hazardous to human populations (291).

Even though the FDA Bureau of Foods is fully sympathetic toward the development of satisfactory developmental and/or neurotoxicological testing methods, it is not yet convinced that these same testing methods are sufficiently mature for the FDA Bureau of Foods to recommend that they be used for routinely screening food additives. The results of one neurobehavioral study supported by the FDA Bureau of Foods serves to highlight some of the difficulties in interpretation of results and application of these results to safety assessment in the regulatory setting (70). In the aforementioned study, aspartame was continuously administered in three dose levels: 2, 4, and 6% of the diet. Data from these subjects were compared with those from other animals receiving normal chow diet (negative controls), hydroxyurea at 550 mg/kg on the 12th day of gestation (positive controls), and phenylalanine at 3% of the diet. The subjects fed 6% aspartame suffered untoward effects, such as delayed development of the startle response and forward locomotion, eye opening, righting, and swimming activity, along with evidence of hypoactivity. It should be noted, however, that the responses of the subjects exposed to 3% phenylalanine were essentially identical (70). This concordance of results between aspartame and phenylalanine is not especially surprising because approximately 50% of aspartame is made up of phenylalanine. High levels of phenylalanine have been shown previously to adversely affect embryonic development (112).

Thus, although it may appear at first that there is a neurotoxicity problem with aspartame, a closer examination reveals that the adverse effects are due to the subjects being exposed to very high levels of phenylalanine, an amino acid found in large amounts in the protein we eat every day. Moreover, it is important to realize the dosages required to produce these effects in animals are many times greater than the projected levels of aspartame consumption in humans. Whatever neurotoxicological test series is utilized, it should be able to discriminate between the toxic effects observed following administration of normal food constituents (such as phenylalanine) and the food additive (such as aspartame). Otherwise, the selectivity as well as the meaning of the testing results will be open to spirited debate. In a regulatory setting, where the FDA is expected to apply the results of scientific safety assessment to legal actions (e.g., interim listing), the evidence against a compound should not be too equivocal or there is a high likelihood that attempts at legal action will not succeed.

As stated above, although it would be desirable to have available specific screening tests for neurotoxicological effects to be used during the initial testing of food additives, it is not clear that these testing paradigms are sufficiently developed at this time to warrant their routine application. At this time, standardization of test batteries for assessing neurobehavioral toxicity could discourage further test development and perhaps result in failure to detect certain unique properties of new types of substances. The Bureau of Foods remains interested in the development of test methods for the routine detection of neurobehavioral effects, but as yet no definitive or widely accepted battery of tests exists (291). Until some degree of scientific consensus concerning such neurotoxicological testing develops, the FDA will be unlikely to initiate specific recommendations regarding such testing. However, if the results of short- or long-term feeding studies provide some evidence of neurotoxicological effect or if evidence in the scientific literature indicates that a structurally or functionally similar compound mediates neurotoxicity, then further testing would be requested. The additional testing would be conducted in order to develop data on the probable no-toxicological effect dose for the food additive compound, with the hope of providing information on the mechanism of toxicological response and its applicability to humans.

Within the general field of toxicological testing, the FDA Bureau of Foods views the development of behavioral teratological or neurotoxicological testing as one of the most important and urgent areas for future improvement. We await with keen interest the creation of testing paradigms that can be recommended for routine measurement of the neurotoxicological potential of food additive substances.

REFERENCES

1. Aaron, H. L. (1966): Letter from Consumers Union to Food and Drug Administration Dec. 6. Bureau of Foods Files, Washington, D.C.
2. Aberg, B., Ekman, L., Falk, R., Grietz, V., Persson, G., and Sniks, J. O. (1969): Metabolism of methylmercury (^{203}Hg) compounds in man. *Arch. Environ. Health*, 19:478–484.
3. Abraham, R. W., Dougherty, W., Goldberg, L., and Coulston, F. (1971): The response of the hypothalmus to high doses of MSG in mice and monkeys. Cytochemistry and ultrastructural study of lysosomal changes. *Exp. Mol. Pathol.*, 15:43–60.
4. Abraham, R., Swart, J., Goldberg, L., and Coulston, F. (1975): Electron microscopic observations of hypothalami in neonatal rhesus monkeys *(Macaca mulatta)* after administration of monosodium-L-glutamate. *Exp. Mol. Pathol.*, 23:203–213.
5. Airoldi, L., Bizi, A., Salmona, M., and Garrattini, S. (1979): Attempts to establish safety margin for neurotoxicity of monosodium glutamate. In: *Glutamic Acid: Advances in Biochemistry and Physiology*, edited by L. J. Filer, Jr., S. Garattini, M. R. Kare, W. A. Reynolds, and R. J. Wurtman, pp. 321–331. Raven Press, New York.
6. Alexander, J., and Norseth, T. (1979): The effect of selenium on the biliary excretion and organ distribution of mercury in the rat after exposure to methylmercuric chloride. *Acta Pharmacol. Toxicol.*, 44:168–176.
7. American Cyanamid Co. (1960): Food Additive Petition No. 1B–0249, FDA Bureau of Foods files, Washington, D.C.
8. Amin-Zaki, L., Elhassani, S., Majeed, M., Clarkson, T., Doherty, R., and Greenwood, M. (1974): Studies of infants post-natally exposed to methylmercury. *J. Pediatr.*, 85:81–84.
9. Amin-Zaki, L., Majeed, M., Clarkson, T., and Greenwood, M. (1978): Methylmercury poisoning in Iraqui children: Clinical observations over two years. *Br. Med. J.*, 1:613–616.
10. Amin-Zaki, L., Majeed, M., Elhassani, S., Clarkson, T., Greenwood, M., and Doherty, R. (1979): Prenatal methylmercury poisoning. Clinical observations over five years. *Am. J. Dis. Child.*, 133:172–177.
11. Andersen, C. J., Keiding, N. R., and Nielsen, A. B. (1964): False elevation of serum protein-bound-iodine caused by red colored drugs or foods. *Scand. J. Clin. Lab. Invest.*, 16:249.
12. Anonymous (1981): Acrylamide-acrylic acid resins and acrylate-acrylamide resins. *Code of Federal Regulations*, 21:Sections 173.5 and 176.110.
13. Anonymous (1981): *Action Levels for Poisonous or Deleterious Substances in Human Food and Animal Feed*. FDA Bureau of Foods, Industry Programs Branch, Washington, D.C.
14. Anonymous (1981): Administrative practices and procedures. *Code of Federal Regulations*, 21:Part 10.
15. Anonymous (1980): *Bureau of Foods Exceptions to the Decision of the Public Board of Inquiry on Aspartame*, pp. 1–41. Docket Number 75F-0355. FDA Documents Management Branch, Rockville, Md.
16. Anonymous (1981): Chemicals used in washing or to assist in lye peeling of fruits and vegetables. *Code of Federal Regulations*, 21:Section 173.315.
17. Anonymous (1980): Commissioner's Decision on Cyclamate. *Fed. Reg.*, 45:61477–61481.
18. Anonymous (1971): Definitions and procedural and interpretive regulations—eligibility of substances for classification as generally recognized as safe in foods. *Fed. Reg.*, 36:12093.
19. Anonymous (1970): Eligibility of substances for classification as generally recognized as safe in food. *Fed. Reg.*, 35:18623–18624.
20. Anonymous (1977): Evaluation of health aspects of GRAS food ingredients: Lessons learned and questions unanswered. *Fed. Proc.*, 36:2519–2562.
21. Anonymous (1966): *FDA Guidelines for Chemistry and Technology Requirements of Food Additive Petitions*. Dockets Management Branch, Food and Drug Administration, Rockville, Maryland.

22. Anonymous (1980): *Federal Food, Drug, and Cosmetic Act*, as amended. U.S. Government Printing Office, Washington, D.C.
23. Anonymous (1981): Food additives. *Code of Federal Regulations*, 21: Part 170.
24. Anonymous (1981): Food additives petitions. *Code of Federal Regulations*, 21:Part 171.
25. Anonymous (1974): Food additives permitted in food for human consumption—Aspartame. *Fed. Reg.*, 39:27317–27320.
26. Anonymous (1971): Food and Drug Administration Advisory Committee on Protocols for Safety Evaluation: Panel on Carcinogenesis report on cancer testing in the safety evaluation of food additives and pesticides. *Toxicol. Appl. Pharmacol.*, 20:417–428.
27. Anonymous (1971): *Food Colors*. Committee of Food Protection, Food and Nutrition Board, National Research Council/National Academy of Sciences, Washington, D.C.
28. Anonymous (1981): Formal evidentiary public hearing. *Code of Federal Regulations*, 21:Part 12.
29. Anonymous (1958): House of Representatives Report No. 2284, 85th Congress, Second Session.
30. Anonymous (1978): IARC Monograph Programme on the Evaluation of the Carcinogenic Risk of Chemicals to Humans, Preamble. In: *Some N-Nitroso Compounds, Vol. 17*, pp. 11–34. International Agency for Research on Cancer, Lyon, France.
31. Anonymous (1975): Letters dated April 28 and April 29 from General Foods Corporation and G. D. Searle and Co. to FDA Bureau of Foods. Docket Number 75F-0355. FDA Documents Management Branch, Rockville, Maryland.
32. Anonymous (1980): Levels of free amino acids in lactating women following ingestion of the sweetener aspartame. *Nutr. Rev.*, 38:183–184.
33. Anonymous (1973): Notice of filing of food additive petition, G. D. Searle and Co., Chicago, Illinois. *Fed. Reg.*, 38:5921.
34. Anonymous (1973): President's Science Advisory Committee, Panel on *Chemicals and Health*. Chapter 8, pp. 63–76. National Science Foundation, Washington, D.C.
35. Anonymous (1959): *Principles and Procedures for Evaluating the Safety of Food Additives*. Food Protection Committee, Food and Nutrition Board, National Academy of Sciences, Publication No. 750, Washington, D.C.
36. Anonymous (1959): *Problems in the Evaluation of Carcinogenic Hazard from the Use of Food Additives*. Food Protection Committee, Food and Nutrition Board, National Academy of Sciences/ National Research Council, Publication No. 749, Washington, D.C.
37. Anonymous (1981): Public hearing before a board of inquiry. *Code of Federal Regulations*, 21:Part 13.
38. Anonymous (1981): Public hearing before a public advisory committee. *Code of Federal Regulations*, 21:Part 14.
39. Anonymous (1981): Public hearing before the Commissioner. *Code of Federal Regulations*, 21:Part 15.
40. Anonymous (1981): Regulatory hearing before the Food and Drug Administration. *Code of Federal Regulations*, 21:Part 16.
41. Anonymous (1974): Report of a WHO Scientific Group. Assessment of the carcinogenicity and mutagenicity of chemicals. *WHO Tech. Rep. Ser.*, 546:1–19.
42. Anonymous (1979): Report of the Interagency Regulatory Liaison Group, Work Group on Risk Assessment. Scientific bases for identification of potential carcinogens and estimation of risks. *J. Natl. Cancer Inst.*, 63:243–268.
43. Anonymous (1977): Report of the Subcommittee on Environmental Carcinogenesis, National Cancer Advisory Board. General criteria for assessing the evidence for carcinogenicity of chemical substances. *J. Natl. Cancer Inst.*, 58:461–465.
44. Anonymous (1980): *Risk Assessment/Safety Evaluation of Food Chemicals*. Food and Nutrition Board, Assembly of Life Sciences, National Academy of Sciences, National Academy Press, Washington, D.C.
45. Anonymous (1980): Statement of position, rebuttal points and proposed findings and conclusions of the Bureau of Foods, pp. 1–148. Docket Number 75F-0355. FDA Documents Management Branch, Rockville, Md.
46. Anonymous (1975): Stay of effectiveness of food additive regulation—Aspartame. *Fed. Reg.*, 40:56907.
47. Anonymous (1981): *Strategies to Determine Needs & Priorities for Toxicity Testing, Vol. 1, Design*. Board on Toxicology and Environmental Health Hazards, Assembly of Life Sciences, National Academy Press, Washington, D.C.

48. Anonymous (1973): *The Use of Chemicals in Food Production, Processing, Storage, and Distribution*, Committee on Food Protection, Food and Nutrition Board, Division of Biology and Agriculture, National Academy of Sciences/National Research Council, Washington, D.C.
49. Anonymous (1973): *Toxicants Occurring Naturally in Foods, 2nd edition*, Committee of Food Protection, Food and Nutrition Board, National Research Council/National Academy of Sciences, Washington, D.C.
50. Anonymous (1965): Toxicological evaluation of iodine release from erythrosine BS. *BIBRA*, 4:450–455.
51. Anonymous (1982): *Toxicological Principles for the Safety Assessment of Direct Food Additives*, Food and Drug Administration. Bureau of Foods, Washington, D.C.
52. Anonymous (1981): Unavoidable contaminants in food for human consumption and food-packaging material. *Code of Federal Regulations*, 21:Part 109.
53. Anonymous (1982): *United States of America, Comment to the ad hoc Working Group on Food Additives Intake*, 15th Session of the Food Chemicals Codex Committee on Food Additives. Dockets Management Branch, Food and Drug Administration, Rockville, Maryland.
54. Augustine, G. J., and Levitan, H. (1978): PVC- and postjunctional actions of erythrosine B. *Neurosci. Abstr.*, 4:367.
55. Bakir, F., Damluji, S., Amin-Zaki, L., Murtadha, M., Khalidi, A., Al-Rawi, N., Tikriti, S., Dhahir, H., Clarkson, T., Smith, J., and Doherty, R. (1973): Methylmercury poisoning in Iraq. *Science*, 181:230–241.
56. Bakke, J. L., Lawrence, N., Bennett, J., Robinson, S., and Bowers, C. Y. (1978): Late endocrine effects of administering monosodium glutamate to neonatal rats. *Neuroendocrinology*, 26:220–228.
57. Barsano, C. P. (1981): Environmental factors altering thyroid function and their assessment. *Environ. Health Perspect.*, 38:71–82.
58. Berlin, M. (1979): Mercury. In: *Handbook on the Toxicology of Metals*, edited by L. Friberg, G. Nordberg, and V. Vouk, pp. 503–530. Elsevier/North-Holland Biomedical Press, New York.
59. Berlin, M., Carlson, J., and Norseth, T. (1975): Dose-dependence of methylmercury metabolism. A study of distribution: Biotransformation and excretion in the squirrel monkey. *Arch. Environ. Health*, 30:307–313.
60. Berlin, M., Grant, C., Hellberg, J., Hellstrom, J., and Schutz, A. (1975): Neurotoxicity of methylmercury in squirrel monkeys. *Arch. Environ. Health*, 30:340–348.
61. Berlin, M., and Ullberg, S. (1963): Accumulation and retention of mercury in the mouse. III. An autoradiographic comparison of methylmercuric dicyandiamide with inorganic mercury. *Arch. Environ. Health*, 6:610–616.
62. Berstein, R., Hangen, H. F., and Frey, H. (1975): Thyroid function during erythrosine ingestion in doses encountered in therapy with conventional antibiotics. *Scand. J. Clin. Lab. Invest.*, 35:49–52.
63. Birke, G., Johnels, A., Plantin, L.-O., Sjostrand, B., Skerfuing, S., and Westermark, T. (1972): Studies on humans exposed to methylmercury through fish consumption. *Arch. Environ. Health*, 25:77–91.
64. Blackstone, S., Harley, R., and Hughes, R. (1974): Some inter-relationships between vitamin C (L-ascorbic acid) and mercury in the guinea-pig. *Food Cosmet. Toxicol.*, 12:511–516.
65. Bondy, S. C. (1979): Rapid screening of neurotoxic agents by *in vivo* and *in vitro* means. In: *The Effects of Foods and Drugs on the Development and Function of the Nervous System: Methods of Predicting Toxicity*, edited by R. M. Gryder and V. H. Frankos, pp. 133–143. *Proceedings of the 5th FDA Science Symposium*, October 10–12.
66. Bora, S. S., Radichevich, I., and Werner, S. C. (1969): Artifactual elevation of PBI from an iodinated dye used to stain medicinal capsules pink. *J. Clin. Endocrin. Metab.*, 29:1269–1271.
67. Bornhausen, M., Musch, H., and Greim, H. (1980): Operant behavior performance changes in rats after prenatal methylmercury exposure. *Toxicol. Appl. Pharmacol.*, 56:305–310.
68. Bowie, W. C. (1972): A history on the summary of the erythrosine project. FDA, Bureau of Foods. *Unpublished.*
69. Bowie, W. C., Wallace, W. C., and Lindstrom, H. V. (1966): Some clinical manifestations of erythrosine in rats. *Fed. Proc.*, 25:556.
70. Brunner, R. L., Vorhees, C. V., Kinney, L., and Butcher, R. E. (1979): Aspartame: Assessment of developmental psychotoxicity of a new artificial sweetener. *Neurobehav. Toxicol.*, 1:79–86.

71. Buckman Laboratories, Inc. (1970): Food Additive Petition Number 2B-2717, FDA Bureau of Foods Files, Washington, D.C.
72. Bull, R., and Lutkenhoff, S. (1975): Changes in the metabolic responses of brain tissue to stimulation, *in vitro*, produced by *in vivo* administration of methylmercury. *Neuropharmacology*, 14:351.
73. Burnett, C. M., Agersborg, H. P. K., Borzelleca, J. F., Eagle, E., Ebert, A. G., Pierce, E. C., Kirschman, J. C., and Scala, R. A. (1974): Multigeneration reproduction studies with certified colors in rats. *Toxicol. Appl. Pharmacol.*, 29:21.
74. Butcher, R. E., Vorhees, C. V., Wootten, V., Brunner, R. L., and Sobotka, T. J. (1979): A survey of early tests for the developmental psychotoxicity of food additives and related compounds. In: *The Effects of Foods and Drugs in the Development and Function of the Nervous System: Methods for Predicting Toxicity*, edited by R. M. Gryder and V. H. Frankos, pp. 62–69. *Proceedings of the 5th FDA Science Symposium*, October 10–12.
75. Butterworth, K. R., Gaunt, I. F., Grasso, P., and Gangolli, S. D. (1976): Acute and short-term toxicity studies on erythrosine BS in rodents. *Food Cosmet. Toxicol.*, 14:525–532.
76. Butterworth, K. R., Gaunt, I. F., Grasso, P., and Gangolli, S. D. (1976): Short-term toxicity of erythrosine BS in pigs. *Food Cosmet. Toxicol.*, 14:532–537.
77. Carlson, J. (1977): Selectivity of food colors for different organic acid transport systems in rat renal cortex. *Acta Pharmacol. Toxicol.*, 91:384–391.
78. Carroll, E. J., and Levitan, H. (1978): Fertilization in the sea violin, *Strongylocentrotas purpuratas*, is blocked by fluorescein dyes. *Dev. Biol.*, 63:432–440.
79. Carroll, E. J., and Levitan, H. (1978): Fertilization is inhibited in five diverse animal phyla by erythrosine B. *Dev. Biol.*, 64:329–331.
80. Cavanagh, J., and Chen, F. (1971): Amino acid incorporation in protein during the "silent phase" before organ-mercury and *p*-bromophenylacetylurea neuropathy in the rat. *Acta Neuropathol.*, 19:216–224.
81. Chang, L. (1977): Neurotoxic effects of mercury—A review. *Environ. Res.*, 14:329–373.
82. Chang, L., Desnoyers, P., and Hartmann, H. (1972): Quantitative cytochemical studies of RNA in experimental mercury poisoning. I. Changes in RNA content. *J. Neuropathol. Exp. Neurol.*, 31:489–501.
83. Chang, L., and Hartmann, H. (1972): Electron microscopic histochemical study on the localization and distribution of mercury in the nervous system after mercury intoxication. *Exp. Neurol.*, 35:122–137.
84. Chang, L., and Hartmann, H. (1972): Ultrastructural studies of the nervous system after mercury intoxication. I. Pathological changes in the nerve cell bodies. *Acta Neuropathol.*, 20:122–138.
85. Chang, L., and Hartmann, H. (1972): Ultrastructural studies of the nervous system after mercury intoxication. II. Pathological changes in the nerve fibers. *Acta Neuropathol.*, 20:316–334.
86. Chang, L., Ware, R., and Desnoyers, P. (1973): A histochemical study on some enzyme changes in the kidney, liver and brain after chronic mercury intoxication in the rat. *Food Cosmet. Toxicol.*, 11:283–286.
87. Choi, B., Cho, K., and Lapham, L. (1981): Effects of methylmercury on human fetal neurons and astrocytes *in vitro*: A time-lapse cinematographic phase and electron microscopic study. *Environ. Res.*, 24:61–74.
88. Cikrt, M., and Tichy, M. (1974): Biliary excretion of phenyl- and methylmercury chlorides and their enterohepatic circulation in rats. *Environ. Res.*, 8:71–81.
89. Clarkson, T. (1971): Epidemiological and experimental aspects of lead and mercury contamination of food. *Food Cosmet. Toxicol.*, 9:229–243.
90. Clemens, J. A., Roush, M. E., and Shaar, C. J. (1977): Effect of glutamate lesions of the arcuate nucleus on the neuroendocrine system in rats. *Soc. Neurosci. Abstr.*, 3:341.
91. Clem, J. D. (1974): Management of the Paralytic Shellfish Poison Problem in United States. In: *Proceedings of the First International Conference on Toxic Dinoflagellate Blooms*, edited by V. R. LoCicero, pp. 459–471. Massachusetts Science and Technology Foundation, Cambridge.
92. Collins, T. F. X., and Long, E. L. (1976): Effects of chronic oral administration of erythrosine in the Mongolian gerbil. *Food Cosmet. Toxicol.*, 14:233–248.
93. Cooperman, E. M. (1978): Hyperactivity and diet. *Can. Med. Assoc. J.*, 119:113–114.
94. Corkea, P., and Welsh, R. A. (1960): The effect of excessive iodine intake on the thyroid gland of the rat. *Arch. Pathol.*, 70:247–251.

95. Dagle, G. E., Zwicker, G. M., and Renne, R. A. (1979): Morphology of spontaneous brain tumors in the rat. *Vet. Pathol.*, 16:318–324.
96. Dale, B., and Yentsch, C. M. (1978): Red tide and paralytic shellfish poisoning. *Oceanus*, 21:41–49.
97. Daniel, J. W. (1962): The excretion and metabolism of edible food colors. *Toxicol. Appl. Pharmacol.*, 4:572–594.
98. Davis, P. J. (1966): Factors affecting the determination of serum protein-bound iodine. *Am. J. Med.*, 40:918–940.
99. Derlan, L. K. (1974): Outbreak of food poisoning due to alkylmercury fungicide on southern Ghana state farm. *Arch. Environ. Health*, 28:49–53.
100. Dickinson, D., and Raven, T. W. (1962): Stability of erythrosine in artifically coloured canned cherries. *J. Sci. Food Agric.*, 13:650.
101. Dow Chemical Co. (1961): Food Additive Petition No. 1B-0388, Polyacrylamides-incidental to their use as a flocculant or filter retention aid in the manufacture of paper and paperboard. FDA Bureau of Foods files, Washington, D.C.
102. Dow Chemicals Co. (1962): Food Additive Petition No. 1B-1019, Polyacrylamide as a flocculant used in clarification of sugar cane juice, FDA Bureau of Foods, Washington, D.C.
103. Duke, J. A. (1977): Phytotoxin tables. *Crit. Rev. Toxicol.*, 5:198–238.
104. Edwards, P. M. (1976): The insensitivity of the developing rat fetus to the toxic effects of acrylamide. *Chem. Biol. Interact.*, 12:13–18.
105. Evans, H., Garman, R., and Weiss, B. (1972): Methylmercury: Exposure duration and regional distribution as determinants of neurotoxicity in nonhuman primates. *Toxicol. Appl. Pharmacol.*, 41:15–33.
106. Evans, M. H. (1975): Saxitoxin and related poisons: their actions on man and other mammals. In: *Proceedings of the First International Conference on Toxic Dinoflagellate Blooms*, edited by V. R. LoCicero, pp. 337–345. Massachusetts Science and Technology Foundation, Cambridge.
107. Fassett, D. W. (1963): Organic acids and related compounds. In: *Industrial Hygiene and Toxicology, Vol. II: Toxicology*, edited by F. A. Patty and D. W. Fassett, pp. 1775–1833. Interscience Publishers, New York.
108. Feingold, B. (1975): *Why Your Child is Hyperactive*. Random House, New York.
109. Ferguson, H. B., Rapoport, J. L., and Weingartner, H. (1981): Food dyes and impairment of performance in hyperactive children. *Science*, 211:410–411.
110. Fitzgerald, J. E., Schardein, J. L., and Kurtz, S. M. (1974): Spontaneous tumors of the nervous system in albino rats. *J. Natl. Cancer Inst.*, 52:265–273.
111. Floyd, R. A. (1980): Erythrosine B (Red Dye No. 3)-mediated oxidation-reduction in brain membranes. *Biochem. Biophys. Res. Commun.*, 96:1305–1311.
112. Frankenburg, W. K., Duncan, B. R., Coffelt, R. W., Koch, R., Coldwell, J. G., and Son, C. D. (1968): Maternal phenylketonuria: Implications for growth and development. *J. Pediatr.*, 73:560–566.
113. Friedman, R., and Alfin-Slater, R. B. (1982): Those natural toxins in foods. *Prof. Nutr.*, Winter: 6–8.
114. Fullerton, P. M., and Barnes, J. M. (1966): Peripheral neuropathy in rats produced by acrylamide. *Br. J. Ind. Med.*, 23:210–221.
115. Gage, J. (1964): Distribution and excretion of methyl and phenyl mercury salts. *Br. J. Ind. Med.*, 21:197–202.
116. Gage, J. (1975): Mechanisms for the biodegradation of organic mercury compounds: The actions of ascorbate and of soluble proteins. *Toxicol. Appl. Pharmacol.*, 32:225–238.
117. Gallagher, P., and Lee, R. (1980): The role of biotransformation in organic mercury neurotoxicity. *Toxicology*, 15:129–134.
118. Galton, V., and Pitt-Rivers, R. (1959): The effect of excessive iodine on the thyroid of the rat. *Endocrinology*, 64:835–839.
119. Gangolli, S. D., Grasso, P., and Goldberg, L. (1967): Physical factors determining the early local tissue reactions produced by food colourings and other compounds injected subcutaneously. *Food Cosmet. Toxicol.*, 5:601–606.
120. Ganther, H. (1978): Modification of methylmercury toxicity and metabolism by selenium and vitamin E: Possible mechanism. *Environ. Health Perspect.*, 25:71–76.
121. Garattini, S. (1979): An evaluation of the neurotoxic effects of glutamic acid. In: *Nutrition and*

the Brain, Vol. 4, edited by R. J. Wurtman and J. Wurtman, pp. 79–124. Raven Press, New York.

122. Gart, J. J., Chu, K. C., and Tarone, R. E. (1979): Statistical issues in interpretation of chronic bioassay tests for carcinogenicity. *J. Natl. Cancer Inst.*, 62:957–974.
123. Gilbert, C., and Gillman, J. (1958): Spontaneous neoplasms in the albino rat. *S. Afr. J. Med. Sci.*, 23:257–272.
124. Goldberg, A. (1980): Mechanisms of neurotoxicity as studied in tissue culture systems. *Toxicology*, 17:201–208.
125. Goldberg, L. (1967): The toxicology of artificial colouring materials. *J. Soc. Cosmet. Chem.*, 18:421–432.
126. Goldenring, J. R., Batter, D. K., and Shaynitz, B. A. (1981): Effect of chronic erythrosine B administration on developing rats. *Neurobehav. Toxicol. Teratol.*, 3:57–58.
127. Goldenring, J. R., Wool, R. S., Shaynitz, B. A., Batter, D. K., Cohen, D. J., Young, G. J., and Teicher, M. H. (1980): Effects of continuous gastric infusion of food dyes in developing rat pups. *Life Sci.*, 27:1897–1904.
128. Guerin, M. (1954): Tumeurs spontanées du rat. In: *Tumeurs Spontanées des Animaux de Laboratoire*, edited by A. LeGrand, pp. 130–131, Paris.
129. Haas, S. (1970): Contamination of protein-bound iodine by pink gelatin capsules colored with erythrosine. *Ann. Intern. Med.*, 72:549–552.
130. Hallerman, H. (1967): Letter of Consumers Union, May 29. FDA Bureau of Foods Files, Washington, D.C.
131. Hanin, I. (1978): Central neurotransmitter function and its behavioral correlates in man. *Environ. Health Perspect.*, 26:135–141.
132. Hansen, W. H., Davis, K. J., Graham, S. L., Perry, C. H., and Jacobson, K. H. (1973): Long-term toxicity studies of erythrosine. II. Effects on haematology and thyroxine and protein-bound iodine in rats. *Food Cosmet. Toxicol.*, 11:535–545.
133. Hansen, W. H., Znickey, R. E., Brouwer, J. B., and Fitzhugh, O. G. (1973): Long-term toxicity studies of erythrosine. I. Effects in rats and dogs. *Food Cosmet. Toxicol.*, 11:527–534.
134. Haq, F. V. (1963): Agrosan poisoning in man. *Br. Med. J.*, 1:1579–1582.
135. Harley, J. P., Matthews, C. G., and Eichman, P. (1978): Synthetic food colors and hyperactivity in children: A double-blind challenge experiment. *Pediatrics*, 62:975–983.
136. Harley, J. P., Ray, R. S., and Tomasi, L., Eichman, P. L., Matthews, C. G., Chun, R., Cleeland, C. S., and Tratsman, E. (1978): Hyperkinetics and food additives: Testing the Feingold hypothesis. *Pediatrics*, 61:818–828.
137. Hattan, D. G. (1980): *Transcript of Public Hearing on Aspartame, Vol. 1*, pp. 60–61. Docket Number 75F-0355. FDA Documents Management Branch, Rockville, Maryland.
138. Hattan, D. G. (1980): *Transcript of Public Hearing on Aspartame, Vol. 3*, pp. 189–197. Docket Number 75F-0355. FDA Documents Management Branch, Rockville, Maryland.
139. Haveland-Smith, R. B., and Combes, R. D. (1980): Genotoxicity of the food colors Red 2G and Brown F.K. in bacterial systems. Use of structurally related dyes and azo reduction. *Food Cosmet. Toxicol.*, 18:223–228.
140. Hayes, A. H., Jr. (1981): Aspartame: Commissioner's final decision. *Fed. Reg.*, 46:38284–38308.
141. Herman, S., Klein, R., Talley, F., and Krigman, M. (1973): An ultrastructural study of methyl-mercury-induced primary sensory neuropathy in the rat. *Lab. Invest.*, 28:104–118.
142. Heywood, R., and Worden, A. N. (1979): Glutamate toxicity in laboratory animals. In: *Glutamic Acid: Advances in Biochemistry and Physiology*, edited by L. J. Filer, Jr., S. Garattini, M. R. Kare, W. A. Reynolds, and R. J. Wurtman, pp. 203–215. Raven Press, New York.
143. Hightower, D. (1981): The bioavailability of iodine from erythrosine and iodophores. Erythrosine I and erythrosine II. FDA Contract No. 223-79-2279, Bureau of Foods files, Washington, D.C.
144. Holtz, A. (1967): Memorandum of April 7, to Petitions Control Branch, relative to structure of acrylamide polymers, FDA Bureau of Foods Files, Washington, D.C.
145. Holzwarth-McBride, M. A., Hurst, E. M., and Knigge, K. M. (1976): Monsodium glutamate-induced lesions of the arcuate nucleus. I. Endocrine deficiency and ultrastructure of the median eminence. *Anat. Rec.*, 186:185–196.
146. Hopkins, H. (1978): The GRAS list revisited. *FDA Consumer*, 12(4):13–15.
147. Howland, D. (1981): The etiology of acrylamide neuropathy; enolase, phosphofructokinase, and glyceraldehyde-3-phosphate dehydrogenase activities in peripheral nerve, spinal cord, brain, and skeletal muscle of acrylamide-intoxicated cats. *Toxicol. Appl. Pharmacol.*, 609:324–333.

148. Hunter, D., Bomford, R., and Russell, D. (1940): Poisoning by methylmercury compounds. *Q. J. Med.*, 9:193–217.
149. Hutt, P. B. (1975): Letter of January 22 to Mr. James Turner of Legal Action for Buyer's Education and Labeling. Docket Number 75F-0355. FDA Documents Management Branch, Rockville, Maryland.
150. Iga, T., Anazu, S., and Nogami, H. (1971): Pharmacokinetic study of biliary excretion. III. Comparison of excretion behavior in xanthene dyes, fluorescein and bromosulphthalein. *Chem. Pharm. Bull.*, 19:297–308.
151. Ishii, H., Koshimizu, T., Usami, S., and Fujimoto, T. (1981): Toxicity of Aspartame and its diketopiperazine for Wistar rats by dietary administration for 104 weeks. *Toxicology*, 21:91–94.
152. Iverson, F., and Hierlihy, S. (1974): Biotransformation of methylmercury in the guinea pig. *Bull. Environ. Contam. Toxicol.*, 11:85–91.
153. Jacobs, J., Carmichael, N., and Cavanagh, J. (1977): Ultrastructural changes in the nervous system of rabbits poisoned with methylmercury. *Toxicol. Appl. Pharmacol.*, 39:249–261.
154. Jensen, S., and Jernelov, A. (1969): Biological methylation of mercury in aquatic organisms. *Nature*, 223:753–754.
155. Joiner, F., and Hupp, E. (1979): Development and methylmercury effects on brain protein synthesis. *Arch. Environ. Contam. Toxicol.*, 8:465–470.
156. Kao, C. Y. (1975): Cardiovascular actions of saxitoxin. In: *Proceedings of the First International Conference on Toxic Dinoflagellate Blooms*, edited by V. R. LoCicero, pp. 347–353. Massachusetts Science and Technology Foundation, Cambridge.
157. Kasuya, M. (1975): The effect of vitamin E on the toxicity of alkyl mercurials on nervous tissue in culture. *Toxicol. Appl. Pharmacol.*, 32:347–354.
158. Kelman, B., Steinmetz, S., Walter, B., and Sasser, L. (1980): Absorption of methylmercury by the fetal guinea pig during mid to late gestation. *Teratology*, 21:161–165.
159. Kennedy, D. (1979): Action level for mercury in fish, shellfish, crustaceans and other aquatic animals. *Fed. Reg.*, 44:3990–3993.
160. Kennedy, D. (1977): Letter of November 3 to G. D. Searle and Co. Docket Number 75F-0355. FDA Documents Management Branch, Rockville, Maryland.
161. Khera, K., and Tabacova, S. (1973): Effects of methylmercuric chloride on the progeny of mice and rats treated before or during gestation. *Food Cosmet. Toxicol.*, 11:245–254.
162. Koch, R., Blaskovics, M. E., Wenz, E., Fishler, K., and Schaffler, G. (1974): Hyperphenylalaninemia and phenylketonuria. In: *Heritable Disorders of Amino Acid Metabolism*, edited by W. Nyhan, pp. 109–140. John Wiley, New York.
163. Kojima, K., and Fujita, M. (1973): Summary of recent studies in Japan on methylmercury poisoning. *Toxicology*, 1:43–62.
164. Kokoski, C. J. (1979): Memorandum of March 16 to N. Singletary. Docket Number 75F-0355. FDA Documents Management Branch, Rockville, Maryland.
165. Kokoski, C. J. (1980): *Transcript of Public Hearing on Aspartame, Vol. 1*, p. 16. Docket Number 75F-0355. FDA Documents Management Branch, Rockville, Maryland.
166. Kuperman, A. S. (1958): Effects of acrylamide on the central nervous system of the cat. *J. Pharmacol. Exp. Ther.*, 123:180–192.
167. Lafferman, J. A., and Silbergeld, E. K. (1979): Erythrosine B inhibits dopamine transport in rat caudate synaptosomes. *Science*, 205:410–412.
168. Lamperti, A., and Blaha, G. (1976): The effects of neonatally administered monosodium glutamate on the reproductive system of adult hamsters. *Biol. Reprod.*, 14:362–369.
169. Leonard, B. E. (1979): Pharmacological and biochemical aspects of hyperkinetic disorders. *Neuropharmacology*, 18:923–929.
170. Levitan, H. (1979): Food colors. In: *The Effects of Foods and Drugs on the Development and Function of The Nervous System: Methods For Predicting Toxicity*, edited by R. M. Gryder and V. H. Frankos, pp. 185–191. *Proceeding of the 5th FDA Science Symposium*, October 10–12.
171. Levitan, H. (1977): Food, drug and cosmetic dyes: Biological effects related to lipid solubility. *Proc. Natl. Acad. Sci. USA*, 74:2914–2918.
172. Levitan, H., Zilyan, Z., Smith, Q. R., and Rapaport, S. I. (1981): Brain uptake of erythrosin B, a food dye, in adult rats. *Soc. Neurosci. Abstr.*, 7:949.
173. Lipton, M. A., Nemeroff, C. B., and Mailman, R. B. (1979): Hyperkinesis and food additives. In: *Nutrition and the Brain, Vol. 4*, edited by R. J. Wurtman and J. J. Wurtman, pp. 1–28. Raven Press, New York.

174. Logan, W. J., and Swanson, J. M. (1979): Erythrosin B inhibition of neurotransmitter accumulation by rat brain homogenate. *Science*, 206:363–364.
175. Luschei, E., Mottet, N., and Shaw, C. M. (1977): Chronic methylmercury exposure in the monkey *(Macaca mulatta)*. *Arch. Environ. Health*, 32:126–131.
176. Lutty, G. A. (1978): The acute intravenous toxicity of biological stains, dyes and other fluorescent substances. *Toxicol. Appl. Pharmacol.*, 44:225–249.
177. Magos, L., Peristianis, G., Clarkson, T., Brown, A., Preston, S., and Snowden, R. (1981): Comparative study of the sensitivity of male and female rats to methylmercury. *Arch. Toxicol.*, 48:11–20.
178. Magos, L., Peristianis, G., Clarkson, T., and Snowden, R. (1980): The effect of lactation on methylmercury intoxication. *Arch. Toxicol.*, 45:143–148.
179. Magos, L., and Webb, M. (1977): The effect of selenium on the brain uptake of methylmercury. *Arch. Toxicol.*, 38:201–207.
180. Mailman, R. B., Ferris, R. M., Tang, F. L. M., Vogel, R. A., Kilts, C. D., Lipton, M. A., Smith, D. A., Mueller, R. A., and Breese, G. R. (1980): Erythrosine (Red No. 3) and its nonspecific biochemical actions: What relation to behavioral changes? *Science*, 207:535–566.
181. Marighan, R., Boucard, M., and Geis, C. (1964): Influence possible de l'erythroise sur le metabolism thyroidien. *Pharm. Montpellier*, 24:127–130.
182. Marmion, D. M. (1979): *Handbook of U.S. Colorants for Foods, Drugs and Cosmetics*. Wiley-Interscience, New York.
183. Marnaha, J., and Prabad, K. N. (1981): Hypothyroidism elicits electrophysiological noradrenergic subsensitivity in rat cerebellum. *Science*, 214:675–677.
184. Marsh, D., Myers, G., Clarkson, T., Amin-Zaki, L., Tikriti, S., and Majeed, M. (1980): Fetal methylmercury poisoning: Clinical and toxicological data on 29 cases. *Ann. Neurol.*, 7:348–353.
185. Matsumoto, H., Susuki, A., and Marita, C. (1967): Preventive effect of penicillamine on the brain defect of fetal rat poisoned transplacentally with methylmercury. *Life Sci.*, 6:2321.
186. Mawdesley-Thomas, L. E., and Newman, A. J., (1974): Some observations on spontaneously occurring tumours of the central nervous system of Sprague-Dawley derived rats. *J. Pathol.*, 112:107–116.
187. McCollister, D. C., Oyen, F., and Rowe, V. K. (1964): Toxicology of acrylamide. *Toxicol. Appl. Pharmacol.*, 6:172–181.
188. McFarren, E. F. (1971): Assay and control of marine biotoxins. *Food Technol.*, 25:38–48.
189. McLaughlin, J. M. (1967): Letter to Consumer Union, Jan. 25. FDA Bureau of Foods Files, Washington, D.C.
190. Merrill, R. (1976): Letter of October 5 to J. W. Olney. Docket Number 75F-0355. FDA Documents Management Branch, Rockville, Maryland.
191. Merrill, R. (1975): Letter to J. Turner and J. W. Olney on August 14. Docket Number 75F-0355. FDA Documents Management Branch, Rockville, Maryland.
192. Merrill, R. (1978): Regulating carcinogens in food: A legislator's guide to the food safety provisions of the Federal Food, Drug and Cosmetic Act. *Mich. Law Rev.*, 77:171–250.
193. Munro, I., Nera, E., Charbonneau, S., Junkins, B., and Zawidzka, Z. (1980): Chronic toxicity of methylmercury in the rat. *J. Environ. Pathol. Toxicol.*, 3:437–447.
194. Nagasawa, H., Yanai, R., and Kikuyama, S. (1974): Irreversible inhibition of pituitary prolactin and growth hormone secretion and of mammary gland development in mice by monosodium glutamate administered neonatally. *Acta Endocrinol.*, 75:249–259.
195. Narahashi, T. (1975): Mode of action of dinoflagellate toxins on nerve membranes. In: *Proceedings of the First International Conference on Toxic Dinoflagellate Blooms*, edited by V. R. LoCicero, pp. 395–402. Massachusetts Science and Technology Foundation, Cambridge.
196. Nauta, W., Lampert, P., and Young, V. (1980): Aspartame—Decision of the Public Board of Inquiry, pp. 1–52. Docket Number 75F-0355. FDA Documents Management Branch, Rockville, Maryland.
197. Nemeroff, C. B., Grant, L. D., Harrell, L. E., Bisette, G., Ervin, G. N., and Prange, A. J., Jr. (1977): Growth, endocrinological and behavioral deficits after monosodium L-glutamate in the neonatal rat: Possible involvement of arcuate dopamine neuron damage. *Psychoneuroendocrinology*, 2:279–296.
198. Nemeroff, C. B., Konkol, R. J., Bissette, G., Youngblood, W., Martin, J. B., Brazeau, P., Rone, M. S., Prange, A. J., Jr., Breese, G. R., and Kizer, J. S. (1977): Analysis of the disruption in hypothalamic-pituitary regulation in rats treated neonatally with monosodium L-glutamate (MSG):

Evidence for the involvement of tubero-infundibular cholinergic and dopaminergic systems in neuroendocrine regulation. *Endocrinology*, 101:613–622.

199. Newman, A. J., Heywood, R., Plamer, A. K., Barry, D. H., Edwards, F. P., and Worden, A. N. (1973): The administration of monosodium L-glutamate to neonatal and pregnant rhesus monkeys. *Toxicology*, 1:197–204.

200. Newman, A. J., and Mawdesley-Thomas, L. E. (1974): Spontaneous tumours of the central nervous system of laboratory rats. *J. Comp. Pathol.*, 84:39–50.

201. Noonan, J. E., and Meggos, H. (1973): Synthetic food colors. In: *CRC Handbook of Food Additives, 2nd ed., Vol. 2*, edited by T. E. Furia, pp. 339–383. CRC Press, Inc., Boca Raton, Florida.

202. Norseth, T., and Clarkson, T. (1971): Intestinal transport of [203]Hg-labeled methylmercury chloride. *Arch. Environ. Health*, 22:558–577.

203. Nyhan, W. (1980): *Transcript of Public Hearing on Aspartame, Vol. I*, pp. 244–253. Docket Number 75F-0355. FDA Documents Management Branch, Rockville, Maryland.

204. O'Hara, Y., Iwata, S., Ichimura, M., and Sasaoka, M. (1977): Effect of administration routes of MSG on plasma glutamate levels in infant, weanling and adult mice. *J. Toxicol. Sci.*, 2:281–289.

205. O'Hara, Y., and Takasaki, M. (1979): Relationship between plasma glutamate levels and hypothalamic lesions in rodents. *Toxicol. Lett.*, 4:499–505.

206. Ohi, G., Nishigaki, S., Seki, H., Tamura, Y., Maki, T., Konno, H., Ochiai, S., Yamada, H., Shimamura, Y., Mizoguchi, I., and Yogyu, H. (1976): Efficacy of selenium in tuna and selenite in modifying methylmercury intoxication. *Environ. Res.*, 12:49–58.

207. Ohsawa, M., and Magos, L. (1974): The chemical form of the methylmercury complex in the bile of the rat. *Biochem. Pharmacol.*, 23:1903–1905.

208. Olney, J. W. (1976): Brain damage and oral intake of certain amino acids. *Adv. Exp. Med. Biol.*, 69:497–506.

209. Olney, J. W. (1969): Brain lesions, obesity and other disturbances in mice treated with MSG. *Science*, 164:719–721.

210. Olney, J. W. (1979): Excitotoxic amino acids: research applications and safety implications. In: *Glutamic Acid: Advances in Biochemistry and Physiology*, edited by L. J. Filer, Jr., S. Garratini, M. R. Kare, W. A. Reynolds, and R. J. Wurtman, pp. 287–319. Raven Press, New York.

211. Olney, J. W. (1974): Letter of August 16 to Food and Drug Administration Bureau of Foods. Docket Number 75F-0355. FDA Documents Management Branch, Rockville, Maryland.

212. Olney, J. W. (1980): *Transcript of Public Hearing on Aspartame, Vol. 3*, pp. 131–155. Docket Number 75F-0355. FDA Documents Management Branch, Rockville, Maryland.

213. Olney, J. W., Cicero, T. J., Meyer, E. R., and Degubareff, T. (1976): Acute glutamate-induced elevation in serum testosterone and luteinizing hormone. *Brain Res.*, 112:420–424.

214. Olney, J. W., and Ho, C. L. (1970): Brain damage in infant mice following oral intake of glutamate, aspartate or cysteine. *Nature*, 227:609–611.

215. Olney, J. W., Sharpe, L. G., and Feigin, R. D. (1972): Glutamate-induced brain damage in infant primates. *J. Neuropathol. Exp. Neurol.*, 31:464–488.

216. Olson, K., and Boush, G. (1975): Decreased learning capacity in rats exposed prenatally and postnatally to low doses of mercury. *Bull. Environ. Contam. Toxicol.*, 13:73–79.

217. Ordonez, J. V., Carrillo, J., and Miranada, M. (1966): Estudio epidmemiologico de una enfermedad considerada como encefalitis en la region de Los Altos de Guatemala. *Bol. Sanit. Panam.*, 60:510–519.

218. Paterson, R., and Usher, O. (1971): Acute toxicity of methylmercury on glycolytic intermediates and adenine nucleotides of rat brain. *Life Sci.*, 10:121–128.

219. Pekkanen, T., and Sandholm, M. (1971): The effect of experimental methylmercury poisoning on the number of sulfhydryl (SH) groups in the brain, liver and muscle of rat. *Acta Vet. Scand.*, 12:551–559.

220. Pierce, E. C., Agersburg, H. P. K., Borzelleca, J. F., Burnett, C. M., Eagle, E., Ebert, A. G., Kirschman, J. C., and Scala, R. A. (1974): Teratogenic studies with certified colors in rats and rabbits. *Toxicol. Appl. Pharmacol.*, 29:121–122.

221. Pierce, P., Thompson, J., Likosky, W., Nickey, L., Barthel, W., and Hinman, A. (1972): Alkyl mercury poisoning in humans. *JAMA*, 220:1439–1442.

222. Pizzi, W. J., Barnhart, J. E., and Fanslow, D. J. (1977): Monosodium glutamate administration to the newborn reduces reproductive ability in female and male mice. *Science*, 196:452–454.

223. Pletscher, A. (1977): Effect of neuroleptics and other drugs on monoamine uptake by membranes of adrenal chromaffin granules. *Br. J. Pharmacol.*, 59:419–424.
224. Prejean, J. D., Peckham, J. C., Casey, A. E., Griswold, D. P., Weisberger, E. K., and Weisberger, J. H. (1973): Spontaneous tumors in Sprague-Dawley rats and Swiss mice. *Cancer Res.*, 33:2768–2773.
225. Radomski, J. L. (1974): Toxicology of food colors. *Annu. Rev. Pharmacol.*, 14:127–137.
226. Redding, T. W., Schally, A. U., Arimura, A., and Wakabayaski, I. (1977): Effect of monosodium glutamate on some endocrine functions. *Neuroendocrinology*, 8:245–255.
227. Refsvik, T., and Norseth, T. (1975): Methylmercuric compounds in rat bile. *Acta Pharmacol. Toxicol.*, 36:67–78.
228. Reynolds, W. A., Lemkey-Johnston, N., Filer, L. J., Jr., and Pitkin, R. (1971): Monosodium glutamate: Absence of hypothalamic lesions after ingestion by new primates. *Science*, 172:1342–1344.
229. Reynolds, W. A., Lemkey-Johnston, N., and Stegink, L. D. (1979): Morphology of the fetal monkey hypothalamus after *in utero* exposure to monosodium glutamate (MSG). In: *Glutamic Acid: Advances in Biochemistry and Physiology*, edited by L. J. Filer, Jr., S. Garattini, M. R. Kare, W. A. Reynolds, and R. J. Wurtman, pp. 217–230. Raven Press, New York.
230. Rodier, P. M. (1976): Critical periods for behavioral anomalies in mice. *Environ. Health. Perspect.*, 18:79–83.
231. Rodier, P. M. (1979): Rate of post-embryonic development of the rat brain. Memorandum of telephone conversation of August 27 with Dr. David Hattan, HFF-185. Docket Number 75F-0355. FDA Documents Management Branch, Rockville, Maryland.
232. Rodricks, J. V., and Roberts, H. R. (1977): Mycotoxin regulation in the United States. In: *Mycotoxins in Human and Animal Health*, edited by J. V. Rodricks, C. W. Hesseltine, and M. A. Mehlman, pp. 753–758. Pathotox Publishers, Park Forest South, Illinois.
233. Rosenberg, L., and Scriver, C. (1974): Phenylalanine metabolism and the hyperphenylalaninemias. In: *Diseases of Metabolism*, edited by P. Bondy and L. Rosenberg, pp. 589–610. W. B. Saunders, Philadelphia.
234. Rowland, I., Davies, M., and Evans, J. (1980): Tissue content of mercury in rats given methylmercuric chloride orally: Influence of intestinal flora. *Arch. Environ. Health*, 35:155–160.
235. Rustam, H., and Hamdi, T. (1974): Methylmercury poisoning in Iraq. *Brain*, 97:499–510.
236. Sandbach, W. (1966): Letter from Consumers Union, Dec. 6. FDA Bureau of Foods Files, Washington, D.C.
237. Saxena, K. M., Chapman, E. M., and Pryles, C. V. (1962): Minimal dosage of iodide required to suppress uptake of iodine-131 by normal thyroid. *Science*, 138:430–431.
238. Schainker, B., and Olney, J. W. (1974): Glutamate-type hypothalamic-pituitary syndrome in mice treated with aspartate or cysteate in infancy. *J. Neural Transm.*, 35:207–215.
239. Schantz, E. J., McFarren, E. F., Schafer, M. C., and Lewis, K. H. (1958): Purified shellfish poison for bioassay standardization. *J. Assoc. Off. Anal. Chem.*, 41:160–178.
240. Schardein, J. L., Fitzgerald, J. E., and Kaump, D. H. (1968): Spontaneous tumors in Holtzman-source rats of various ages. *Pathol. Vet.*, 5:238–252.
241. Schmidt, A. (1974): Action level for mercury in fish and shellfish. *Fed. Reg.*, 39:42738–42740.
242. Schmidt, A. (1975): Statement of July 10 before Senate Subcommittee on Health, and Administrative Practice and Procedure. Docket Number 75F-0355. FDA Documents Management Branch, Rockville, Maryland.
243. Shaw, C. M., Mattet, N., Body, R., and Luschel, E. (1975): Variability of neuropathologic lesions in experimental encephalopathy in primates. *Am. J. Pathol.*, 80:451–469.
244. Shimizu, Y. (1978): Dinoflagellate toxins. In: *Marine Natural Products, Vol. 1*, edited by P. J. Scheuer, pp. 1–42. Academic Press, New York.
245. Silbergeld, E. K. (1979): Detection of neurotoxicity using neurochemical methods. In: *The Effects of Foods and Drugs on the Development and Function of the Nervous System: Methods for Predicting Toxicity*, edited by R. M. Gryder and V. H. Frankos, pp. 99–105. *Proceedings of the 5th FDA Science Symposium*, October 10–12.
246. Silbergeld, E. K. (1981): Erythrosine B is a specific inhibitor of high affinity ^{3}H-oubain binding and ion transport in rat brain. *Neuropharmacology*, 20:87–90.
247. Simpson, R., Horwitz, W., and Roy, C. (1974): Surveys of mercury levels in fish and other foods. *Pestic. Monit. J.*, 7:127–138.

248. Singh, M., and Graichen, C. (1974): Determination of FD & C Red No. 3 (erythrosine) in rat blood serum. *J. Assoc. Off. Anal. Chem.*, 56:1458–1459.
249. Singletary, N. (1979): Letter of April 10 to J. Turner and J. W. Olney. Docket Number 75F-0355. FDA Documents Management Branch, Rockville, Maryland.
250. Skerfving, S. (1972): Mercury in fish—Some toxicological considerations. *Food Cosmet. Toxicol.*, 10:545–556.
251. Skerfving, S. (1974): Methylmercury exposure, mercury levels in blood and hair and health status in Swedes consuming contaminated fish. *Toxicology*, 2:3–23.
252. Snyder, R. (1971): Congenital mercury poisoning. *N. Engl. J. Med.*, 284:1014–1016.
253. Snyder, S. H., and Meyerhoff, J. L. (1973): How amphetamine acts in minimal brain dysfunction. *Ann. NY Acad. Sci.*, 208:310–320.
254. Sobotka, T. J. (1978): Hyperkinesis and food additives: A review of experimental work. *FDA Bylines*, 4:165–176.
255. Sobotka, T. J. (1979): Update on studies of the relationship between hyperkinesis in children and food additives. *FDA Bylines*, 7:343–351.
256. Sommer, H., and Meyer, K. F. (1932): Paralytic shellfish poisoning. *Arch. Pathol.*, 24:560.
257. Somjen, G., Herman, S., and Klein, R. (1973): Electrophysiology of methylmercury poisoning. *J. Pharmacol. Exp. Ther.*, 186:579–592.
258. Somjen, G., Herman, S., Klein, R., Brubaker, P., Briner, W., Goodrich, J., Krigman, M., and Haseman, J. (1973): The uptake of methylmercury (^{203}Hg) in different tissues related to its neurotoxic effects. *J. Pharmacol. Exp. Ther.*, 187:602–611.
259. Spencer, P. S., and Schaumberg, H. H. (1974): A review of acrylamide neurotoxicity, II. Experimental animal neurotoxicity and pathologic mechanisms. *Can. J. Neurol. Sci.*, 1:152–169.
260. Spencer, P. S., and Schaumberg, H. H. (1974): A review of acrylamide neurotoxicity. I. Properties, uses and human exposure. *Can. J. Neurol. Sci.*, 1:143–150.
261. Spyker, J., Sparber, S., and Goldberg, A. (1972): Subtle consequences of methylmercury exposure: Behavioral deviations in offspring of treated mothers. *Science*, 77:621–623.
262. Stegink, L. D. (1980): *Transcript of Public Hearing on Aspartame, Vol. 1*, pp. 92–96. Docket Number 75F-0355. FDA Documents Management Branch, Rockville, Maryland.
263. Stegink, L. D. (1980): *Transcript of Public Hearing on Aspartame, Vol. III*, pp. 72–86. Docket Number 75F-0355. FDA Documents Management Branch, Rockville, Maryland.
264. Stegink, L. D., Filer, L. J., Jr., and Baker, G. L. (1981): Plasma and erythrocyte concentrations of free amino acids in adult humans administered abuse doses of aspartame. *J. Toxicol. Environ. Health*, 7:291–305.
265. Stegink, L. D., Filer, L. J., Baker, G. L., Brummel, M. C., and Tephly, T. R. (1978): Aspartame metabolism in human subjects. In: *Health and Sugar Substitutes, Proceedings of ERGOB Conference*, Geneva, pp. 165–169. Karger, Basel, Switzerland.
266. Stegink, L. D., Pitkin, R. M., Reynolds, W. A., Brummel, M. C., and Filer, L. J., Jr. (1979): Placental transfer of asparate and its metabolites in the primate. *Metabolism*, 28:669–676.
267. Stegink, L. D., Reynolds, W. A., Filer, L. J., Jr., Daabees, T. T., Baker, G. L., and Pitkin, R. (1979): Comparative metabolism of glutamate in mouse, monkey and man. In: *Glutamic Acid: Advances in Biochemistry and Physiology*, edited by L. J. Filer, Jr., S. Garattini, M. R. Kare, W. A. Reynolds, and R. J. Wurtman, pp. 85–102. Raven Press, New York.
268. Stegink, L. D., Reynolds, W. A., Filer, L. J., Jr., Pitkin, R., Boaz, D., and Brummel, M. (1975): Monosodium glutamate metabolism in the neonatal monkey. *Am. J. Physiol.*, 229:246–250.
269. Stillings, B., Lagally, H., Bauersfeld, P., and Soares, J. (1974): Effect of cystine, selenium, and fish protein on the toxicity and metabolism of methylmercury in rats. *Toxicol. Appl. Pharmacol.*, 30:243–254.
270. Strichartz, G. R. (1975): The binding of saxitoxin to nerve tissue and its antagonism by various agents. In: *Proceedings of the First International Conference on Toxic Dinoflagellate Blooms*, edited by V. R. LoCicero, pp. 403–412. Massachusetts Science and Technology Foundation, Cambridge.
271. Sved, A. F., and Fernstrom, J. D. (1979): Effects of glutamate administration and pituitary function. In: *Glutamic Acid: Advances in Biochemistry and Physiology*, edited by L. J. Filer, Jr., S. Garattini, M. R. Kare, W. A. Reynolds, and R. J. Wurtman, pp. 277–285. Raven Press, New York.
272. Swanson, J. M., Kelly, J. J., and McConahey, N. M. (1981): Neurologic aspects of thyroid dysfunction. *Mayo Clin. Proc.*, 56:504–512.

273. Swanson, J. M., and Kinsbourne, M. (1980): Food dyes impair performance of hyperactive children in a laboratory learning test. *Science*, 207:1485–1487.
274. Swanson, J. M., and Logan, W. L. (1979): Effects of food dyes on neurotransmitter accumulation in rat brain homogenate and on the behavior of hyperactive children. In: *The Effects of Foods and Drugs on the Development and Function of the Nervous System: Methods for Predicting Toxicity*, edited by R. M. Gryder and V. H. Frankos, pp. 182–184. *Proceedings of the 5th FDA Science Symposium, October 10–12.*
275. Syversen, T. (1974): Biotransformation of Hg-203 labelled methylmercuric chloride in rat brain measured by specific determination of Hg^{2+}. *Acta Pharmacol. Toxicol.*, 35:277–283.
276. Takasaki, Y. (1978): Studies on brain lesion by administration of MSG to mice. I. Brain lesions in infant mice caused by administration of MSG. *Toxicology*, 9:293–305.
277. Takasaki, Y., Matsuzawa, Y., O'Hara, Y., Yonetani, S., and Ichimira, M. (1979): Toxicological studies of monosodium L-glutamate in rodents: Relationship between routes of administration and neurotoxicity. In: *Glutamic Acid: Advances in Biochemistry and Physiology*, edited by L. J. Filer, Jr., S. Garattini, M. R. Kare, W. A. Reynolds, and R. J. Wurtman, pp. 255–277. Raven Press, New York.
278. Takeuchi, T., and Eto, K. (1977): Pathology and pathogenesis of Minamata disease. In: *Minamata Disease*, edited by T. T. Subaki and K. Irukoyama, pp. 103–142. Elsevier Scientific Publishing Company, New York.
279. Tate and Lyle, Ltd. (1973): *Food Additive Petition Number 3A-2904*. FDA Bureau of Foods Files, Washington, D.C.
280. Terry, L. C., Epelbaum, J., Brazeau, P., and Martin, J. B. (1977): Monosodium glutamate: Acute and chronic effects on growth hormone (GH), prolactin (PRL) and somatostatin (SRIF) in the rat. *Fed. Proc.*, 36:364.
281. Thompson, S. W., Huseby, R. A., Fox, M. A., Davis, C. L., and Hunt, R. D. (1961): Spontaneous tumors in the Sprague-Dawley rat. *J. Natl. Cancer Inst.*, 27:1037–1057.
282. Trentini, G. P., Botticelli, A., and Botticelli, C. S. (1974): Effect of monosodium glutamate on the endocrine glands and on the reproductive function of the rat. *Fertil. Steril.*, 25:478–483.
283. Tsubaki, T., Shirakawa, K., Hirota, K., Kanbayashi, K., Iwata, K., Ino, H., Mizukosni, K., Horada, Y., Tatetsu, S., Harada, M., Inoue, T., Tsukayama, T., Minami, R., Hattori, E., and Kabashima, K. (1977): Clinical aspects of Minamata Disease. In: *Minamata Disease*, edited by T. Tsubaki and K. Irukoyama, pp. 143–268. Elsevier Scientific Publishing Company, New York.
284. Tsuzuki, Y. (1981): Effect of chronic methylmercury exposure on activities of neurotransmitter enzymes in rat cerebellum. *Toxicol. Appl. Pharmacol.*, 60:379–381.
285. Turner, J., and Meyer, K. (1976): *Letter of November 15 to R. Merrill*. Docket Number 75F-0355. FDA Documents Management Branch, Rockville, Maryland.
286. Typhmas, H., and Trites, R. (1979): Food allergy in children with hyperactivity, learning disabilities and/or minimal brain dysfunction. *Ann. Allerg.*, 42:22–27.
287. Umeda, M. (1956): Experimental study of xanthene dyes as carcinogenic agents. *Gann*, 47:51–78.
288. Verity, M., Brown, W., and Cheung, M. (1975): Organic mercurial encephalopathy *in vivo* and *in vitro* effects of methylmercury on synaptosomal respiration. *J. Neurochem.*, 25:759–766.
289. Vorhees, C. V., Brunner, R. L., Wooten, V., and Butcher, R. E. (1981): *Developmental Psychotoxicity of Selected Food Additives and Related Compounds in Rats: Report on Dietary Red No. 3 (Repeat)*. USFDA Contract No. 223–75–2030.
290. Vorhees, C. V., Brunner, R. L., Wooten, V., and Butcher, R. E. (1983): *Psychotoxicity of Selected Food Additives and Related Compounds; Report on FD & C Red No. 3 (Erythrosine)*. USFDA Contract No. 233-75-2030 *(In press)*.
291. Vorhees, C. V., and Butcher, R. E. (1982): Behavioral teratogenicity. In: *Developmental Toxicology*, edited by K. Snell, pp. 247–298. Groom Helm Press, London.
292. Vorhees, C. V., Butcher, R. E., Brunner, R. L., and Sobotka, T. J. (1979): A developmental test battery for neurobehavioral toxicity in rats: A preliminary analysis using monosodium glutamate, calcium carrageenan, and hydroxyurea. *Toxicol. Appl. Pharmacol.*, 50:267–282.
293. Vought, R. L., Brown, F. A., and Wolff, J. (1972): Erythrosine: An adventitious source of iodine. *J. Clin. Endocrinol.*, 34:747–752.
294. Waliszewski, T. (1952): Chromatographic and biologic study of food coloring with special reference to erythrosine. *Acta Pol. Pharm.*, 9:127–132.

295. Waterman, N., and Lignac, G. O. E. (1958): The influence of the feeding of a number of food colors on the occurence of tumors in mice. *Acta Physiol. Pharmacol. Neerlandica*, 7:35–55.
296. Webb, J. M., Fonda, M., and Brouwer, E. A. (1962): Metabolism and excretion patterns of fluorescein and certain halogenated fluorescein dyes in rats. *J. Pharmacol. Exp. Ther.*, 137:141–147.
297. Weisberger, E. K. (1979): Natural carcinogenic products. *Environ. Sci. Technol.*, 13:278–281.
298. Weiss, G., and Hechtman (1971): The hyperactive child syndrome. *Science*, 205:1348–1354.
299. Weiss, B., Williams, J. H., Margen, S., Abrams, B., Cran, B., Citron, L. J., Cox, C., Mackibben, J., Ogar, D., and Schultz, S. (1980): Behavioral responses to artificial food colors. *Science*, 207:1487–1489.
300. Wen, C. P., Hayes, K. K., and Gershoff, S. M. (1973): Effects of dietary supplementation of monosodium glutamate on infant monkeys, weanling rats and suckling mice. *Am. J. Clin. Nutr.*, 26:803–813.
301. Willes, R., Truelove, J., and Nera, E. (1978): Neurotoxic response of infant monkeys to methylmercury. *Toxicology*, 9:125–135.
302. Willheim, R., and Ivy, A. C. (1953): A preliminary study concerning the possibility of dietary carcinogenesis. *Gastroenterology*, 23:1–19.
303. Williams, J. I., Cram, D. M., Tausig, F. T., and Webster, E. (1978): Relative effects of drugs and diet on hyperactive behaviors: An experimental study. *Pediatrics*, 61:811–817.
304. Willis, R. A. (1967): Incidence of gliomas. In: *Pathology of Tumours*, edited by R. A. Willis, pp. 819–830. Appleton-Century-Crofts, New York.
305. Wills, J. H., Serrone, D. M., and Coulston, F. (1981): A 7-month study of ingestion of sodium cyclamate by human volunteers. *J. Regulat. Toxicol. Pharmacol.*, 1:163–176.
306. Wolff, J. (1969): Iodide goiter and the pharmacologic effects of excess iodide. *Am. J. Med.*, 47:101–117.
307. Yankell, S. L., and Loux, J. J. (1977): Acute testing of erythrosine and sodium fluorescein in mice and rats. *J. Periodontol.*, 48:228–231.
308. Yonetani, S., and Matsuzawa, Y. (1978): Effect of monosodium glutamate on serum luteinizing hormone and testosterone in adult male rats. *Toxicol. Lett.*, 1:207–211.
309. Yoshino, Y., Mozai, T., and Nikao, K. (1966): Biochemical changes in the rats poisoned with an alkylmercury compound, with special reference to the inhibition of protein synthesis in brain cortex slices. *J. Neurochem.*, 13:1223–1230.
310. Yoshino, Y., Mozai, T., and Nikao, K. (1966): Distribution of mercury in the brain and its subcellular units in experimental organic mercury poisonings. *J. Neurochem.*, 13:397.

Editor's note (see footnote 7, page 46): Of course, consumption of the protein also contributes to the plasma large amounts of other neutral amino acids (e.g., leucine, valine, tyrosine) that compete with circulating phenylalanine for uptake into the brain. A mole of phenylalanine consumed as aspartame would be expected to cause a much greater increase in brain phenylalanine than a mole of phenylalanine consumed as a constituent of dietary protein. This is especially so if the subject concurrently consumes insulin-releasing carbohydrates—which lower plasma levels of the other neutral amino acids.

Nutrition and the Brain, Vol. 6 edited by
R. J. Wurtman and J. J. Wurtman.
Raven Press, New York © 1983.

Assessing Behavioral and Cognitive Effects of Diet in Pediatric Populations

Judith M. Rumsey and Judith L. Rapoport

Unit on Childhood Mental Illness, Biological Psychiatry Branch, National Institute of Mental Health, Bethesda, Maryland 20205

I. INTRODUCTION

Early interest in the relationship between diet and behavior centered on malnutrition, which, by the 1950s, was recognized as a disease with essential similarities throughout its worldwide distribution (219). In the 1960s attention turned to the cognitive development of malnourished infants in developing countries, and more recently, to the effects of early malnutrition secondary to medical disorders in nondeprived populations. Concurrently, growing concerns among consumers and professionals have focused attention on the possible behavioral toxicity of food additives that constitute part of the typical American diet (e.g., caffeine, artificial dyes). Much of this concern has focused on children, in whom adverse behavioral effects may interfere with learning and development.

Although American regulatory agencies routinely test drugs and food additives for acute toxicity, teratogenicity, and carcinogenicity, their determinations of safety do not generally involve testing for behavioral toxicity. The limitations inherent in extrapolating from animal studies to human behavior necessitate the development of rigorous paradigms and evaluation methods for use with human subjects. Current methodologies for studying behavioral and cognitive effects in children have been developed, to a great extent, within pediatric psychopharmacology. The increased administration of stimulant drugs to hyperactive children in the 1960s and the increased interest in methods for assessing subject responses in the 1970s (239) provided insights and tests that may be useful in resolving the most pressing current concerns regarding behavioral toxicity—the hypothesized link between food additives and hyperactivity in children.

This chapter reviews certain methodological considerations in the conducting of behavioral and cognitive nutritional research, and surveys a wide range of behavioral and cognitive measures available for research use. Knowledge gained from research in pediatric psychopharmacology provides a basis for discussion of the relative merits of various research strategies and measures. The literature relating various dietary and nondietary substances (e.g., lead, drugs) to behavior and cognition is surveyed with respect to issues of toxicity and methodology. Finally, the malnutrition literature is reviewed with respect to major methodological and theoretical issues.

II. CONSIDERATIONS OF METHOD

A. Considerations in Designing and Administering Dietary (or Drug) Treatments

1. Dosages

Definitions of high versus low dosages are dependent on available, but sometimes inadequate, epidemiological data. The strategy of using high dosages to enhance the probability of identifying behavioral effects is popular. Data from records of subjects' food intakes can be compared with those from nutritional surveys to evaluate the representativeness of various research samples. Such data may also provide a crude check on the adequacy of available epidemiological data. Optimal therapeutic dosages are generally best determined by comparisons made across groups receiving different dosages. Dose–response curves are best studied in crossover designs, in which each subject receives various dosages at different times.

2. *Duration and Timing*

The possibility of cumulative effects of dietary substances, similar to those seen with drugs, makes the duration of treatment important. A "washout" period may be required to rid the body of active compounds between treatments. The lack of knowledge regarding the pharmacokinetics of compounds such as food dyes raises the possibility that crossover studies may employ treatments of insufficient duration (193). The timing of food challenges with respect to trials on elimination diets, considered important in allergy testing, may also be important in testing substances such as artificial food dyes, which are suspected of acting like allergens.

3. *Double-Blind Control Trials*

The importance of double-blind, controlled conditions is well illustrated in the behavioral–nutritional literature. Dramatic improvement in hyperactivity seen in uncontrolled, nonblind situations is vastly reduced in double-blind, controlled studies of the Feingold elimination diet. Possible contributors to what appears to be a large placebo effect include altered family interaction, demand characteristics (experimenter and subject expectations), and high spontaneous remission rates for some childhood behavioral disorders.

Where dietary manipulations are restricted to the consumption of challenge substances, the subjects should be unable to discriminate between drinks or foods containing the active substance and placebo on the basis of taste or appearance to ensure experimental blindness. Where treatments involve the entire diet, they are likely to prove particularly difficult to disguise and equate.

To equate the numerous nonspecific factors that may contribute to a placebo effect, two or more "experimental" diets should be compared. Parental expectations should include the possibility that dietary manipulation may prove either therapeutic or detrimental, an expectation that is unlikely to be aroused if one diet is presented as experimental and the other as a control or comparison diet. Specific labels associated with highly publicized diets, e.g., the Feingold diet, should, of course, be avoided. The time spent by parents shopping, preparing food, and monitoring their child's compliance and any infractions should be equated. Diets should be equally palatable, easy to follow, nutritious, and plausible as effective treatments. Nonoverlapping diets that include foods from the same food groupings and categories are desirable for obviating speculations about the identities of the critical elements in the diets.

The difficulties encountered in achieving this type of control have prompted some investigators to supply families with all of the food to be consumed during the research period (99), and others (211) to hospitalize children for study.

4. Monitoring Compliance

Compliance and nutrient intake are best monitored with daily diaries or checklists. Such running records are then available for nutritional analyses (total intake of calories and essential nutrients). Chemical methods for quantifying the substance that is biologically active and available (e.g., salivary caffeine concentrations) are also useful.

5. Recordkeeping

In addition to dietary compliance and any infractions, records should reflect total nutritional intake, duration of treatment, dosages, any changes in dose of experimental substances, concurrent medications, any changes in drug regimen, and intercurrent illnesses. Ease of compliance might also be recorded periodically throughout treatment as a check on the comparability of dietary manipulations. Routine recording of medical, social, and demographic information on families and children may prove useful in retrospective attempts to identify variables discriminating responders and nonresponders (46).

B. Subject Selection and Description

Psychiatric interviews, direct behavioral observations, history, and reports of teachers and parents may all contribute to the varied data base involved in child diagnosis and subject selection. The process of selection (methods used and inclusionary and exclusionary criteria) should be standardized and clearly and adequately described. Where quantitative criteria are involved, e.g., the use of cutoff scores on behavioral rating scales, they should be specified. Interobserver or interrater reliabilities are also relevant, especially for symptoms such as anxiety and depression, which historically have been poorly defined.

Transient symptoms and environmental factors may distort outcome measures and should be carefully considered in the selection process. High spontaneous remission rates in some childhood disorders (68) may grossly inflate estimates of treatment efficacy. Environmental factors have been shown to affect outcomes substantially, particularly long-term outcomes, in studies of high-risk and nutritionally deprived children (5,184,204,243). Children from emotionally nonsupportive home environments have shown less improvement in hyperactivity with dietary manipulations than those with less negative home experiences (46).

Where effects are observed in only a minority of subjects, special attention might be given to subject characteristics (e.g., age, genetic characteristics, autonomic responsivity) that may discriminate responders and nonresponders.

C. Subject Attrition

Subjects who drop out of studies because of unusual reactions create legitimate concern that the strongest drug or dietary effects may be missed. This problem has been encountered in the study of food additives, where indications that only a small number of children are responders magnify concerns for the consequences of diminishing small subject groups even further. The question of who drops out and the circumstances (treatments) under which he or she drops out warrant investigation. Impressed by parental reports of extreme adverse reactions to double-blind challenges (e.g., severe destructiveness and uncontrollable behavior), Conners (46) found such reactions were actually associated with placebo challenges in some children, illustrating the danger of making assumptions in such situations.

D. Subject Heterogeneity

1. Sources of Heterogeneity

Careful selection of homogeneous samples, generally important and difficult, is complicated by the heterogeneity seen in child populations. Greater heterogeneity may characterize diagnostic categories within child psychiatry, where theoretical and empirical bases are less certain than in adult psychiatry. The more limited behavioral repertoires available to children may contribute to a single behavioral syndrome being associated with a variety of etiological factors.

Children's behaviors tend to vary across situations. Only weak correlations are noted between measures of behavior at home and at school, for example (140,182). Behavioral disorders that are restricted to particular settings may differ in important respects from those displayed generally. Pervasive hyperactivity, for example, is likely to be persistent and to be accompanied by cognitive deficits (189), factors shown to influence the responses of subjects to treatment with stimulant drugs (38–40).

Age and developmental status contribute to the problem of heterogeneity and may interact with drug or dietary effects. When studying young children or infants, particularly when developmental skills constitute dependent variables (as they often do in nutritional research), the investigator needs to examine prenatal history, gestational age, birth history, and early developmental history. Prenatal variables may weakly predict neurological, academic, and behavioral status primarily up to age 7 (171,184) and may assume a more powerful predictive role within disadvantaged socioeconomic environments (228,230).

Where great developmental variability exists within a behavioral syndrome (e.g., autism), developmental and cognitive status should be systematically considered with respect to treatment effects and the selection of control subjects. Differences between clinical populations and normal controls may reflect either immaturity (developmental lags) or qualitative abnormalities (biochemical abnormalities, lesions), and differentiating between the two types of problems requires consideration of the developmental dimension.

Prior dietary status, another element of heterogeneity, may be important specifically with respect to tolerance and withdrawal effects (as suggested by the literature on caffeine) and, more generally, in evaluating responses to comprehensive dietary treatments. Any experimental diet may constitute a significant change from past nutrient intake. Unintended changes in total caloric intake or in the intake of specific nutrients may influence behavior. Adequate dietary records will allow the consequences of changes in these factors to be differentiated from those caused by varying the dietary factor under investigation.

2. Strategies for Dealing with Heterogeneity

Strategies for dealing with subject heterogeneity include the use of crossover and single-case designs and the use of subject characteristics as independent variables. Crossover designs, in which the subject serves as his own control, are helpful in reducing error variance. Baseline periods and measures aid in controlling or adjusting for initial differences between subjects; they also provide time for discontinuing medications or other confounding treatments. At the same time, they introduce the problem of practice effects and order effects. Treatment order, therefore, must be counterbalanced or, where precluded by large numbers of treatment conditions, randomized or otherwise equated through the use of Latin squares or lattice designs (242).

Single-case designs (reversal designs, multiple baseline designs) may prove helpful where a small minority of subjects are expected to show effects or where rare disorders and/or great heterogeneity preclude using group designs or the matching of control subjects on relevant dimensions (e.g., autism). Herson and Barlow's (103) book on single-case experimental designs is a helpful guide to the methodological problems, controls, and statistical questions involved in the use of such designs.

The strategy of using subject characteristics (e.g., diagnoses, personality traits, physiological characteristics) as independent variables has been employed by several investigators to look at interactions between drugs and subject characteristics in hyperactive children. Subgroups formed on the basis of behavioral symptoms (79) and neurophysiological measures—skin conductance, cortical evoked potentials, and EEGs (186,187)—have, for example been reported to respond differently to stimulant drug treatment.

E. Assessing Cognition and Behavior

1. Terminology

The meaning of the terms "behavior," "cognition," and "attention," as used here, correspond to their general usage in clinical studies. Some cognitive psychologists might argue against a distinction between assessing behavior and assessing cognition, which must be evaluated via its behavioral manifestations. "Behavior," as used here, refers to overt, directly observable actions. Although assessed through one's performance on certain tasks, "cognition" involves inferences about internal processing of information that is not directly observable. "Attention" refers to orientation to and focus on a stimulus to receive information. Cognition, on the other hand, refers to a later stage in which information is actively manipulated.

2. How Thoroughly Should One Assess Cognition and Behavior?

The answer will, of course, depend on many factors, including cost and time considerations and the subtlety and nature of the anticipated effects. Subtle effects may be missed by inadequate "screening" evaluations, whereas the probability of finding significant effects by chance will be increased as the number of measures increases. Care should be taken to avoid overinterpreting restricted cognitive measures. Screening for intelligence with limited measures such as the Peabody Picture Vocabulary Test (PPVT) may be misleading. Scores derived from this measure basically tap receptive vocabulary, not global intelligence or even language abilities in general.

3. Attentional Changes or Basic Intellectual or Cognitive Changes

In using cognitive measures, particularly with children who show attentional deficits, care must be taken to distinguish between improvements attributable to attentional enhancement or improved control (decreased impulsivity) and those that may stem from alterations in later stages of information processing *per se*. Barkley (8) concluded that the inconsistent changes seen on cognitive measures in response to stimulant drugs reflect attentional effects rather than effects on basic intellectual or cognitive processing. However, Weingartner et al.'s (222) recent reports of enhanced cognition, independent of attentional improvement in normal and hyperactive children, would seem to challenge this view. In any event, the investigator should be aware that a wide variety of cognitive measures, particularly those with a substantial learning or memory component, may be affected by attentional deficits or distractibility.

F. Examining the Scope of Possible Dietary Effects

Alterations in diet may stimulate a series of changes involving biological substrates, learning, social interactions, and so forth. Winick (243) for example, has proposed that malnutrition may produce adverse effects on cognitive development by altering the developing organism's interaction with his environment. Whalen and Henker (237,238) have hypothesized that although stimulant drugs may have some beneficial effects (decreased impulsivity, improved attention) they may actually have adverse effects on the child's personal belief systems, which, in turn, can interfere with school achievement.

Developmental variations may be noted in the expression of effects. Behavioral abnormalities and cognitive deficits may be expressed differently with age-related biological changes (e.g., postnatal maturation of the brain) and with differing social contexts and demands (e.g., borderline intelligence may be more handicapping during school years than subsequently, depending on environmental factors). Cumulative effects may cause initially mild disabilities to appear more severe (e.g., learning disabled children may fall farther behind their age peers as they grow older).

Qualitative differences in response may be seen as well. Gittelman-Klein and Klein (85) found little correspondence between behavioral changes and improvements on psychometric tests in children treated with methylphenidate. Weingartner et al. (221) recently reported enhanced learning in a subgroup of hyperactive children given stimulant medications and a dissociation between these "learning responders" and "clinical responders" (those who showed improvements measured by teachers' and parents' behavioral ratings). Such qualitative variations in response—effects on activity, impulsivity, attention, learning—suggest a danger in prematurely restricting the breadth of the behavior variables to be measured.

III. MAJOR BEHAVIORAL AND COGNITIVE MEASURES

A. Reliability and Validity Requirements

To be useful, any measurement must possess reliability—that is, stability or consistency over time (test–retest reliability) or across examiners (interrater reliability). Reliability provides a stable background against which to detect effects of treatments or other independent variables and thus sets an upper limit on validity. Validity may be established in several ways—content validity, through representative sampling from some specified behavioral domain; concurrent or predictive validity, through significant correlations with a criterion measure; discriminative and convergent validity, through low correlations with unrelated variables and high correlations with theoretically related variables, respectively; and construct validity, through the gradual accumulation of information from a variety of sources. Validity is established within a specific population. Demonstrated validity in one population does not imply validity in a sample with differing age, sex, or cultural characteristics (5).

B. Basic Types of Measures

Several basic types of measures are available for assessing behavioral and cognitive effects of diet. These include (a) specific behavioral measures based on direct observation, (b) mechanical and electronic devices used to monitor physical activity, (c) behavioral rating scales, (d) laboratory performance measures, (e) psychological and neuropsychological tests, and (f) self-report measures.

C. Specific Behavioral Measures

These measures were developed within the behaviorist tradition, which approaches behavior as an ongoing series of observable stimulus–response sequences. Behavioral analysis, within this model, focuses on direct observations of objectively defined target behaviors and their rates of occurrence. Behaviors are quantified through the use of permanent products, frequency tallies, duration recordings, interval recordings, and time sampling techniques. Permanent products are observable results in behavior (e.g., the number of math problems completed, a count on an activity monitor) from which quantitative inferences about behavior can be drawn. Tallies of the frequency of a behavior's occurrence are generally useful for single, discrete behaviors of low to moderate frequency (e.g., seizures) and short-duration behaviors (e.g., hitting, talking out of turn), whereas duration recordings are more valid indicators of the severity of a problem where duration varies significantly (e.g., out of seat classroom behavior). Interval recordings, records of whether a behavior occurs within a specified time interval, reflect both duration and frequency. Time-sampling procedures are used to record target behavior only at the end of specific time intervals, thereby eliminating the need for continuous monitoring (133).

Interrater reliabilities of 90% and greater are generally considered acceptable. Lower reliabilities generally require refinement of behavioral definitions. The tendency of interobserver reliabilities to drift downward over time requires periodic reliability checks. Validity can be demonstrated through correlations with independent measures of specific behaviors, such as rating scales. Related nontarget behaviors might also be measured to establish validity (64).

Although such measures are designed to be highly objective and reliable, their most frequently cited drawback is the fact that they may not adequately reflect the social context in which behavior normally occurs, thus limiting their relevance and meaningfulness.

Specific behavioral measures have been applied, though not emphasized, in drug research. Werry (231) suggests that the shortage of generally applicable measurement devices, logistical difficulties, and the variable sensitivity of such measures to drug effects may account for this deemphasis. In general, such measures have proven less sensitive to drug effects than behavioral rating scales completed by teachers and parents. Applications and modifications with demonstrated drug sensitivity, however, include the use of diaries, kept by parents, of general categories (e.g., activity shifts, negative interactions) of their children's activity over a number of days (166a,167,173,231); psychologist's counts of limit-setting instructions during sessions (1,166a,173); and playroom measures (grid crossings, actometer) used by Rapoport et al. (166a,173).

Several applications of direct observational/behavioral measures are seen within the nutritional literature. Harley et al. (98) studied the effects of a food coloring challenge, and Harley et al. (99) examined the effects of Feingold's elimination diet on hyperactive and normal children, using classroom observations. While specific behavioral measures and other measures differentiated hyperactive and normal children in both studies, no dietary effects were seen when using these or other measures. Prinz et al. (163) found significant correlations between estimates of sugar consumption and behavioral measures of destructiveness–aggressiveness and restlessness. Single-case studies (97,179,227) have shown effects of the Feingold elimination diet and of a food coloring challenge using such measures. Graves (93,94) found significant differences between well-nourished and malnourished 7- to 18-month-old infants using direct observational measures of attachment and of exploratory behaviors. "Attachment" was defined as all behaviors of the child that were directed toward the mother, such as physically touching the mother, looking toward her, smiling at her, giving her a toy, and the like. "Exploration" consisted of fine and gross manipulations of toys.

D. Mechanical and Electronic Activity Monitors

Various mechanical and electronic devices have been used to measure motor activity directly. Their advantage is in providing an automated alternative to more cumbersome and time-consuming direct observations.

However, while attention and vigilance consistently appear to increase with stimulant medications, changes in activity levels *per se* may be dependent on situational variables (8). "Hyperactivity" as a syndrome, once considered in its more literal sense as excessive movement, has taken on more qualitative connotations of socially inappropriate, impulsive, task-irrelevant, or disruptive behavior (65). Thus the relevance of these measures has been questioned along the same lines as the criticisms of other behavioristic measures. However, recent studies with more sophisticated activity-monitoring devices may reestablish activity as central to the hyperactivity syndrome (162).

Available monitors vary in the degree to which they can be used as naturalistic measures and in the type of movement monitored. Werry (231) reports that correlations between measures provided by different monitors are generally modest, with situational demands having substantial influence on resulting activity values. Situations that restrict activity or place demands on the child (e.g., laboratory testing) generally magnify differences between hyperactive and normal children in comparison with nondemand, free play situations (10).

The actometer (34) (Fig. 1), usually worn on the wrist or ankle, is generally well-suited to use in naturalistic settings. It records activity of the limb within one plane of movement and responds more to acceleration than to the distance of

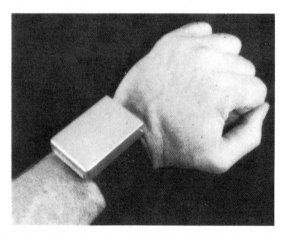

FIG. 1. The activity monitor worn on an adult male wrist. The case is stainless steel, and the strap is 2-in. Velcro.

movement. Data obtained using the actometer and a similar device, the pedometer, have been shown to be drug-sensitive (8,138,166). Wrist, ankle, and locomotor activity, as measured by these devices, appear significantly reduced by stimulants during free play, whereas trunkal activity (actometer worn on back) may not show significant alterations in response to stimulant drugs (8).

One study of food additives (49a) and two studies of caffeine (69,172) have used actometers. Ankle and wrist monitors provided good indicators of responses to a food color challenge, and monitors worn on the back (to measure trunkal activity) showed effects of caffeine in children and adults.

E. Behavioral Rating Scales

Behavioral rating scales have constituted the mainstay of behavioral measures used in pediatric psychopharmacological research. Most of this research has focused on stimulant medication used with children (see Table 1). Highly convenient, efficient, and sensitive, these scales provide algebraic summations of extended observations of children across varied social situations. Scales used in studies of hyperactive children have included the Davids Rating Scales for Hyperkinesis (60), the Werry-Weiss-Peters Activity Rating Scale (231), the Conners Parent and Teacher Questionnaires (36,92), and the Global Clinical Impressions Scale (96). The Conners scale, adopted by the National Institute of Mental Health's (NIMH) Early Clinical Drug Evaluation Unit as part of their children's psychopharmacological battery, has, however, virtually replaced other hyperactivity rating scales. The Global Clinical Impressions Scale, also included in the NIMH Child Battery, is highly recommended as a supplementary measure.

1. The Conners Rating Scales

Current versions of the Conners scales, appropriate for ages 4 through 12 years (215), include a 39-item teacher rating scale, a 28-item teacher rating scale, a 93-item parent rating scale, and a 10-item Abbreviated Parent-Teacher Questionnaire (36,37,41,92). Items are rated on a 4-point scale as applying "not at all" (0 rating) to "a great deal" (3 rating). Long and short versions and mother, father, and teacher ratings all yield a relatively consistent factor structure, similar to those seen in other

TABLE 1. *Stimulant medications used with children*

Drug	Number of daily doses	Range for each dose (mg/kg)
Amphetamines		
Dextroamphetamine	1–3	0.15–0.50
Methamphetamine	1–3	0.15–0.25
Methylphenidate	1–3	0.3–1.0
Magnesium pemoline	1	0.5–2.0
Deanol	1–3	1.0–3.0

children's behavioral rating scales (36,41,92,164,234,236). Factors include conduct problems, inattention, anxiety, hyperactivity, and sociability. Mean scores on these dimensions are typically calculated as part of the scoring procedures.

Normative studies include those of Sprague et al. (199) in Germany, Trites et al. (215) in Canada, Werry and Hawthorne (234) in New Zealand, Werry et al. (236) in the midwestern United States, Kupietz et al. (118) in New York City, and Goyette et al. (92) in the Pittsburgh area. Cutoff scores of 15 and higher on the abbreviated form have been considered indicative of hyperactivity (202). However, variations in norms among samples, even those using subjects from different regions of the United States, suggest a need to rely on regional or local norms (215,234,236).

Test–retest reliabilities for the factor scores are reported to range from 0.72 to 0.91 over a 2-week period (36,250). One-year test–retest reliabilities ranged from 0.35 for anxiety/tension to 0.57 for hyperactivity in one study (214). Higher 1-year reliabilities (0.90) for low scores on hyperactivity (less than 15-point cutoff) suggest greater behavioral variability in children initially rated as hyperactive, and a potential high rate of false-positives.

Interrater reliabilities vary with the type of rater and the specific factor scores. Teachers and parents show only modest levels of agreement on these scales, although both alter their ratings to reflect improved behavior in response to stimulant treatment (8). Teacher ratings produce less independent factor ratings than parent ratings (92). This may suggest that teachers rate children's behavior more globally, that teachers are sensitive to more restricted aspects of behavior, or that the uniformity of the school environment produces less variable behavior. Low interrater and test–retest reliabilities for the anxiety factor may reflect greater difficulty of perception, less sensitivity of this factor, or the scale characteristics of the particular test used (the fact that few items contribute to this factor score).

Demographic influences have also been studied. A higher percentage of boys than girls are rated as having conduct disorders and being hyperactive (92,215,237,250), consistent with clinical experience. Girls initially rated high are more likely than boys rated as high to change categories with a second rating 1 year later, suggesting that this scale is less useful for identifying persistent hyperactivity in girls (214). Younger children are rated more impulsive/hyperactive than older children, and as displaying more conduct problems and fewer psychosomatic symptoms. No significant effects of social class were seen in a normative study of the abbreviated version of this scale (92), although an earlier study (37) reported higher scores for lower-class children on individual items of a longer test version given to parents.

Practice effects (a pronounced decrease in scores) necessitate counterbalancing for order and may restrict the use of the Conners scale as a repeated measure. These effects are seen primarily between the first and second administrations according to Werry and Sprague (235) and may be more marked with the parental version (85,235). The intertest interval may be a crucial determinant of practice effects. Zentall and Barack (250) reported significant practice effects (a decline in scores in the absence of treatment) on the Conners scales when the test was administered after a 2-week interval.

Evidence of validity has been somewhat limited when evaluated in light of this scale's popularity. Until recently, the primary evidence for validity was the scale's demonstrated capacity to discriminate consistently between normal and hyperactive children and its consistent ability to display effects of stimulant drugs (8,36, 52,92,118,237). Recent findings of a high correlation between the Conners Abbreviated Parent-Teacher scale and Davids' scale for hyperactivity (250) provide evidence of concurrent validity. Comparisons of Canadian children who fell above and below a 15-point cutoff for hyperactivity indicated that those with high scores were more likely to be receiving special education and remedial reading and to have been referred more frequently to the Board of Educational Psychology Department (214). Comparisons of those who changed from a high to low score with those who remained above the cutoff showed that the former were more likely to be males and to be less-than-average achievers.

Experimental studies of caffeine, the Feingold diet, and food color challenges have made frequent use of the Conners scale. Studies of the behavioral effects of caffeine on normal and hyperactive children using this scale have produced mixed and inconsistent results (6,42,78,107,170). Although these scales have generally proven more sensitive than other measures (psychological tests, specific behavioral measures, monitored activity) in studies of the Feingold elimination diet and food color challenges, inconsistencies in results are prevalent. Parent ratings sometimes reflect effects in the absence of teacher-rated effects (123,134) and vice versa (50,241). Other findings (e.g., 134) suggest that the Conners scale's narrow focus on a certain subset of behaviors (e.g., hyperactivity) may miss other significant changes that may be affected by diet (e.g., irritability, anxiety, withdrawal, initiative, apathy).

2. Clinical Global Impressions Scale

The Global Clinical Impressions Scale (96) is a 7-point bipolar scale on which a rater (physician, parent, teacher) rates the overall degree and direction of changes in behavior. The physician version has two additional scales—one an efficacy index for therapeutic effects and side effects; the other, for severity of the psychiatric disorder. The physician integrates information available to him/her from all sources, including parent and teacher reports, in making these global ratings. While sensitive to the effects of medications (45,88,235), this scale yields no insight into the nature of the change. Used in conjunction with more specific scales or measures, however, it may provide a check on the adequacy of other measures. This may prove particularly useful when one is uncertain about the quality or subtlety of anticipated changes and may suggest more appropriate measures for future studies.

3. Other Scales

Additional rating scales used in pediatric psychopharmacology have been reviewed by Werry (231) and by Conners (44). Many of the better scales within this field have focused on severe psychopathology or hyperactivity, attention deficits, and aggressive behavior, despite the fact that brain damage or dysfunction in children may be manifested by a variety of other signs and symptoms (16). Scales that reveal other aspects of behavior and that measure more subtle behavioral deviations may prove preferable for assessing milder or more acute effects of nutrition and diet.

4. Laboratory Performance Measures

This category includes tasks involving restricted or specific aspects of cognitive functioning; many of them are similar to clinical neuropsychological measures. Laboratory measures are useful primarily for research purposes, since control groups can compensate for a lack of published normative data. Attentional and learning tasks are among the most drug-sensitive laboratory performance measures.

One of the most widely used and most drug-sensitive measures in this category is the Continuous Performance Test (CPT), which is used to assess attention. The CPT requires continuous monitoring and sustained vigilance to detect target stimuli (e.g., a particular letter or number or a particular sequence, such as "A" followed by "X"). Variations include the use of either auditory or visual stimuli presented at either a constant or variable rate. In the variable rate version, the subject's correct response (pushing a button in response to a target) speeds up the presentation rate, and his errors reduce the speed. Scores include reaction time, number of omission errors, number of commission errors (impulsivity), and interstimulus interval (speed).

Distractible, hyperactive, and impulsive children perform worse than normal children on the CPT, and stimulant medications fairly consistently enhance their accuracy and performance (8,231). Normal children also show stimulant-induced improvement on the CPT (169). McNair (136) lists this task as one of the most highly sensitive to the effects of mild tranquilizers among normal and patient populations. The effects of antidepressants on behaviorally disordered children are unclear (231).

Simple performance measures of vigilance and auditory distractibility have been shown to discriminate between epileptic and normal boys (208), although effects of drugs have not been determined. Barbiturates have been shown to impair auditory vigilance (110,139).

Several experimental studies of caffeine have shown significant positive effects on CPT measures and on other similar vigilance measures (7,28,33,69,172). These findings are balanced by a number of studies that failed to find effects on these measures (42,45,170). Of the three studies of food colorings that used these measures (98,99,123), none found them to be affected by elimination diets or active challenges.

Research using laboratory memory and learning tasks has emphasized verbal association. Paired associative learning has been shown to be facilitated by stimulant medications in behaviorally- and learning-disordered groups (2,231) and in normal children (169). Children with low and average IQs improved more than high-IQ children in several of Conners' studies (47,51). This task is also highly sensitive to the effects of mild tranquilizers in normal and patient populations (136). At least one report (102) has shown that chlorpromazine impairs paired-associate learning.

Short-term memory tasks, though not shown to discriminate between hyperactive and normal children, may be sensitive to stimulant medications (196,198,200–202,232), if not consistently (231,249). Rote memory has been shown to be adversely affected by chlorpromazine (102).

Haloperidol has recently been shown to decrease inappropriate responding and to improve simple discrimination learning in autistic children (27).

The use of laboratory learning tasks in nutritional research is fairly limited. Caffeine failed to affect verbal learning in normal prepubertal boys and college males (69,172) and also failed to affect memory for digits in adults (33). Performance on an associative learning task failed to discriminate between 11- to 17-year-old Ugandan survivors of protein-calorie malnutrition and their controls (105).

F. Psychological Tests

Psychological tests have served as major outcome measures in naturalistic, follow-up studies of malnutrition and have played a lesser role in laboratory studies of drug and dietary effects. While these instruments have been viewed historically as measuring one's hereditary intellectual potential, they are now recognized as measures of abilities that have developed through the interaction of hereditary and environmental factors (108). Measured intelligence (IQ scores) correlates with social class, rural–urban status, birth order, family size, and maternal education and intelligence (188). Academic achievement has served and continues to serve as a measure for validating tests of intelligence. These measures are, in general, characterized by built-in stability over time (high test–retest reliability); this makes them unlikely candidates for displaying sensitivity to relatively subtle effects of brief nutritional or drug interventions, and better candidates for assessing long-term effects of chronic and/or severe nutritional insults (e.g., sustained protein-calorie malnutrition).

1. Infant Developmental Scales

Infant developmental scales, while demonstrating fairly good concurrent validity, show very limited predictive validity. Social class background, parental education, and other characteristics of the home environment may, in fact, predict future IQ scores better than these measures when administered in early infancy. Their predictive utility is much better within clinical than within normal populations (5). Yet, even here, interaction with social–environmental variables appears important. Low scores on infant scales are more likely to be associated with poor intellectual performances later (ages 4 and 10 years) among subjects of low rather than of high socioeconomic status (229,240). These scales focus primarily on sensorimotor skills; items differ qualitatively from those on intelligence tests designed for children of school age (5).

Judged to be among the best available infant scales (59), the Bayley Scales of Infant Development are based on a larger and more representative subject sample than are other infant scales. These scales, appropriate for ages 2 to 30 months of age, include a Motor Scale and a Mental Scale, each of which yields a developmental index. The Mental Scale includes adaptive responses such as attending to visual and auditory stimuli; the manipulation and combination of objects; the ability to follow directions; goal-directed behaviors; and memory, or object constancy. An Infant Behavior Record, completed following the two scales, provides a standard rating of the infant's responsiveness during testing, his emotional reactions, his endurance, and his goal-directedness.

2. Intelligence Tests

Major general cognitive measures include the Stanford-Binet Intelligence Scale, the Wechsler scales, and more recently, the McCarthy Scales of Children's Abilities.

The Stanford-Binet, appropriate for ages 2 to adult, is highly reliable and valid. However, it emphasizes verbal skills and yields only a global measure of intellectual ability—the IQ or Mental Age (5). Advantages include its high interest value (particularly important with young, difficult-to-test children) and its sensitivity at the extreme ranges of intelligence, a factor contributing to its accuracy in measuring degrees of mental retardation. Because of its wide age range, this instrument's use for longitudinal studies allows the investigator to avoid the use of different tests at different ages.

The Wechsler tests include the Wechsler Preschool and Primary Scales of Intelligence (WPPSI), designed for ages 4½ to 6 years of age; the Wechsler Intelligence Scale for Children (WISC); its recent (1974) revision—the WISC-R, for ages 6 to 16; and the Wechsler Adult Intelligence Scale (WAIS), whose revision (the WAIS-R) has just become available. The WISC-R shows considerable similarity of content and factor structure with the WISC, but requires more active inquiry on the part of the examiner and generally yields somewhat lower scores (24). Minority children were included in the new standardization sample.

The Wechsler tests have the advantage of yielding a variety of standardized scores, including a Verbal, Performance, and Full-Scale IQ and individual subtest scores. These scales are most sensitive to the middle ranges of abilities and less sensitive than the Binet at the extremes. The verbal portion correlates more highly with the Binet, whereas the Performance scale places less emphasis on verbal skills (24). These tests may show disparities when used to test children at the extremes of their age ranges, where the forms overlap, and thus may present problems of test crossover in longitudinal research and in some cross-sectional research.

Patterns of scores seen on these instruments have been related to a wide variety of sociocultural and biological variables. Kaufman's (115) book provides an excellent analysis of various score patterns on the WISC-R, including those suggestive of attentional deficits. Kaufman also discusses practice effects on the various subtests and scales, and age × subtest interactions—issues that are highly relevant to longitudinal studies.

More recently, the McCarthy Scales of Children's Abilities, appropriate for ages 2½ to 8½ years of age, have gained in popularity. These scales consist of 18 subtests that yield six scores: verbal, perceptual–motor, quantitative, composite (general cognitive), memory, and motor. The McCarthy Scales combine the use of a summary score, roughly comparable to a deviation IQ score, and a diagnostic profile of abilities. Generally well-constructed and standardized on a sample reflecting the 1970 United States census, the scales have not displayed conspicuous differences between black and white children nor between the sexes in subsequent analyses. Reliability and validity are generally good, although additional work is needed to determine predictive validity and utility of the scales as a diagnostic/prescriptive instrument (24). Kaufman and Kaufman's (116) book is a valuable resource for analyzing and interpreting these scales.

Studies of stimulant drug effects on intelligence test performances, which have most frequently used the WISC, have shown inconsistent effects (231). Barkley (8) interprets this inconsistency as reflecting improved concentration and attention by test subjects, rather than changes in basic intellectual or cognitive processing. Douglas (66) similarly attributes such changes to nonintellectual factors, e.g., improved impulse control. Relationships between stimulant-induced changes on intelligence test performance and improved classroom learning have not generally been demonstrable (231). However, Gittelman et al. (87) recently found small but significant improvements in both academic skils and psychological test performances over a 4-month period in response to a therapeutic combination involving methylphenidate, remedial reading instruction, and individual tutoring, when subjects were compared with members of a placebo group receiving the same educational interventions. The selection of subjects on the basis of poor academic achievement and lack of behavior disorders, the educational interventions provided, and the use of highly sensitive measures all probably contributed to the effects noted in this study. The sensitive measures included the performance subscale of the WISC-R, the CPT, the Visual Sequential Memory subtest of the Illinois Test of Psycholinguistic Abilities (ITPA), Raven's Progressive Matrices, the Matching Familiar Figures Test, and Porteus Mazes, measures with substantial attentional components. The scores on several of these measures also reflect speed in addition to accuracy.

Studies with other drugs are few. McNair (136) compared the sensitivity of 43 performance measures with antianxiety drugs. The studies he reviewed involved a high percentage of normal subjects; only 11% of the studies involved patients. Sixty percent of the studies that used intelligence-type tests demonstrated significant effects of antianxiety drugs. However, it was unclear whether speed or accuracy ("power") was affected. Antidepressants failed to alter IQ scores in two studies of hyperactive children (165,173). Anticonvulsants (phenytoin, phenobarbitone, and primidone) were associated with declining intelligence scores over time in epileptic patients, independent of seizure frequency (213). Chlorpromazine had no immediate effect on Performance IQ in two studies of hyperactive children (224,226) but might have influenced Verbal IQ in such children over time (225). Haloperidol had no effect on the IQ scores of emotionally disturbed children in one study (246).

Small deficiencies in intelligence as assessed by IQ test scores have been linked to elevated serum lead levels, even in asymptomatic children (181).

Studies of malnutrition that have used developmental scales and intelligence tests as outcome measures have generally found significant group differences between malnourished and well-nourished groups at younger ages, primarily preschool ages, and no clear differences in later childhood (130). Interpretation of such findings is complicated by the fact that control subjects also score poorly on these measures (130), and by the frequent use of the scales and tests to examine foreign populations for whom they lack demonstrated validity.

3. Achievement Tests

Standardized achievement tests have played an important role in assessing the skills attained primarily through formal education. These measures are constructed on the basis of content validity so as to reflect levels of basic skill competencies. They vary in the range and level of skills covered—from measures that focus specifically on reading or one other particular content area to those that are more comprehensive in scope, and from those that cover a wide age range to those limited to a narrow range of age and grade levels. Wide-range measures generally sacrifice some precision and sensitivity to change and thus would be expected to prove less useful than narrow-range tests in short-term studies of acute nutritional effects.

Most American school systems have testing programs that use group-administered achievement batteries on a regular basis. The Iowa Tests of Basic Skills, Metropolitan Achievement Tests, and Stanford Achievement Tests are representative achievement batteries covering grades 1 through 8 and, in some cases, kindergarten and grade 9 as well. Though seldom used in nutritional research, they might provide a readily available and highly relevant measure for naturalistic, follow-up research. However, local community norms present a more appropriate basis for comparisons, a complicating factor in studies that sample children from a variety of communities. Administration of these tests to groups may distort their validity as measures of academic skills in children with attentional or behavioral problems and in learning-disabled children.

Among the most widely used individually administered achievement measures are the Wide Range Achievement Test (WRAT) (113) for ages 5 through adult and the Peabody Individual Achievement Test (PIAT) (67) for grades K to 12. Both yield scores for reading, spelling, and math skills, while the PIAT also tests basic knowledge or information. Standardized scores, percentile ranks, and age and grade equivalents can be determined. Age and grade equivalents are ordinal measures. Since they do not constitute interval scales, parametric statistics should not be applied to them.

The reading subtest of the WRAT tests single-word recognition only, whereas the PIAT assesses decoding and comprehension of narrative material. The WRAT subtests are timed. Failure to follow standard administration guidelines regarding time limits will reduce the test's sensitivity. The multiple-choice, untimed format of most of the subtests of the PIAT contrasts with that of the WRAT, which requires the subject to produce (recall) rather than merely recognize or identify correct responses. These limitations and variations may each result in distortions, but this may be more likely to present problems when not supplemented by other achievement measures with populations where discrepancies in abilities are expected (e.g., learning-disabled children). Moreover, these tests, which are designed for a wide age range, may sacrifice precision of measurement when compared with tests that serve a more restricted age range (87).

Achievement tests have generally not been shown to be sensitive to drug effects. Barkley's (8) review reports mixed, but primarily negative, results with respect to the drug sensitivity of these measures. Conners' and Werry's (52) review also concludes that there is little evidence for improvement on measures like the WRAT, which are relatively crude and insensitive, and offer Rie and Rie's (178) hypothesis that stimulants produce only a brief, nonspecific improvement in performance rather than enhancing new learning. Long-term controlled studies of hyperactive children generally fail to show effects of stimulant treatment on academic achievement (9). Rather, these children continue to show educational problems despite positive behavioral changes.

However, Gittelman et al. (87) point out that most of these negative studies have selected children on the basis of their behavioral problems rather than learning disabilities, thereby potentially restricting the range of therapeutic benefits. A second methodological problem has been the inadequacy of drug trials in many of the short-term studies. Several months might be required for a measurable improvement in reading or other academic skills to occur. The variable quality of instruction, negative attitudes toward instruction on the part of students, negative expectations of both students and teachers, and inappropriate levels of instruction for academically deficient students all might mask positive drug effects.

To overcome these difficulties, Gittelman et al. (87) compared the effect of giving subject remedial reading instruction, individual tutoring, and methylphenidate or placebo for 18 weeks, using a between-subjects design. Subjects of ages 7 to 12 were selected on the basis of poor academic performance and lack of current behavioral problems and hyperactivity. Significant drug effects were seen on several academic measures (Davids-Drack phonetic reading test; several mathematics subtests and the social studies subtest of the Stanford Achievement Test), but not on the WRAT or Gray Oral Reading Test, which proved less sensitive. Follow-up of these groups at 2 and 8 months posttreatment found that differences were not maintained in the absence of continued treatment.

Thus, highly sensitive (narrow-range) achievement measures and controlled educational interventions will likely be needed to demonstrate subtle effects of drugs or diets on achievement. Such effects may be more likely to occur when subjects are selected on the basis of academic rather than behavioral criteria. Even here, effects may prove transient.

Within-subject, or crossover, designs might also lend additional sensitivity. Gittleman et al. (87) argued against the use of a crossover design on the basis of an inability to return to baseline performance in reading. However, single-subject designs do not necessitate a level baseline, only one from which predictions can be made. One could compare the slopes or rates of increases in reading skills that characterize placebo and drug manipulations using several designs along with appropriate statistical techniques [e.g., time series analysis (103)].

Overall, achievement measures may prove more useful for long-term follow-up studies, where they should provide a useful supplement to intelligence measures, than for studies on the acute effects of drugs or nutrients.

4. Neuropsychological Tests and Approaches

Traditional psychometric approaches to intelligence testing have emphasized statistical manipulations and analyses to achieve validity. Techniques such as factor analysis have yielded considerable common variance, which provided evidence for a unitary view of intelligence. This view proved highly compatible with the notion of equipotentiality of brain function, espoused by psychologists in the early 1900s. Inferences were drawn from scores chiefly on the basis of population norms— a "level of performance" criterion.

An increasing interest in brain–behavior relationships and a shift away from equipotential toward localizationist views of brain function led to a considerable redefinition of concepts of intelligence and an expansion of inferential bases in testing. Behavior came to be conceptualized as the product of functional systems dependent on the integrity of the brain's connections (132). Intellectual functioning came to be viewed in terms of *specific* components and cognitive processes that arose from localized brain regions and functional pathways.

One example of this theme of specificity includes distinctions made within various theoretical models of memory and learning. These include immediate (sensory), short-term, and long-term (consolidated) memory, retrieval and recognition, episodic and semantic memory, and deliberate and incidental learning, among others (20). Neuropsychological research suggests that memory can be specifically, rather than than globally, impaired in different neurological syndromes (25).

With these conceptual changes, approaches to testing expanded to include the comparison of the two sides of the body and the use of pathognomonic signs and patterns of test performance (intraindividual comparisons), in addition to a normative, or level-of-performance, criterion. The use of such intraindividual comparisons adds a new dimension to our evaluation methods, one that should not be neglected by relying solely on normative comparisons between groups.

Related developments include the identification of limitations of traditional global intellectual measures, increased knowledge of the differential effects of brain insult on certain types of abilities, and increased attention to a new category for conceptualizing behavior—that of learning disability.

It is now recognized that considerable cognitive deficit may coexist with above-average IQ scores. Diffuse brain damage at any age may impair one's ability to solve problems and to learn new, unfamiliar material, while proving much less disruptive to the ability to draw upon stored, previously acquired knowledge and experience (16).

Children may rely more heavily on new learning and problem-solving. Studies of the effects of brain damage on performance in intelligence tests have shown consistent IQ deficits in children, while finding an apparent lack of IQ deficits in many brain-damaged adults. This finding suggests that it may be inappropriate to make statistical adjustments for IQ in examining the effects of nutritional insult on other cognitive tasks and measures in children. Brain-damaged adults appear more able to retain average or above-average IQs, while displaying deficits in new learning and problem-solving, leading Boll (14) to hypothesize that intelligence tests tap different types of abilities in children and adults. The Wechsler vocabulary subtest, shown to be relatively resistent to diffuse cerebral insult in adults, appears much more sensitive in children (16).

Relatively little is known about the effects of various lesions on the child's development of specific cognitive abilities and social–emotional functioning, an important point to keep in mind when attempting to generalize from the adult neuropsychological literature to children. Evidence reviewed by Boll and Barth (16) suggests limitations in generalizing from studies of brain-damaged adults to children with brain insults.

Although intelligence tests, designed with predictive validity in mind, have used achievement scores as criterion measures, substantial discrepancies may be seen in individual cases between achievement as anticipated on the basis of IQ scores and that actually observed. Where achievement falls substantially below that expected on the basis of age, grade, and IQ, the child may be diagnosed as learning-disabled, provided that certain exclusionary criteria are met—namely, the absence of an emotional or sensory basis for the learning problem. The majority of learning-disabled children show language deficits, which may not be reflected in low Verbal IQs. More *specific* tests may be required to identify positive evidence of learning disability (61). Overall, these changes in the conceptualization of intelligence and behavior and in approaches to their assessment would suggest a need to broaden our search for specific cognitive abilities and processes that might be affected by nutritional status or diet.

Two major approaches to neuropsychological measurement include the use of a standard test battery or the use of more individualized test batteries. Advocates of the standard battery approach generally argue the need for a comprehensive study, designed to assess both areas of deficit and intact abilities, and using standard procedures to facilitate research comparisons. This approach is best exemplified by the Halstead-Reitan Neuropsychological Test Battery. This test battery, originally designed for use with adults, has been adapted for use with children aged 9 through 15 (Halstead-Reitan Neuropsychological Battery for Children) and ages 5 through 8 (Reitan-Indiana Neuropsychological Battery for Children). These procedures are described by Boll (15). Recent assessments of the validity of these procedures and their use in combination with other tests are provided by Boll (14,15), Boll and Barth (16), and Filskov and Levi (73).

In the other, more individualized and qualitative approach tests are selected primarily to identify and clarify an individual patient's particular deficits, or those of a particular research population. Both qualitative deviations in the subject's approach to a task and quantitative determinations (i.e., test scores) contribute information about the nature of the deficit.

A large number of neuropsychological tests that are thought to be sensitive to localized or diffuse brain damage are reviewed by Lezak (125), who organizes her review around various intellectual and control functions for which tests exist. Speech and language, visuospatial functions, learning and memory, attention, problem-solving ability, sensory–perceptual functions, motor functions, and behavioral control are all assessed by various particular tests. The psychometric properties of several of these and other psychological tests are reviewed in Buros' *Mental Measurement Yearbook* series.

Barkley (8) concludes that the Porteus Mazes Test and Kagan's Matching Familiar Figures Test, both of which contain a large attentional component, are among the most sensitive to, and predictive of subject responses to, stimulant medications. Tests of left/right orientation, motor control and inhibition, tapping speed, and pegboard tasks are consistently unresponsive to stimulants. Sprague (197) also found the Porteus Mazes to be among the most consistently sensitive measures of performance in the pediatric psychopharmacological literature. He also recommended Reitan's Motor Steadiness Battery. McNair's (136) evaluation of the sensitivity of various performance measures to antianxiety drugs concluded that pegboard and manual dexterity tasks and digit symbol substitution tasks were highly sensitive, i.e, they yielded significant results in 50 to 75% of the studies reviewed. Coordination, memory, writing, tapping, steadiness tasks, and mazes yielded significant results in 25 to 40% of the studies reviewed that used these types of measures. Arithmetic, problem-solving, cancellation, and digit span tasks showed low sensitivity and were significant in only 0 to 20% of the studies reviewed.

Dietary studies that have used a variety of neuropsychological measures to evaluate the effects of artificial food colors (98,99) have failed to find any effects on these or any other measures used (CPT, parent and teacher Conners ratings, direct observations of classroom behavior). The neuropsychological tests did, however, differentiate hyperactive from normal children, as did other measures.

G. Self-Ratings

Self-report ratings have received only limited attention within pediatric psychopharmacology. However, as pediatric psychopharmacological research begins to focus more on internal states—anxiety, depression, mood—such measures are likely to assume a new role and to add a new dimension to this body of research.

The age at which such measures may prove useful is an open question. Children below the fourth grade should probably not be relied on to complete paper and pencil measures independent of oral testing. In children under 8 years of age or the third grade, insufficient introspection, self-awareness, and conceptualization may severely limit the use of even orally administered objective measures (166).

Objective self-report measures of self-concept, anxiety, and locus of control have served as measures of children's personality traits. Other research with children has attempted to differentiate between anxiety as a state and as a personality trait and to measure both aspects with self-report measures.

1. Self-Concept

The Piers-Harris (155) questionnaire, entitled "The Way I Feel About Myself," is one example of a self-report, self-concept measure appropriate for use with children. It consists of 80 items requiring the child to decide whether or not various descriptions apply to him/her (yes/no, true/false format). A manual presents data on reliability and validity, which are adequate for research purposes, norms for grades 4 through 12, correlations with intellectual and achievement measures, and information on factor structure. Seven cluster scores (e.g, intellectual and social status, anxiety, behavior, physical appearance) can be derived in addition to a total score.

2. Locus of Control

Locus of control has been discussed by Whalen and Henker (237,238) with respect to their proposed "social–ecological" approach to child psychopharmacology. Internal locus of control reflects a perception of one's self as responsible for his fate (able to affect environmental events and life outcomes), whereas external control reflects a perception of self as being acted upon by fate, luck, other people, and other environmental forces. Research using the locus of control construct suggests that, in general, people are handicapped by an external orientation, although excessive internality (self-blame) may be pathological. Academic achievement and intellectual performance, variables that are not significantly affected by stimulant medications (8), are directly related to internal locus of control (35,55,101,135,151). On the basis of their study of attitudinal and cognitive correlates of methylphenidate administration, Whalen and Henker (237,238) have hypothesized that stimulant treatment promotes an external orientation that interferes with its long-term benefits as related to behavior and to academic achievement.

Several children's scales with good psychometric characteristics and construct validity have been developed to measure this construct: Nowicki and Strickland's Locus of Control Scale (152) for children beyond the second grade and the Stephens-Delys Reinforcement Contingency Interview (205) for ages 4 to 10 are based on generalized life expectations. The latter permits subscaling for expectations regarding various people significant to the subject, e.g., teacher, mother/father, adults, peers. Crandall et al.'s (54) Intellectual Achievement Responsibility Questionnaire for grades 3 through 12 taps expectations with respect to the academic situation and yields separate scores for the child's successes versus failures.

3. Anxiety

Two self-report anxiety scales have been adapted for use with children. The Children's Manifest Anxiety Scale (CMAS) (30) includes items from the Taylor

Manifest Anxiety Scale and a validity (lie) scale. It has been shown to discriminate between normal and emotionally disturbed children (141) with good reliability and to demonstrate separate factors of cognitive oversensitivity, somatic anxiety symptoms, and impaired concentration (75). This scale has recently been revised and shortened (175). A third-grade reading level is required for self-administration, although the scale is appropriate for grades 1 through 12. Recent factor analysis (176) has yielded primary factors of worry and oversensitivity, fear, and impaired concentration.

The State-Trait Anxiety Inventory for Children (STAIC) (195), developed for elementary school children, consists of a 20-item trait scale to measure stable predispositions and a 20-item state scale to assess momentary, situational aspects of anxiety. Initial study of this instrument with normal children showed good reliability (195). Stress was shown to affect the state scale selectively in normal children (149). However, the state/trait distinction has not been supported by data from studies with emotionally disturbed children (74). Finch and his colleagues hypothesized that developmental differences between these populations and a complicated test format might account for this failure. However, their modification of the scale to a simple yes/no format also failed to achieve the desired validity in a series of studies with normal and abnormal children (74). Numerous inconsistencies prevented any meaningful picture from emerging that might have contributed to construct validity. Factor study of this scale (76) has suggested that trait anxiety may not be as firmly established in emotionally disturbed children as it is in normal children.

While reliability studies with both the CMAS and STAIC have been encouraging and while both instruments distinguish, albeit to a limited extent, between normal and emotionally disturbed children, evidence of construct validity is quite limited. Relationships between anxiety, as measured by these instruments, and other behaviors and constructs are inconsistent and unclear. The validity of the state/trait distinction, particularly with emotionally disturbed children, is questionable. Trait anxiety appears to be multidimensional and subject to interactions with situational factors.

4. Sensitivity of Self-Report Measures to Diet

Several caffeine studies have shown limited effects on self-report ratings. Goldstein's studies with adults (89,90) found effects on alertness, activity, and nervousness using nonstandardized self-report measures. Several caffeine studies with normal children and adults (69,170,172) that have used the revised CMAS (which is sensitive to amphetamines) and a nonstandardized 10-item side effects questionnaire failed to find effects on mood, but found some limited side effects (nervousness, nausea). No effects of caffeine were seen on the revised CMAS in another study of normal boys, ages 8 to 11 (170).

Only one study of food colorings (a single case study) used a self-report rating. Mattes and Gittelman-Klein (134) found a 10-year-old hyperactive boy's self-rating on the Abbreviated Conners Scale (a measure of hyperactivity) sensitive to a double-blind challenge.

The use of such subjective, self-report measures in dietary research may await the development of more valid measures. Anxiety, in particular, appears to be a multidimensional construct (176) that may be especially difficult to measure in children. Theoretical uncertainty with respect to the existence of depression and anxiety in children, the subjective qualities of these emotional states, and their modes of expression may delay the development of truly adequate measures for use with children and encourage additional studies using adults as a temporary alternative.

IV. STUDIES OF SUBSTANCES (DIETARY AND NONDIETARY) WITH POSSIBLE BEHAVIORAL AND COGNITIVE TOXICITY

A. Caffeine

Dietary sources of caffeine include coffee, tea, cocoa, chocolate, and cola beverages, ingested alone or as ingredients in other foods (e.g., puddings, cookies, etc.). A number of prescription and over-the-counter drugs contribute considerably to caffeine consumption as well.

Recent concerns about dietary caffeine have focused on possible relationships to anxiety states, various physical illnesses and symptoms, and birth defects. The Food and Drug Administration (FDA) recently issued warnings to pregnant women about possible adverse effects of caffeine on the developing fetus and expressed concern about the neurobehavioral effects of caffeine consumption by children. The amount of caffeine in colas consumed by children borders on the dose known to produce central nervous stimulation in adults (127). FDA is reconsidering the status of caffeine as a "GRAS" substance (generally recognized as safe), a status that exempts it from premarketing clearances required for food additives. A redefinition of cola beverages to eliminate caffeine as a mandatory ingredient has been proposed.

1. The Nature of Effects on Performance

After comprehensively reviewing the literature on the effects of caffeine on human performance, Weiss and Laties (223) conclude that caffeine enhances a wide range of performances, consistently counteracts decrements associated with fatigue and boredom, and positively affects motivation.

Task variables, particularly complexity, appear to be important contributors to effects seen on both motor and cognitive tasks. Response speed appears facilitated, whereas motor skill, coordination, and steadiness (control) may even be adversely affected. Vigilance and alertness, and perhaps perceptual sensitivity, appear enhanced, whereas no convincing evidence of enhanced cognitive processing is seen (223).

These effects appear compatible with an arousal model. Cognitive performance is a nonmonotonic function of level of arousal within this model (143). Increased arousal may facilitate dominant, automatic, well-learned responses at the expense of others with less "response strength" in a theoretical hierarchy of responses. Thus, less complex tasks requiring more automatic responses may be facilitated; and more complex tasks, adversely affected by increased arousal (inverted U curve).

Where effects are seen in children, they are compatible with this model. Elkins et al. (69) found decreased reaction time and omission errors on the CPT, increased errors of commission, and no facilitation of learning and memory with a 10 mg/kg dose (see Table 2). Caffeine, in fact, tended to worsen free recall. These results suggest an increased tendency to respond rather than enhanced cognitive processing. This contrasts with the tendency of amphetamine to decrease both omission and commission errors (168), perhaps enhancing the selectivity of attentional processes more than caffeine. Campbell et al. (28) found no improvements on reaction time in a small sample of normal children at a low (6 mg/kg) dose.

2. Individual Variability in Response and Prior Dietary Status

Several investigators have been impressed by the individual variability seen in responses to caffeine, although few have directly studied prior dietary status in relationship to this variability in adults (90) and even fewer in children. Caffeine abstainers have generally reported more aversive responses, whereas habitual users have reported positive effects. A recent comprehensive study that compared high- and low-dose habitual adult consumers at two dosages (172), for example, found evidence of greater side effects among low-caffeine consumers.

Using a similar paradigm, Rapoport et al. (170) examined the effects of prior dietary status on children's caffeine responses in a double-blind crossover study. Following a 1-week caffeine-free baseline, 10 boys, ages 8 to 11 years, with low habitual intakes of caffeine (less than 50 mg/day) and nine, also ages 8 to 11 years, with high intakes (300 mg/day or more) received 5 mg/kg of caffeine or its placebo twice a day, each for 2 weeks. The order of drug–placebo treatments was counterbalanced such that approximately half the subjects were first placed on caffeine, followed by placebo, and half received placebo treatment prior to caffeine treatment. Weekly test measures included a side effects and anxiety scale (revised CMAS) completed by both children and parents, CPT, reaction time, and physiological measures (skin conductance, heart rate, blood pressure, and pulse). Parent and teacher ratings (using an abbreviated Conners scale) were collected at the end of each 2-week treatment period. Saliva samples were used to monitor caffeine concentrations. At baseline, low-dose consumers displayed significantly more autonomic reactivity on skin conductance measures, and some differences in behavioral ratings were seen. A discriminant analysis of the Conners ratings indicated the high users were most distinguished by the item "demands must be met immediately—easily frustrated."

Saliva concentrations were similarly altered by caffeine in the two groups: They rose from a mean of 0.10 mg/ml (SD = 0.08) on placebo to a mean of 4.63 mg/

TABLE 2. Analysis of variance of cognitive and behavioral performance ratings of 19 normal children after caffeine or placebo

Performance measure	Placebo		3 mg/kg of Caffeine		10 mg/kg of Caffeine		F[a]	Significance
	Mean	SD	Mean	SD	Mean	SD		
Vigilance measures								
Reaction time (sec)	309.40	84.80	293.2	63.8	288.2	88.4	3.86	p = 0.03
Continuous Performance Test								
Number of omission errors	9.63	3.77	8.37	2.83	7.63	2.89	7.76	p = 0.05
Number of commission errors	11.84	5.99	11.50	11.99	18.32	39.54	.74	n.s.
Interstimulus interval (msec)	550	225	471	176	452	189	3.23	n.s.
Cognitive measure								
Free recall (total correct)	4.31	3.38	4.15	3.84	3.05	3.74	2.45	p = 0.10
Activity measure								
Movements per 2 hr	416	95	398	115	472	128	3.56	p = 0.05

[a]df = 2, 36 for all measures.

ml (SD = 1.70) on caffeine in the low-consuming group, and from a mean of 0.34 mg/ml (SD = 0.69) to 3.47 mg/ml (SD = 3.69) in the high-consuming group. Low-dose consumers showed a significant increase in skin conductance after caffeine, while this measure showed a nonsignificant decrease among high-intake consumers. Low-dose consumers reported increased side effects (headaches, nausea, nervousness, insomnia) in response to caffeine, whereas high-dose consumers reported more side effects on placebo. However, this latter effect was confined to one order of treatment (placebo followed by caffeine), raising the possibility of withdrawal effects. No drug effects were seen on the other measures.

Consistent relationships between caffeine response and prior dietary history appeared confined to self-reported side effects. However, the failure of vigilance measures to show expected drug effects in this study suggests that the tests used may not have been sufficiently sensitive to discern possible effects of prior diet on the performance measures.

Whether differences between high- and low-dose consumers reflect differences in drug tolerance or differences in initial preferences based on subjective responses is unclear. High-dose consumers might represent a different, perhaps more impulsive, population who respond to questionnaires differently than do low-dose consumers. This appears unlikely, however, as other questionnaire responses failed to differentiate high- and low-dose consumers. Another possibility is that high-dose consumers were experiencing withdrawal symptoms during placebo periods. As symptoms of caffeine withdrawal resemble those of caffeinism, this could obscure differences between caffeine and placebo periods. This hypothesis would be best tested by repeating this study following a prolonged period of abstinence. Caffeine interacts with a variety of receptors, and differential receptor number and/or sensitivity might conceivably influence dietary preferences. Alterations in neurotransmitter concentrations have been demonstrated to influence dietary choice in rats (247), and in man (248a,248b).

3. Relationship to Psychiatric Symptoms—Cause or Cure?

Anxiety symptoms associated with caffeine ingestion—"caffeinism"—are well recognized in adults (4). Nevertheless, adults consume caffeine for certain beneficial effects, such as improved alertness, energy, relaxation, and mood (89,90,148). Studies with children have explored both possible therapeutic and possible adverse behavioral effects.

a. Hyperactive children

Schnackenberg (190) compared the effects of caffeine and methylphenidate on hyperactive children in an uncontrolled, nonblind crossover paradigm. Both parent and teacher ratings and reports reflected significant behavioral improvements with caffeine, when compared with placebo, that did not differ significantly from those observed after methylphenidate. Apparently stimulated by this study, several better controlled studies were performed, which failed to replicate its major finding. Caffeine has generally failed to produce significant improvements over placebo treatments in hyperactive children assessed using parent and teacher behavioral ratings or objective psychological tests (45,77,82,107). Firestone et al. (77) did find improved parent and teacher ratings of hyperactive children treated with caffeine compared with placebo, but this effect was confined to one order of treatment, suggesting a practice effect. Other measures failed to reflect any difference.

Where therapeutic trials with methylphenidate and/or d-amphetamine were also studied, these drugs caused significant changes and were superior to caffeine (6,77,82,95,107).

Conners (45) found dose-related effects of caffeine in the visual-evoked responses of hyperactive children in the absence of behavioral effects (CPT performance, seat activity and movement) using a double-blind crossover design. He concluded that the clinical failure of caffeine could not be explained by a lack of central effects and suggested the possibility that the central effects of caffeine may be too shortlived to affect clinical improvements.

Only one study (28) has directly compared the responses of normal and hyperactive children to caffeine. Effects of a single dose of caffeine on simple and choice reaction time measures were studied. The simple reaction time measure required the subject to press a switch when a light came on, whereas the choice reaction time task required the subject to decide whether two letters projected onto a screen were the same or different and to respond with the dominant or nondominant hand accordingly. Only choice reaction time differentiated normal from hyperactive children (normal children performed better on this task). Caffeine enhanced accuracy on choice reaction time in hyperactive children and thus helped normalize their performance.

Overall, evidence for the therapeutic efficacy of caffeine in this population is not convincing. No controlled studies have shown it to compare favorably with stimulant medications, and evidence of normalizing effects is limited to this last study.

b. Normal Children

Rapoport and her colleagues have studied the effects of caffeine on mood, anxiety, side effects, and autonomic reactions in normal prepubertal boys using a variety of measures in double-blind crossover paradigms. Elkins et al. (69) examined the effects of single 3 mg/kg and 10 mg/kg doses and placebo using a mood scale, behavioral ratings of psychiatric symptoms by an observer, and a 10-item side effects questionnaire. Only one of four observational ratings ("fidgety") showed an effect of caffeine. Those few children who reported increased side effects were characterized by an absence of caffeine in their diet.

In a subsequent study, Rapoport et al. (170) again found similarly limited effects. An anxiety scale and observer ratings of psychiatric symptoms failed to reveal effects, whereas children's self-reports showed an increase in only one item on the side-effects list: "nervous and jittery"—which increased in response to a single dose of caffeine.

A comparison of the effects of caffeine administration (3 mg/kg and 10 mg/kg) to normal boys (ages 10.6 years $\pm$ 2.5 years) and male college students (ages 21.7 years $\pm$ 3.4 years) (170) showed similar salivary caffeine concentrations at each dosage and similar dose-dependent increases in autonomic reactivity. Adults reported more side effects, whereas children increased their motor activity in response to caffeine. Only children showed a significant increase in speech rate and improved attention (CPT, RT measures), both of which were limited to a higher dose.

These observed differences in motor effects versus verbally reported side effects may reflect either differences in biological effects or differences in expression, with children expressing effects more through this motor activity and adults, more verbally. Similar differences have been seen in response to amphetamines (168). Adults reported more side effects, whereas children showed a more consistent pattern of behavioral change in response to d-amphetamine, suggesting a degree of generalizability.

A final study (170) selected children (mean age 9.8 $\pm$ 1.8 years) on the basis of high (300 mg/day +) versus low (50 mg/day) prior dietary consumption and extended dietary treatment to include 2 weeks each of 10 mg/kg/day of caffeine and a placebo. Caffeine increased autonomic reactivity only in low-dose consumers. The side effects rated by the parents showed considerable sensitivity to caffeine; however, only the children consuming the low dose reported increased side effects with caffeine. Neither the Conners scale nor the revised CMAS showed effects of caffeine, the latter perhaps reflecting general difficulties involved in measuring anxiety in children.

This limited evidence of side effects stimulated by caffeine and increased autonomic arousal (reflected in increased skin conductance) in low-dose consumers suggests the possibility that anxiety symptoms may be stimulated in children by caffeine. Spontaneous skin conductance, a common index of autonomic arousal, has been found to be markedly elevated in clinical anxiety patients (126).

B. Artificial Food Additives

1. Feingold's Hypothesis

Dr. Feingold, a pediatrician and former professor of allergy at the Kaiser-Permanente Medical Center in San Francisco, was the first to propose that food additives and salicylates play a significant causative role in hyperactivity and associated learning and behavioral problems. He initially developed this hypothesis on the basis of his clinical experiences with patients who were sensitive to aspirin and salicylates and who seemed to benefit behaviorally from the dietary elimination of food colorings with a salicylate radical. Drawing analogies from these early experiences, Feingold hypothesized that similar symptoms in hyperactive children might respond to his elimination diet, which came to be known as the Feingold or

"K-P" (Kaiser-Permanente) diet (70,71). Feingold claimed success rates of about 50% in hyperkinetic populations. He attributed failures to possible genetically linked sensitivities to these artificial food colorings, to possible irreversible damage from long-term exposure, and to infractions, inasmuch as perfect compliance was held to be essential. The enthusiasm generated by widespread early publicity probably did more to stimulate experimental research relating diet and behavior than any other single event.

2. The Feingold Diet

The diet itself, described in Dr. Feingold's (70) popular book, *Why Your Child is Hyperactive*, is highly restrictive and demanding. Permissible foods include fresh meats, fish, and vegetables, many of which require home preparation. Offending foods include two groups—those Feingold felt contained natural salicylates (tomatoes, cucumbers, and nearly all common fruits) and those containing synthetic additives (baked goods, lunch meats, convenience foods, most desserts and candies, most commercial beverages, condiments, and colored margarine), as well as pediatric medications and vitamins containing artificial colors and flavors and aspirin. In most cases, the entire family adopts the diet to avoid possible infractions and the perception by the child that he/she is being discriminated against.

Two scientific panels set up to study the diet's efficacy—the National Advisory Committee on Hyperkinesis and Food Additives (144), sponsored by the Nutrition Foundation, and the Food and Drug Administration's Interagency Collaborative Group on Hyperkinesis (112)—criticized the diet for its lack of a scientific biochemical and nutritional rationale and the lack of proof of long-term safety. No chemical basis, e.g., identifiable chemical substances to be eliminated, was defined. Instead the diet appeared to be based on the assumption that the body could discriminate chemically identical compounds on the basis of their artificial source and that such chemically heterogeneous compounds as artificial colorings and salicylates would have similar effects. Even Feingold's assumptions regarding the occurrence of salicylic acid in various foods appeared erroneous (111).

3. Consumption of Food Additives and Salicylates by Hyperactive Children

The amount of food additives and salicylates consumed by hyperactive children has received little attention, possibly because Feingold hypothesized that adverse reactions would occur only in vulnerable individuals (those with genetic predispositions or allergies). However, some correlation between exposure to these substances and symptoms within susceptible individuals might be expected in the event that hyperactivity and food additives actually were linked.

Palmer et al. (154) however, failed to find differences in dietary habits between hyperactive boys ($n = 79$) and normal controls ($n = 23$) using a parent questionnaire designed to give particular attention to the foods in question. No differences were seen within the hyperactive population between those taking stimulant medications and those not treated with stimulants.

4. Allergy in Hyperactive Children

Palmer et al.'s (154) survey found a 20% incidence of allergy in their hyperactive sample, compared with a 25% incidence reported for the general population of age peers. However, Tryphonas and Trites (216) found a high number of allergies in a subgroup of 90 hyperactive children who were selected from a large pool of children referred to a hospital neuropsychological laboratory for evaluation. Children were tested with 43 food extracts using Radioallergosorbent (RAST) tests, which measure the degree of antibody reaction to specific allergens. Whereas most of the hyperactive children tested were not found to have allergies, some children in this group had a larger number of allergies than a contrast group of nonhyperactive, learning-disabled children. Teachers' ratings using the Conners scale showed a significant positive correlation with the number of allergies identified, suggesting the possibility of a cumulative effect and a possible contribution of unidentified food allergies to some hyperactivity.

While children in general show more cytotoxic reactions to food colorings than adults, such reactions in individuals are not related to responses to an elimination diet or to responses to challenges with artificial colors (46). Moreover, dose–response studies are needed to clarify the issue of adequate dosage.

5. Uncontrolled Studies of the Feingold Elimination Diet's Efficacy

Anecdotal reports (18,53,206) and nonblind studies of hyperactive children (104,153,174,183) have been highly positive and supportive of Feingold's claims of success. However, methodological problems, including, but not limited to, the lack of assessment of prior dietary status, lack of adequate compliance monitoring, lack of objective assessment instruments, failure to control for practice effects, and failures to perform statistical tests, pose severe restrictions on the scientific inferences that can be drawn from these studies.

6. Controlled Studies of the Feingold Elimination Diet

a. Hyperactive children

Controlled studies on the effects of the Feingold diet on hyperactive children have been reviewed by Lipton et al. (129). Major published efforts include the double-blind, crossover studies of Conners et al. (50) and Harley et al. (99). Similarities include careful diagnosis, drug-free baselines, comparison of two diets, each implemented for 3 to 4 weeks and counterbalanced for order, and careful monitoring of compliance with diet diaries. Both studied children ages 6 through 12, and Harley et al. also studied 10 preschool children. Measures in both studies included parent and teacher Conners ratings. Conners et al. also included a Clinical Global Impressions Scale, while Harley et al. (99) supplemented their behavioral ratings with classroom and laboratory observations and neuropsychological tests. Teacher ratings reflected significant improvements on the Feingold diet in the Conners study. Only four or five children were thought by both parents and teachers to have improved. More trials of the Feingold diet than placebo were rated as improved on global impressions. Although all of Harley's measures have been shown to discriminate between hyperactive and normal children, only parent ratings showed the effect of the Feingold diet. Moreover, this measure interacted with treatment order in the school-age sample, suggesting a practice effect. Although parent ratings of *preschool* children were significantly affected by the Feingold diet independent of order, this finding was not bolstered by changes in teacher ratings or test performances. The lack of validity data for 3- to 5-year-olds on the Conners scale further complicates the interpretation of these results. The inconsistencies seen in these careful, well-controlled studies failed to provide convincing support for the diet's efficacy, yet suggest the possibility that some subgroup of children might show significant behavioral effects when so treated. The Conners scales generally proved to be the most sensitive of the measures used.

b. Mentally retarded subjects

Harner and Lopp-Foiles (100) examined the effects of the Feingold elimination diet on 30 mentally retarded residential patients, ages 4 to 25 years, in a double-blind crossover design. No effects were demonstrated on nurses' and teachers' ratings on the Abbreviated Conners Scale.

7. Challenge Studies

a. Hyperactive children

The preceding studies prompted a shift in research strategy. In traditional allergy testing, active challenges are used to control for possible confounding effects of medical problems other than allergy itself, which could account for cross-sensitivities to food colorings (185). Following exclusionary diets, "challenge" testing with specific foods or allergens is performed to affirm that a causal link between adverse reactions and specific substances does, in fact, exist. The National Advisory Committee on Hyperactivity and Food Additives (144) recommended the use of this two-stage strategy for the testing of food colorings.

The three studies that employed both an elimination diet and active challenge with hyperactive children (123,211,241) yielded inconsistent findings similar to those seen in controlled studies of the elimination diet. This prompted other investigators to attempt to maximize the probability of finding effects with challenges by selecting for study children already thought to be responsive to the Feingold diet.

Group studies employing this strategy of selecting only diet-responsive children for challenge studies include those of Harley et al. (98), Levy and Hobbes (124), Goyette et al. (91), and Conners et al. (50). Harley et al. (98) found no significant effects on any of a wide range of measures. The other studies, too, failed to find statistically significant challenge effects, but hypothesized, on the basis of post hoc examinations of data, that younger children might be more responsive (91,124) and that effects might be short-lived (91). Further attempts to demonstrate effects in younger children (91) have not proved successful. However, time-limited effects (1 hr postchallenge) have been demonstrated on a laboratory visual-motor tracking task in a small number of children whose parents' behavioral ratings failed to reflect corresponding effects (46).

Single-case designs might be considered a further refinement of these attempts to increase the probability of identifying effects that may be limited to a minority of children. In this vein, Mattes and Gittelman-Klein (134) studied a 10-year-old hyperactive child, reported by parents to be highly diet-responsive, over 10 weeks of multiple double-blind crossovers. Only the mother's, not the teacher's, Conners ratings showed some related variability. Most impressive was the fact that the mother was able to identify the nature of the challenge on 8 of 10 weeks based on the child's irritability and fidgetiness, symptoms perhaps not well measured by the Conners scales.

Rose (179) studied two 8-year-old hyperactive girls, who had discontinued medications in favor of dietary maintenance, using classroom behavioral observations and a tartrazine challenge in a double-blind crossover. Significant adverse effects were seen on out-of-seat and on-task behavior, but not on aggression, which was a low-frequency problem.

b. Normal children

One group (227) studied 22 children, ages 2 through 7 years, whose parents reported behavioral responsivity to the elimination diet. The authors reported that none of these children suffered from clinically significant medical or psychiatric problems, but failed to describe the basis on which this was determined. Parents of each child identified several aversive and positive target behaviors that they believed were sensitive to diet. These were monitored daily throughout the 8-week, double-blind, food-coloring challenge and placebo crossover periods. These individually tailor-made behavioral measures were analyzed as 22 single case studies. Two children showed a significant challenge effect.

8. Summary of Clinical Research and Needs

Attempts to modify experimental paradigms to maximize their sensitivity to any limited and subtle effects that food colorings may have on behavior have failed to support Feingold's hypothesis. Clinical studies have not linked food colorings to hyperactivity. While a small percentage of children may show improvements on the Feingold diet, the percentage of this subgroup that also responds to an active challenge of food colorings appears severely limited, suggesting that factors other than food colorings account for observed "dietary" responses.

Successful demonstrations of challenge responses in a limited number of single-case studies, however, suggest that these designs may offer the greatest flexibility and sensitivity needed to objectify the relatively limited and subtle effects of diet. They also caution against the danger of overrelying on readily available, sometimes inadequate, behavioral measures. The emphasis on ratings of hyperactivity, in particular, may need to be broadened to encompass more subtle qualitative fluctuations in symptoms such as irritability and restlessness.

However, the most pressing current need is for a theory to guide future investigations. The applicability of the allergy model has not been supported by immunologic or challenge tests. No compelling hypotheses have been advanced to separate the nonresponding majority from the minority of children who appear sensitive to artificial food colorings. Testing for sensitivity to specific colorings or a group of chemically related colorings may prove more useful for theory construction and validation.

Some evidence in the experimental animal literature suggests that artificial food colors, particularly erythrosin (FD & C Red #3), are neurotoxins. Silbergeld and Andersen (193) cite effects of diminished habituation to the test environment in rats as a possible indication of hyperactivity or greater distractibility. They propose Na-dependent ATPase, known to be under genetic control, as a site of action for erythrosin B. These investigators, in accordance with their hypothesized genetic basis for neurotoxicity of food dyes, favor clinical research designed to assess the range of responses, including unusual reactions, in selected subgroups of hyperactive children, and the contribution of genetic variability to such responses.

C. Sugar

Sucrose is not recognized as posing a health hazard apart from its contribution to tooth decay [Select Committee on GRAS Substances (SCOGS), 1976]. However, concern on the part of consumer groups about its behavioral toxicity is growing. While the SCOGS committee based its conclusions on available evidence that some individuals consume more than 15% of their calories as sucrose, more recent reports suggest that some 10-year-olds may consume a much greater proportion of their calories as sucrose (Center for Science in the Public Interest, *personal communication*, 1981).

The Center for Science in the Public Interest, a nonprofit, medically oriented, consumer interest group, has expressed concern, based on clinical observations, that dietary sugar may be associated with hyperkinesis and hypoglycemia. They cite a report (119) of abnormal glucose tolerance curves in a majority of hyperactive children, of excessive intakes of refined carbohydrates in hypoglycemic patients, and of alterations in mental and psychological function when glucose levels drop (137). Finally, they point out that many parent advocates of the Feingold diet consciously restrict sugar intake beyond the restrictions inherent in the diet itself and suggest that this may contribute to positive results reported by Feingold association members. Scientific research on the effects of the Feingold diet, however, suggests that the highly positive effects experienced by parents cannot be attributed to the diet itself. Neither is there any compelling evidence of a relationship between blood glucose and behavior in children (with the exception of rare medical conditions). Only one clinical study has appeared in the scientific literature that bears directly on the hypothesized link between sugar and hyperkinesis.

Prinz et al.'s (163) recent correlational study explored the possibility of a link between sugar and hyperactivity. These investigators collected 7-day dietary records on 28 hyperactive children, ages 4 to 7, and 26 matched controls and videotaped their behavior when left alone in a playroom. Destructive and aggressive behaviors, restlessness, and activity as measured by quadrant changes (activity) constituted the behavioral categories measured. Scores from a structured parent interview, the "Cognitive Home Environment Scale," were used in partial correlational analyses.

Hyperactive subjects scored higher on the Werry-Weiss-Peters Activity Scale and showed significantly more quadrant changes and aggressive-destructive behavior than controls. Restlessness did not differentiate these two groups. Hyperactive and control children consumed comparable amounts of sugar and qualitatively similar diets. The major dietary difference seen was quantitative—hyperactive children consumed significantly fewer grams of food per day.

Within the hyperactive group, significant moderate positive correlations were seen between dietary ratios involving sugar and carbohydrate content (ratios of sugar products to "nutritional foods," sugar products plus refined carbohydrates to "nutritional foods," and carbohydrates to protein) and aggressive–destructive behavior. "Nutritional foods" were defined to include most foods and beverages that are neither sugar products nor refined carbohydrates. This included meats, vegetables, fresh fruits, dairy products, and whole-grain breads. Activity *per se* failed to correlate significantly with diet. Within the control group, activity showed significant positive correlations with the above dietary ratios. Partial correlations using socioeconomic status, maternal education level, and the measure of home stimulation did not alter these relationships. The percentage of foods not allowed by the Feingold diet failed to correlate significantly with any behavioral index. Although these correlational relationships do not permit inferences regarding causality, they do provide a basis for pursuing experimental studies.

Diets that are low in protein and high in carbohydrates have been associated with increases in spontaneous activity in rats (32). However, associations between heightened activity and high carbohydrate diets, even if demonstrated in children, are difficult to interpret as carbohydrates affect not only blood sugar levels, but neurotransmitters like serotonin as well (248).

D. Lead

The most important and comprehensive work linking elevated lead levels and and impaired cognitive and behavioral functioning in children is that of Needleman and his colleagues (145–147). Their series of studies using dentine lead levels (which reflect the duration of exposure to lead) suggest small intellectual deficits associated with high lead in the general population, whose exposure may be primarily airborne. Teachers' behavioral ratings became systematically more negative with increasing dentine lead, except for two of 11 items—"disorganized" and "hyperactive"—which failed to differentiate the two most extreme groups. Thus, hyperactivity was not implicated. The threshold for toxicity suggested by this work

(20 μg/g + 0.65 SD) stands far below that suggested by other methodologically sound investigations.

Questions are raised by the failure of these studies to identify other sources of lead exposure and by the failure to covary measures of pica, which correlated with lead level but were unassociated with teacher behavioral ratings. Pica, the eating of nonfood substances (e.g., paint, plaster, dirt, clay, paper), is common in infants and particularly common among iron-deficient and culturally deprived infants. The increased frequency of pica in retarded and disturbed children (11) may result in a greater exposure to lead in such children. Despite these criticisms, Needleman's studies certainly warrant serious attempts at replication.

Rutter (181) has reviewed evidence linking raised lead levels and impaired cognitive and behavioral functioning in children. Among the methodological considerations he discusses are the desirability of serial assessments of blood lead levels or other measures (such as dentine lead) that reflect duration of exposure, or chronicity, and the need to clarify causality in these correlational studies, since lead exposure, like malnutrition, is nonrandomly distributed.

Clinic-type studies, though contradictory, suggest that blood lead levels persistently raised above 60 μg/100 ml are probably associated, on the average, with a 3- to 4-point reduction in IQ, even among asymptomatic children. Greater decrements and behavioral deviations are seen in children suffering lead encephalopathy. Chronic lead levels in the lower range (40 to 60) and acute peaks of 60 and above may also have adverse sequalae, but the evidence here is less conclusive. Studies of mentally retarded and hyperactive children have consistently shown higher than normal lead levels, but the insufficiency of the data regarding pica, the source of exposure to lead, and other background variables preclude inferences about the direction of causality in these correlational studies (181).

Another strategy applied to the question of the behavioral toxicity of lead is to study children living near smelters. Lead exposure in these children is extrinsic to their personal characteristics. However, geographical location can vary with socioeconomic status. Thus, control subjects should be carefully matched for socioeconomic factors. Four of six studies carefully reviewed by Rutter (181) suggest small (1 to 5 IQ points) intellectual deficits associated with raised lead levels in the 40 to 80 μg/100 ml range.

Chelation studies, in which the effects on intelligence and/or behavior of medical interventions to reduce body lead are studied, approximate an experimental paradigm and represent an improvement over correlational methodologies. Rutter (181) has aptly pointed out that the validity of such studies depends on (a) the use of contrasting interventions to ensure that any gains can be specifically attributed to decreased lead levels, rather than nonspecific therapeutic efforts, and (b) the use of control groups or baselines to determine whether alterations in the dependent measures exceed random fluctuations and maturational and experiential effects. While several chelation studies have been reported, their failure to meet these methodological criteria and their small population samples make it impossible to draw conclusions.

E. Phenobarbital

Anticonvulsant drugs, though inadequately studied, have been implicated with respect to behavioral and cognitive toxicity (207). Much of the evidence on their psychological effects (good or bad) is clinical. Relatively few well-controlled studies are available.

Adverse effects may represent toxicity associated with high dosages or blood levels, side effects at therapeutic dosages, or idiosyncratic responses, unrelated to dose or blood levels. Although it is important to classify the complications of these drugs, inadequate information concerning dosage and serum levels makes this impossible in many reports. Many adverse reactions—sedation, confusion, and mood changes—may be nonspecific by drug. Drug-specific reactions are encountered occasionally, however, perhaps the best example being the irritability, depression, and hyperactivity encountered in children treated with barbiturates (207).

Wolf et al. (244) noted side effects of irritability, lethargy, and particularly hyperactivity in a substantial percentage of child patients receiving phenobarbital and noted a resumption of normal behavior when the drug was discontinued. Wolf and Forsythe (245) found, in an uncontrolled study, that approximately 40% of over 100 children treated with phenobarbital following a first febrile seizure developed a behavioral disturbance, usually hyperactivity, compared with 18% of those not treated with medication. Behavioral symptoms improved with the discontinuance of phenobarbital in 100% of the treated children as compared with 52% of the untreated children. These behavioral disturbances failed to correlate with blood drug levels or with other characteristics of the child. Nonblind parental reports constituted the dependent "measure." No behavioral rating scales, teacher reports, or placebo controls were used, however, thus restricting the confidence that can be placed in these findings. Conners et al. (49) have reported that disturbed and, particularly, hyperactive children may be more likely to suffer adverse effects.

High blood levels of phenobarbital (above 60 μg/ml) result in confusional states, neurological signs, and clear intellectual deterioration (207). Clinical studies at lower doses have provided some conflicting evidence with respect to adverse effects on intellectual performance (31,212,218). Trimble (213), however, after reviewing the limited literature on the cognitive effects of phenobarbital, concludes that the drug does appear to have adverse effects, as evidenced by declining intelligence scores over time. The dosage at which this occurs was not specified.

Studies with humans using laboratory tests show adverse effects more consistently (207). Stores (207) sees the somewhat discrepant findings between clinical and laboratory studies as consistent with other pediatric psychopharmacological findings and questions the validity of laboratory tests for naturalistic situations. He recommends that studies of the behavioral and cognitive effects of anticonvulsants take into account the type of epilepsy (including EEG pattern), sex, and age. All have been shown to interact with anticonvulsants in affecting behavior and learning (207). Intellectual level and the presence of gross structural brain pathology (58,131) also need to be considered in study design. Social environmental circumstances, too, should be studied for their contributions to drug effects.

V. MALNUTRITION

A. Early Findings and Issues

The bulk of the research on malnutrition consists of retrospective naturalistic field studies in underdeveloped countries that stand in sharp contrast with the experimental studies discussed elsewhere in this chapter. This literature is so broad and the methodological problems associated with it so diverse as to preclude truly adequate coverage. Only some of the major methodological considerations will be outlined here.

Several good reviews of research on the cognitive and behavioral consequences of malnutrition are available. Studies of the behavioral and cognitive effects of protein-calorie malnutrition have been comprehensively reviewed by Pollitt and Thomson (160), Lloyd-Still (130), Hurwitz (109), Brozek (21), and Winick (243). Brozek (22) lists and indexes special conferences that have helped bring together the widely scattered world literature on this topic. Leibel et al. (121) and Pollitt and Leibel (157) have reviewed the behavioral and cognitive effects of iron deficiency. Pollitt et al. (156) have reviewed the literature pertaining to the effects of eating breakfast versus brief morning fasting on school children.

1. Classifications of Malnutrition

Malnutrition is a broad category, which is best subdivided for research and discussion purposes. Primary malnutrition, attributable to inadequate food intake, may be contrasted with malnutrition that is secondary to disorders such as cystic fibrosis, pyloric stenosis, and other gastrointestinal disturbances that interfere with the digestion and absorption of nutrients. General deficiencies of protein and/or calories (protein-calorie malnutrition) may also be contrasted with specific nutritional deficiencies, such as iron or vitamin deficiencies.

Severe protein-calorie malnutrition takes two forms—marasmus and kwashiorkor. Marasmus results from insufficient intake of both proteins and calories, generally affects infants under 1 year of age, and is characterized by marked growth failure, severe muscle wasting, loss of subcutaneous fat, wizened facial features, and a protuberant abdomen. Kwashiorkor results from starchy diets inadequate in proteins, generally occurs later (from 1 to 3 years of age), and is more likely to be acute than chronic. Muscle wasting, edema, palpable liver enlargement with fatty infiltration and tissue damage, depigmentation of the skin, and dermatosis are characteristic. Serum protein levels are depressed in kwashiorkor, while nearly normal in marasmus (150). These two conditions are actually continuous rather than discrete and thus the term "marasmic-kwashiorkor" is sometimes used for clinical states falling between the extremes.

2. Cognitive and Behavioral Findings Associated with Protein-Calorie Malnutrition

Clinical symptoms associated with general malnutrition are well documented and include lethargy, apathy, irritability, deficient environmental exploration, and emotional lability. While there is general agreement that early protein-calorie malnutrition is associated with cognitive and behavioral deficits, at least up to school age, close associations between malnutrition and several nonnutritional factors complicate interpretation of this relationship. Possible confounding factors include poverty, poor housing and sanitation, frequent illnesses and infections, general poor health, inadequate prenatal care, ignorance that contributes to the ineffective use of resources, and nonsupportive and nonstimulating environments for cognitive development. Where socioeconomic and other environmental conditions are more favorable, effects of malnutrition appear to be minimal or nonexistent (243). With increasing age (school age and up) and socioeconomic status, differences between malnourished children and controls are seen less consistently (130).

3. Types of Variables that Require Study

This apparent interaction between environment and early nutritional insult is consistent with findings that environment plays an important role in determining the outcome of infants whose prenatal and birth histories place them at risk for learning and cognitive deficits (12). Low scores on infant developmental scales are more likely to lead to poor intellectual performances at later ages in the context of low socioeconomic status (229,240).

Observed associations between disadvantaged environments, poorer health, malnutrition, and cognitive and behavioral deficits necessitate that several elements be addressed and measured. Health and developmental status *prior* to malnutrition (e.g., prenatal history, differences in gestational age and birth weights) is especially relevant when young children or infants are being studied. Nutritional status (the quality, severity, and duration of malnutrition) should preferably be assessed directly rather than inferred from anthropometric indices alone. Physical and social environments should be assessed, since differences in stability, living conditions, economic disadvantage, maternal education, and literacy are seen between families with and without severely malnourished children, even within the same general community and social class (177). Finally, cognitive and behavioral status need to be assessed using measures of demonstrated validity for the culture being examined.

4. Measuring Nutritional Status

Nutritional status may be assessed through dietary surveys, biochemical tests, clinical signs of malnutrition, and anthropometric indices. Lloyd-Still (130) lists the biochemical measures that may be useful in certain types of malnutrition. Retrospective studies should ideally obtain this sort of information from medical records.

This ideal is often unattainable, however. Many retrospective studies infer past nutritional status from anthropometric measures in the absence of early records. The use of anthropometric age norms is not infrequently precluded by unknown and indeterminable birthdates when children in developing countries are studied (191).

Height is heavily influenced by the duration of malnutrition, whereas weight is more sensitive to current nutritional status and the severity of past undernutrition (130).

Head circumference is, in general, a good indirect indicator of brain weight (210), although ventricular dilatation and atrophy may distort this measure (142,217). Compensatory, "catch-up" growth may also contribute to error in the absence of serial measures (203).

5. Measuring and Controlling Social–Environmental Variables

a. Environmental scales

The relationship between social class background and other social-environmental variables (e.g, urban–rural status, birth order, family size, maternal education and intelligence) and measured intelligence is well documented and widely recognized. Richardson's (177) finding of social–environmental discriminators of families with and without malnourished children within the same community and social class level suggests that some direct assessment of environmental quality is desirable. However, instruments for assessing environmental variations, beyond indices of socioeconomic class, are quite limited. One example of such a measure is Caldwell's (26) home observation scale, designed to capture everyday variations in the young child's environment. The items were designed to reflect the frequency and stability of adult contact, degree of developmental and vocal stimulation, restrictions on motor and exploratory behavior, emotional climate, availability of play material, and parental concern with achievement. Cravioto and DeLicardie (56) found that this scale discriminated the environments of malnourished Mexican children, ages 6 months to 3 years, and their nonmalnourished controls.

b. Sibling control subjects

The limited availability and added work involved in the use of such scales would seem to make siblings of malnourished children attractive as controls. While potentially useful in controlling many problematic variables, some limitations and complicating factors should be considered. Index children and their siblings may differ in important ways, including age, sex, paternity, and experience with hospitalization. The higher frequency of many developmental and learning problems in boys argues for taking sex into account when using sibling controls. Prolonged hospitalization may interfere with attachment behavior (17) and reduce active interaction with the environment. The duration of hospitalization may interact with age and the severity of malnutrition, variables that have been related to the magnitude of the effects of malnutrition (57). In addition, there is considerable evidence to suggest that in studies of primary malnutrition siblings may often be subclinically malnourished (130,243). If large differences in nutritional status are seen among siblings, the question of selective parental neglect becomes relevant. The most reasonable practice may be the inclusion of both a sibling group and another matched-control group.

6. *Assessing Cognition and Behavior*

a. *Test validity and culture*

The reliance on cognitive measures borrowed from Western industrialized nations and minimally adapted for use in underdeveloped countries constitutes a major weakness of naturalistic studies in this area. Validity requires that the sample on which a test is developed be representative of the population in which the test is to be used for drawing inferences (3). Translation of test content or instructions, the collection of normative data, and the use of nonverbal measures or tests of specific cognitive functions or processes assumed to be biologically based and universal (e.g., memory, attention, perception) (13,19,56) have all been used to adapt tests for use in other cultures. All of these approaches are inadequate as substitutes for demonstrated validity. Cross-cultural research has shown considerable variation in specific areas of sensorimotor and cognitive development, as early as infancy, which fail to correspond to any simple concept of degree of advancement or industrialization (122).

Three approaches appropriately used to assess cultural fairness or test bias include: (a) item analysis, (b) examination of practice effects, and (c) statistical tests of differential validity. Item wording and content can be examined to judge whether different groups may have varying exposure to specific content or may interpret their meanings differently because of variations in dialect. Items or tasks that are shown to be heavily affected by practice may be expected to lack validity as indicators of general cognitive ability. However, the ultimate test of bias rests with empirical measures of differential validity. A measure is equally valid for two groups if, regardless of whether or not the normative distributions are similar, it predicts some criterion performance with equal accuracy. Conversely, a test is biased if, despite equal score distributions for two groups, it predicts performance on some criterion with differential accuracy.

The identification of appropriate criterion measures against which to validate cognitive measures may present special problems in developing countries. American intelligence tests have been designed to predict academic achievement and are more limited in their capacity to predict occupational success and nonacademic skills (188). Free mandatory public elementary- and secondary-level education, an open, socially mobile society, and direct links between literacy, academic learning, educational credentials, and job requirements all lend validity to the use of academic achievement as an appropriate criterion variable. However, the lack of free and mandatory public education, restrictions on mobility imposed by caste, and a generally diminished role of academic learning and formal education all constitute factors that negate the appropriateness of academic achievement as a criterion measure. An appropriate criterion should reflect achievements that require adaptive abilities within the culture and that are relatively open to all of its members.

The cross-cultural literature suggests several major strategies for assessing cognitive development in other countries (122). One might take the psychometric approach of selecting a variety of measures of diverse cognitive abilities that are well researched and understood in terms of their correlations with independent measures. The measures might then be applied to a new culture on the premise that response biases contributed by each would help cancel each other out and achieve convergent validation. Intercorrelations among measures could be examined and compared with those in the original culture. Alternatively, a theoretically based approach such as that of Bruner (23), which assumes invariant stages of cognitive development, might be used to examine rates of development. A third approach, described by Gay and Cole (83), would start by examining descriptions of cognition within the culture, e.g., conventional modes of thought used by adults for adaptation, ways in which logical relationships are expressed, ways that children acquire knowledge and conventional cognitive patterns, and the nature of education. Research instruments would then be designed to tap differences in cognitive functioning suggested by such descriptions. These would be administered to adults and children for the purpose of making age comparisons with which to assess the direction and rate of cognitive development over time within the culture.

One illustration of an attempt to attain cultural validation of cognitive tests is provided by Klein et al. (117), who explored indigenous concepts of intelligence and their correspondence with the preschool psychological tests that they were using. These investigators interviewed adults about their concepts of intelligence, examining how they talked about intelligence, the words used, and the behavioral characteristics attributed to smart children (rapidity of movement, good memory, and independence). The adults interviewed demonstrated a high level of agreement in their judgments of the relative smartness of ten 7-year-old boys. These highly reliable judgments showed significant correlations with tests of embedded figures, verbal analogies, and memory for designs. A vocabulary measure failed to correlate with the adults' judgments of intelligence. Thus, a number of the tests used were linked to the culture's concept of intelligence, while at least one was shown to be unrelated to this concept.

b. Nonintellectual influences on performance

Insuring cooperation and maximal performance may be difficult when testing young children whose behavior is often influenced by their physiological states (hunger, fatigue, illness). Older children may be influenced by varying social expectations in cultures where testing does not constitute a part of the child's normal experience. A general lack of familiarity with active problem-solving tasks, in which the child is expected to develop or create his or her own answer, may exist where schools emphasize rote learning. Expectations regarding compliance may vary with sex in certain cultures and thereby differentially influence subgroups of children. Practice or warm-up sessions may help alleviate such problems (122).

Malnutrition may adversely affect sustained attention and active exploration, factors that may affect performance on cognitive measures (120). Graves (93,94) used direct behavioral observations to study attachment and exploration in malnourished infants, ages 7 to 18 months. Malnourished infants manipulated toys less and initiated less interaction with their mothers than did their well-nourished age-

and sex-matched controls. Lasky and Klein (1980) examined visual preferences for novel stimuli in malnourished infants, 5 to 7 months of age. Following a 60-sec display of a photograph of a human face, test stimuli—the familiar photograph and a novel photograph of a face—were presented simultaneously for 10 sec. The time each infant visually fixated on each photograph was measured. The malnourished infants showed no preference for the novel face. These results contrasted with the novelty preferences displayed by well-nourished infants of the same age and from the same community. A second study directly compared 32 malnourished and 32 well-nourished infants, 5 to 7 months of age, using the same task. However, one additional calculation was made—that of a cumulative fixation time for the initial exposure to the standard stimulus, the familiar face. This initial fixation time determined the exposure; both groups were required to actually look at the stimulus for a total of 30 sec prior to the testing for novelty preference. When malnourished infants actually attended to the face for the same amount of time as the well-nourished infants, they, too, showed a preference for the novel face. The malnourished infants fixated on the standard stimulus for a lower proportion of time (p < 0.06) than did the well-nourished controls, suggesting greater differences in active orientation to and attention to stimuli than in later stages of cognitive processing. Care should be taken to design test procedures capable of providing some assessment of attentional processes that can be used to examine and interpret results on cognitive measures. Apparent improvements in intellectual status over time may actually reflect improvements in attention.

7. Mechanism of Action

In addition to focusing on outcomes, attention might also be directed toward the mechanisms through which malnutrition exerts its effects and toward the process of recovery. Winick (243) has discussed the difficulty of altering nutrition without affecting environment and other variables in animal studies. He proposes that decrements in learning or performance in malnourished rats may be attributed to decreased exploration and heightened emotionality. When fed a low-protein diet, nonhuman primates show a decrease in play, sexual behavior, curiosity, and puzzle solving and increased aggression, effects that reverse with the introduction of food rewards. Thus, many of the changes seen might be interpreted as motivational and attentional in nature. However, delays in reflex development and physical development (e.g., eye opening, incisor eruption) seen in malnourished animals may also restrict their interactions with the environment and their opportunities for learning.

Early environmental isolation alone may result in behavioral and biological effects similar to those seen with malnutrition. Isolation can decrease cell division, myelination, and dendritic proliferation in rats. Enriched environmental stimulation is capable of reversing some of these biological effects in rats (243). Thus, malnutrition may achieve its ultimate effects on the brain and on behavior by altering the organism's interaction with the environment. The task of separating the effects of malnutrition from those of environment may prove impossible. A focus on their interactive influences may provide a meaningful direction for future research.

B. Recent Studies of Restricted Nutritional Deficiencies

1. Breakfast

Pollitt and his colleagues (156) have reviewed the limited literature pertaining to effects of morning feedings on emotional, cognitive, and physical components of behavior of school children. The morning feedings studied have ranged from mid-morning feedings of milk or orange juice to various breakfasts, such as cereal and milk or bacon and eggs. Although these studies have not yielded a uniform set of results, they have found some indications that short-term hunger from skipping breakfast may have some adverse effects on emotional behavior, arithmetic and reading ability, and physical work output. Studies of long-term effects of school lunch and breakfast programs have focused on a more uniform set of dependent measures—school grades, achievement, and attendance—but these too have failed to yield a uniform set of results. Inferences are severely limited by the failure to monitor many important moderating variables (prior nutritional status, degree of participation in feeding programs, food intakes on the day of achievement testing, teacher expectations) and other methodological weaknesses. Also, the effects of breakfasts with differing nutrient contents (e.g, high in protein versus high in carbohydrates) have not been compared systematically, as would be desirable.

Pollitt et al. (159) recently studied the effects of skipping breakfast on problem solving in 9–11-year-old, well-nourished children. They hypothesized that behavioral effects of fasting were more likely to be detectable in children as compared with adults, because of greater metabolic stress induced by the child's higher metabolic rates per unit of brain weight, and limited availability of glucogenic amino acids for hepatic gluconeogenesis. Two groups of children and two treatment orders of breakfast versus no breakfast were used. Breakfast consisted of waffles and syrup, margarine, orange juice, and milk (total calories = 535 kcal; 15 g protein, 20 g fat, and 75 g carbohydrate). Blood samples were taken the evening before and the morning of treatment (breakfast or no breakfast) and cognitive testing and assayed for D-(−)-3-hydroxybutyrate, L-(+)-lactate, and glucose. Free fatty acid determinations were made. Cognitive tests included the Peabody Picture Vocabulary Test, Matching Familiar Figures Test, CPT, and Hagen Central-Incidental Task (HCI) and were administered at 11:00 a.m.

Significant changes in β-hydroxybutyrate and glucose, but not in lactate, were seen in the no breakfast condition. Noon values for β-hydroxybutyrate, lactate, and free fatty acids, but not glucose, differed significantly between breakfast and no breakfast conditions. Because of the lack of differences in blood glucose between conditions, the authors analyzed breakfast–no breakfast difference scores as a function of changes in glucose level. Subjects with large changes in glucose showed greater increases in MFF errors when skipping breakfast. CPT and HCI memory test failed to show effects. Because of significant moderate correlations between PPVT and MFF scores, the authors also used PPVT scores as an independent variable in examining MFF performance. Subjects who fell below the median on the PPVT performed significantly better under the breakfast as compared with no breakfast condition. The authors interpreted these subtle findings as evidence that brief fasting induces changes in arousal that influence cognitive function.

2. Iron

Pollitt and Leibel (157) have reviewed research pertaining to the effects of iron deficiency on human behavior. They discuss compensatory mechanisms that come into play to preserve tissue oxygenation when threatened by decreasing hemoglobin levels and point out the failure of the majority of studies to control properly for the effects of these mechanisms in evaluating behavioral correlates specific to various types of anemia.

Clinical reports focus on subjective complaints of fatigue, weakness and impaired concentration, and irritability and anorexia in children. Pagophagia (pathological craving for ice) is associated with iron deficiency, though not necessarily with anemia. Other symptoms may also result from metabolic correlates other than anemia.

Reports of studies with children, most of which are published in proceedings of conferences, provide information that is insufficient for evaluating methodologic rigor. In reviewing the more detailed available reports (106,209,220), Pollitt and Leibel conclude that inferences about the effects of iron deficiency on cognitive performance are precluded by *ex post facto* designs that failed to take prior environment into account. Evidence suggests that there are socioeconomic correlates of iron deficiency (114). One longitudinal study of infants suffering from iron deficiency anemia, which controlled for social class (29), reported a greater incidence of soft neurological signs such as clumsiness, poorer attentiveness and more hyperactivity in index children, compared with controls, ages 6 to 7, and possible small differences in IQ, although it was unclear whether these differences were statistically significant.

More recently, Pollitt et al. (158) reported reversible changes in cognitive performance in mildly iron-deficient 3- to 6-year-olds in Cambridge, Massachusetts. These children and a group of matched controls were tested on three discrimination learning tasks prior to and following the index group's return to a normal iron status. Results suggested that impairments were confined to the reception of information (attentional processes) rather than internal processing or retrieval of information.

Following this, Pollitt and his associates (161) applied this paradigm to children with severe iron deficiency anemia and matched control subjects (mean age, 4 years) in Guatemala. Children were tested with a similar battery of discrimination and oddity learning tasks, whose stimuli were altered to fit the local culture. Similar distributions of test scores characterized the Guatemalan and American samples in pilot work. However, only the oddity learning task showed significant group differences. A wide range of performances and overlap between groups were seen on the discrimination learning tasks. Following 4 months of iron treatment, group differences in biochemical and hematological determinations and on the oddity learning task disappeared. The authors tentatively concluded that iron deficiency impairs attention, though not necessarily in a linear fashion relating to severity of the deficiency.

3. Chloride

The physiologic importance of chloride and metabolic consequences of chloride deficiency (metabolic alkalosis, potassium depletion) are reviewed and discussed by Simopoulos and Bartter (194). This essential nutrient is present in such a wide variety of foods that its deficiency is seldom encountered in healthy individuals. Individuals placed on low-sodium diets because of heart, kidney, or liver disease may, however, require an alternative source of chloride.

Healthy infants have become increasingly dependent on a single food source—formula—for their nutrition. In past years, infants more often received baby food early in life and, these commercial baby foods contained considerable sodium (128). However, solid foods now contain less salt (72) and are introduced later in infancy (80), increasing the risk of chloride deficiency.

A number of cases of a "Bartter-like" syndrome were reported to the Center for Disease Control in 1979, which surveyed the country in its case-finding efforts. Bartter's syndrome is a rare disorder with hypokalemia that severely and irreversibly retards growth and may impair mental development (84). Hypochloremia in Bartter's syndrome is associated with high urinary chloride excretion, a finding not characteristic of these infants (180). The feeding history of the high number of identified cases implicated Neo-Mull-Soy formula, one of a number of soy formulas frequently prescribed for infants allergic to breast or cow's milk. Further investigative efforts suggested that this formula became chloride deficient, unknown to its producers, sometime between October of 1978 and 1979.

A number of infants were fed this deficient formula for 2 to 7 months prior to diagnosis. Most were diagnosed under 7 months of age. A large number suffered metabolic alkalosis and symptoms of lethargy, anorexia, vomiting, diarrhea, hematuria, and growth failure, which reversed with dietary changes (128,180). Preliminary growth data on these infants suggests significant effects on weight and head circumference and a lesser effect on height, which may be only partially reversible (180). Preliminary studies of effects on cognitive and motor development have yielded conflicting results, possibly due to small population samples, variations in assessment techniques and methodology, and numerous potential confounding variables. However, there is some suggestion of adverse effects, particularly on cognitive development, related to the length of time on the formula and age at which infants began this diet (H. Moss, *personal communication*, 1981).

Additional study of these infants and children has been mandated by Congress. Potentially confounding variables include the difficulty of ascertaining the onset and duration of chloride deficient feedings, the complications of neonatal risk factors, the question of whether some associated predisposition toward abnormal renal function was necessary to the development of metabolic alkalosis, possible geographic factors (a higher incidence of allergy in certain regions), problems in measuring cognitive development in the infancy period, and environmental factors, such as the stress experienced by mothers of these infants. In addition, the publicity associated with the formula's deficiency had a substantial impact and appears to have resulted in considerable developmental intervention (infant stimulation programs), which further complicates design needs.

VI. CONCLUSIONS

Methodologies for examining therapeutic effects of nutrients and other food constituents are perhaps better developed than those for identifying toxic effects. The relatively subtle nature of findings in toxicity or malnutrition studies—where exposure is limited to low dosages, limited insults, or brief periods of time—will require thoughtfully designed, well-controlled studies and sensitive measures. Among the measures reviewed, behavioral rating scales, certain laboratory vigilance and learning tasks, and tests with attentional and efficiency components appear to offer considerable promise for studies of toxicity. Psychological tests or other measures with built-in stability will generally prove more useful in studies of longer-term or more chronic effects. Other measures may become more useful when employed in intervention paradigms designed to provide greater control and sensitivity. New instruments may be needed to measure effectively symptoms like apathy, irritability, and decreased initiative.

Developmental aspects of behavioral expression and cognitive growth need to be carefully assessed. Deficits associated with toxicity or malnutrition may be differentially expressed with age; thus a comparison of effects across various age groups of identical or similar measures may disclose different processes across ages. The difficulty level of a task represents one obvious variable that may vary with age. Given the evidence that arousal, which interacts with cognitive complexity, may contribute to test results, future investigations might systematically vary difficulty or complexity within a task when comparing different age groups. Differential validity of intellectual measures as indicators of cerebral dysfunction is another example of this problem. Both short-term and long-term studies will be needed to assess possible cumulative effects, as well as the reversibility of effects or recovery.

The clarification of causal relationships will require attention to social–environmental variables that invariably influence children's behavior and cognitive development. Identifying sources of toxicity, controlling for subject and other environmental characteristics, and consistent dose–response relationships will add validity to claims of causality. Intervention studies that attempt to reverse adverse effects may also clarify causal relationships and provide more sensitive paradigms for studying therapeutic effects.

REFERENCES

1. Abikoff, H., Gittelman-Klein, R., and Klein, D. (1977): Validation of a classroom observation code for hyperactive children. *J. Clin. Consult. Psychol.*, 45:772–783.
2. Aman, M. G. (1980): Psychotropic drugs and learning problems: A selective review. *J. Learn. Disabil.*, 13:36–46.
3. American Psychological Association (1974): *Standards for Educational and Psychological Tests*. Washington, D.C.
4. American Psychiatric Association (1980): *Diagnostic and Statistical Manual of Mental Disorders*, 3rd edition. Washington, D.C.
5. Anastasi, A. (1976): *Psychological Testing*, 4th edition. Macmillan, New York.
6. Arnold, L. E., Christopher, J., Huestis, R., and Smeltzer, D. J. (1978): Methylphenidate vs. dextroamphetamine vs. caffeine in minimal brain dysfunction. *Arch. Gen. Psychiatry*, 35:463–475.
7. Baker, W. J., and Theologus, G. C. (1972): Effects of caffeine on visual monitoring. *J. Appl. Psychol.*, 56(5):422–427.
8. Barkley, R. A. (1977): A review of stimulant drug research with hyperactive children. *J. Child Psychol. Psychiatry*, 18:137–165.
9. Barkley, R., and Cunningham, C. (1978): Do stimulant drugs improve the academic performance of hyperkinetic children? A review of outcome research. *Clin. Pediatr.*, 17(17):85–92.
10. Barkley, R., and Ullman, D. (1975): A comparison of objective measures of activity and distractibility in hyperkinetic and non-hyperkinetic children. *J. Abnorm. Child Psychol.*, 3:231–244.
11. Bicknell, D. J. (1975): Pica: A childhood syndrome. IRMMH Monograph No. 3. Butterworths, London.
12. Birch, H. G., and Gussow, J. D. (1970): *Disadvantaged Children: Health, Nutrition and School Failure*. Harcourt, Brace & World, New York.
13. Birch, H. G., and Lefford, G. A. (1963): Intersensory development in children. *Monogr. Res. Child Dev.*, 28(5):1–48.
14. Boll, T. J. (1978): Diagnosing brain impairment. In: *Clinical Diagnosis of Mental Disorders: A Handbook*, edited by B. Wolman. Plenum Press, New York.
15. Boll, T. J. (1981): The Halstead-Reitan Neuropsychological Battery. In: *Handbook of Clinical Neuropsychology*, edited by S. B. Filskov and T. J. Boll. John Wiley, New York.
16. Boll, T. J., and Barth, J. T. (1981): Neuropsychology of brain damage in children. In: *Handbook of Clinical Neuropsychology*, edited by S. B. Filskov and T. J. Boll. John Wiley, New York.
17. Bowlby, J. (1960): Separation anxiety. *Int. J. Psychoanal.*, 41:89–113.
18. Brenner, A. (1977): A study of the efficacy of the Feingold diet on hyperkinetic children. *Clin. Res.*, 16(7):652–656.
19. Brockman, L., and Riccuiti, H. (1971): Severe protein-calorie malnutrition and cognitive development in infancy and early childhood. *Dev. Psychol.*, 4:312–319.
20. Brown, A. L. (1979): Theories of memory and the problems of development: Activity, growth, and knowledge. In: *Levels of Processing and Memory*, edited by F. D. Craik and L. Cermak. Lawrence Frelbaum Association, Hillsdale, New York.
21. Brozek, J. (1978): Nutrition, malnutrition and behavior. *Annu. Rev. Psychol.*, 29:157–177.
22. Brozek, J. (1978): Malnutrition and behavior. *J. Am. Diet. Assoc.*, 72(1):17–23.
23. Bruner, J. S., Oliver, R. R., and Greenfield, P. (1966): *Studies in Cognitive Growth*. John Wiley, New York.
24. Buros, O. K. (Ed.) (1978): *The Eighth Mental Measurements Yearbook*. Gryphon Press, Highland Park, New Jersey.
25. Butters, N. (1979): Amnesic disorders. In: *Clinical Neuropsychology*, edited by K. M. Heilman and F. Valenstein. Oxford University Press, New York.
26. Caldwell, B. M. (1974): The malnourishing environment. In: *Proceedings of the Symposia of the Swedish Nutrition Foundation: XII. Early Malnutrition and Mental Development*, edited by J. Cravioto, L. Hambraeus, and B. Vahlquist. Almquist & Wiksell, Uppsala, Sweden.
27. Campbell, M., Anderson, L. T., Cohen, I. L., Perry, R., Small, A. M., et al. (1982): Haloperidol in autistic children: Effects on learning, behavior and abnormal involuntary movements. Paper presented at the NIMH-NCDEU Annual Meeting, Key Biscayne, Florida, May 25–28, 1981. *Psychopharmacol.*, 18(No. 1):110–111.
28. Campbell, C., Reichard, C., and Eldes, S. T. (1977): Effects of caffeine on reaction time in hyperkinetic and normal children. *Am. J. Psychiatry*, 134(2):144–148.

29. Cantwell, R. J. (1974): The long-term neurological sequelae of anemia in infancy. *Pediatr. Res.*, 8:342.
30. Castenada, A., McCandless, B. R., and Palermo, D. S. (1956): The children's form of the manifest anxiety scale. *Child Dev.*, 27:317–326.
31. Chaundry, M., and Pond, D. (1961): Mental deterioration in epileptic children. *J. Neurol. Neurosurg. Psychiatry*, 24:213–219.
32. Chiel, H. J., and Wurtman, R. J. (1981): Short-term variations in diet composition change the pattern of spontaneous motor activity in rats. *Science*, 213:676–678.
33. Clubley, M., Bye, C. E., Henson, T. A., et al. (1979): Effects of caffeine and cyclizine alone and in combination on human performance, subjective effects and EEG activity. *Br. J. Clin. Pharmacol.*, 7(2):157–163.
34. Colburn, T., Smith, B. M., Guarini, J., et al. (1976): An ambulatory activity monitor with solid-state memory. *ISA Trans.*, 14:149–154.
35. Coleman, J. S., Campbell, E. Q., Hobson, C. J., et al. (1966): *Equality of Educational Opportunity.* Government Printing Office, Washington, D.C. (Superintendent of Documents, Catalog No. FS 5.238:38001).
36. Conners, C. K. (1969): A teacher rating scale for use in drug studies with children. *Am. J. Psychiatry*, 126(6):884–888.
37. Conners, C. K. (1970): Symptom patterns in hyperkinetic, neurotic and normal children. *Child Dev.*, 41:667–682.
38. Conners, C. K. (1970): Stimulant drugs and cortical evoked responses in learning and behavior disorders in children. In: *Drugs, Development, and Cerebral Function*, edited by W. L. Smith. Charles C Thomas, Springfield.
39. Conners, C. K. (1971): Recent drug studies with hyperkinetic children. *J. Learn. Disabil.*, 4:478–483.
40. Conners, C. K. (1972): Psychological effects of stimulant drugs in children with minimal brain dysfunction. *Pediatrics*, 49:702–708.
41. Conners, C. K. (1973): Rating scales for use in drug studies with children. Special Issue: *Pharmacotherapy with Children. Psychopharmacol. Bull.* 24–83.
42. Conners, C. K. (1975): A placebo crossover study of caffeine treatment of hyperkinetic children. *Int. J. Ment. Health*, 4:132–143.
43. Conners, C. K. (1977): Methodological considerations in drug research with children. In: *Psychopharmacology in Childhood and Adolescence*, edited by J. M. Wiener. Basic Books, New York.
44. Conners, C. K. (1979): Global rating scales for childhood psychopharmacology. In: *Guidelines for the Clinical Evaluation of Psychoactive Drugs in Infants and Children.* Food and Drug Administration, DHEW, Rockville, Maryland.
45. Conners, C. K. (1979): The acute effects of caffeine on evoked response, vigilance, and activity level in hyperkinetic children. *J. Abnorm. Child Psychol.*, 7(2):145–151.
46. Conners, C. K. (1980): *Food Additives and Hyperactive Children.* Plenum Press, New York.
47. Conners, C. K., and Eisenberg, L. (1963): The effects of methylphenidate on symptomatology and learning in disturbed children. *Am. J. Psychiatry*, 120:458–464.
48. Conners, C. K., Eisenberg, L., and Sharpe, L. (1963): Effects of methylphenidate (Ritalin) on paired-associate learning and Porteus maze performance in emotionally disturbed children. *J. Consult. Psychol.*, 28:14–22.
49. Conners, C. K., Eisenberg, L., and Sharpe, L. (1965): A controlled study of the differential application of outpatient psychiatric treatment for children. *Jpn. J. Child Psychiatry*, 6:125–132.
49a. Conners, C. K., Goyette, C. H., and Newman, E. B. (1980): Dose-time effect of artificial colors in hyperactive children. *J. Learn. Disabil.*, 13(9):512–516.
50. Conners, C. K., Goyette, C. H., Southwick, D. A., et al. (1976): Food additives and hyperkinesis: A controlled double blind experiment. *Pediatrics*, 58(2):154–166.
51. Conners, C. K., and Rothschild, G. (1968): Drugs and learning in children. In: *Learning Disorders, Vol. 3*, edited by J. Hellmuth, pp. 191–223. Special Child Publications, Seattle.
52. Conners, C. K., and Werry, J. S. (1979): Pharmacotherapy. In: *Psychopathological Disorders in Childhood*, edited by H. C. Quay and J. S. Werry. John Wiley & Sons, New York.
53. Cook, P. S., and Woodhill, J. M. (1976): The Feingold dietary treatment of the hyperkinetic syndrome. *Med. J. Aust.*, 2(3):85–90.

54. Crandall, V. C., Katkovsky, W., and Crandall, V. J. (1965): Children's beliefs in their control of reinforcements in intellectual-academic achievement situations. *Child Dev.*, 36:91–109.
55. Crandall, V. C., Katkovsky, W., and Preston, A. (1962): Motivational and ability determinants of young children's intellectual and achievement behaviors. *Child Dev.*, 33:643–661.
56. Cravioto, J., and DeLicardie, E. (1972): Environmental correlates of severe clinical malnutrition and language development in survivors from kwashiorkor or marasmus. In: *Nutrition, the Nervous System, and Behavior.* Pan American Health Organization, Washington, D.C.
57. Cravioto, J., and Robles, B. (1965): Evolution of adaptive and motor behaviour during rehabilitation from kwashiorkor. *Am. J. Orthopsychiatry*, 35:449–464.
58. Dalby, M. (1971): Antiepileptic and psychotropic effects of carbamazepine (Tegretol) in the treatment of psychomotor epilepsy. *Epilepsia*, 12:325–334.
59. Damarin, F. (1978): Bayley Scales of Infant Development. In: *Mental Measurements Yearbook*, edited by O. K. Buros. Gryphon Press, Highland Park, New Jersey.
60. Davids, A. (1971): An objective instrument for assessing hyperkinesis in children. *J. Learn. Disabil.*, 4:499–501.
61. Denckla, M. B. (1979): Childhood learning disabilities. In: *Clinical Neuropsychology*, edited by K. M. Heilman. Oxford University Press, New York.
62. Dobbing, J., and Sands, J. (1971): Vulnerability of developing brain. IX. The effect of nutritional growth retardation on the timing of the brain growth spurt. *Biol. Neonate*, 19:363–378.
63. Dobbing, J., and Sands, J. (1973): Quantitative growth and development of human brain. *Arch. Dis. Child.*, 48:757–767.
64. Doke, L. A. (1976): Assessment of children's behavioral deficits. In: *Behavioral Assessment*, edited by M. Hersen and A. S. Bellack. Pergamon Press, New York.
65. Douglas, V. I. (1972): Stop, look and listen: The problem of sustained attention and impulse control in hyperactive and normal children. *Can. J. Behav. Sci.*, 4:259–282.
66. Douglas, V. (1974): Differences between normal and hyperkinetic children. In: *Clinical Use of Stimulant Drugs in Children*, edited by C. Conners. Excerpta Medica, Amsterdam.
67. Dunn, L. M. (1970): *Peabody Individual Achievement Test.* American Guidance Service, Circle Pines, Minnesota.
68. Eisenberg, L., Gilbert, A., Cytryn, L., and Molling, P. A. (1976): The effectiveness of psychotherapy alone and in conjunction with perphenazine or placebo in the treatment of neurotic and hyperkinetic children. *Am. J. Psychiatry*, 117:1088–1093.
69. Elkins, R. N., Rapoport, J. L., Zahn, T. P., Buchsbaum, M. S., et al. (1981): Acute effects of caffeine in normal prepubertal boys. *Am. J. Psychiatry*, 138(2):178–183.
70. Feingold, B. F. (1975): *Why Your Child is Hyperactive.* Random House, New York.
71. Feingold, B. F. (1976): Hyperkinesis and learning disabilities linked to the ingestion of artificial food colors and flavors. *J. Learn. Disabil.*, 9:551–559.
72. Filer, L. (1971): Salt in infant foods. *Nutr. Rev.*, 29:27–30.
73. Filskov, S. B., and Leli, D. A. (1981): Assessment of the individual in neuropsychological practice. In: *Handbook of Clinical Neuropsychology*, edited by S. B. Fikskov and T. J. Boll. John Wiley, New York.
74. Finch, A. J., and Kendall, P. C. (1979): The measurement of anxiety in children: Research findings and methodological problems. In: *Clinical Treatment and Research in Child Psychopathology*, edited by A. J. Finch, Jr. and P. C. Kendall. Spectrum, New York.
75. Finch, A. J., Kendall, P. C., and Montgomery, L. E. (1974): Multi-dimensionality of anxiety in children: Factor structure of the Children's Manifest Anxiety Scale. *J. Abnorm. Child Psychol.*, 2:331–336.
76. Finch, A. J., Kendall, P. C., and Montgomery, L. E. (1976): Qualitative difference in the experience of state-trait anxiety in emotionally disturbed and normal children. *J. Personal. Assess.*, 40:522–530.
77. Firestone, P., Davey, J., Goodman, J. T., and Peters, S. (1978): The effects of caffeine and methylphenidate on hyperactive children. *J. Am. Acad. Child Psychiatry*, 17(3):445–456.
78. Firestone, P., Poitras-Wright, H., and Douglas, V. (1978): The effects of caffeine on hyperactive children. *J. Learn. Disabil.*, 11(3):133–141.
79. Fish, B. (1971): The one child, one drug myth of stimulants in hyperkinesis. *Arch. Gen. Psychiatry*, 25:193–209.
80. Fomon, S. L., Filer, L. J., Anderson, T. A., and Ziegler, E. E. (1979): Recommendations for feeding normal infants. *Pediatrics*, 63:52–59.

81. Franks, H. M., Hagedorn, H., Hensley, V. R., Hensley, W. J., and Starmer, G. A. (1975): The effect of caffeine on human performance, alone and in combination with ethanol. *Psychopharmacologia*, 45:177.
82. Garfinkel, B. D., Webster, C. D., and Sloman, L. (1975): Methylphenidate and caffeine in the treatment of children with minimal brain dysfunction. *Am. J. Psychiatry*, 132(7):723–728.
83. Gay, J., and Cole, M. (1967): *The New Mathematics and an Old Culture.* Holt, Rinehart & Winston, New York.
84. Gill, J. R. (1980): Bartter's syndrome. *Annu. Rev. Med.*, 31:405–419.
85. Gittelman-Klein, R., and Klein, D. F. (1975): Are behavioral and psychometric changes related in methylphenidate-treated, hyperactive children? *Int. J. Mental Health*, 4:182–198.
86. Gittelman-Klein, R., Klein, D., Abikoff, H., Katz, S., Gloisten, A., and Kates, W. (1976): Relative efficacy of methylphenidate and behavior modification in hyperkinetic children: An interim report. *J. Abnorm. Child Psychol.*, 4:361–380.
87. Gittelman, R., Klein, D. F., and Feingold, I. (1983): Children with reading disorders: II. Effects of methylphenidate in combination with reading remediation. *J. Child Psychol. Psychiatry (in press).*
88. Gittelman-Klein, R., Klein, D., Katz, S., Saraf, K., and Pollack, E. (1976): Comparative effects of methylphenidate and thioridazine in hyperkinetic children. I. Clinical results. *Arch. Gen. Psychiatry*, 33:1217–1231.
89. Goldstein, A., and Kaizer, S. (1969): Psychotropic effects of caffeine in man. III. A questionnaire survey of coffee drinking and its effects in a group of housewives. *Clin. Pharmacol. Ther.*, 10(4):477–488.
90. Goldstein, A., Kaizer, S., and Whitby, O. (1969): Psychotropic effects of caffeine in man. IV. Quantitative and qualitative differences associated with habituation to coffee. *Clin. Pharmacol. Ther.*, 10(4):489–497.
91. Goyette, C. H., Conners, C. K., Petti, T. A., and Curtis, L. E. (1978): Effects of artificial colors on hyperkinetic children: A double-blind challenge study. *Psychopharmacol. Bull.*, 14(2):39–40.
92. Goyette, C. H., Conners, C. K., and Ulrich, R. F. (1978): Normative data on Revised Conners Parent and Teacher Rating Scales. *J. Abnorm. Child Psychol.*, 6(2):221–236.
93. Graves, P. L. (1976): Nutrition, infant behavior, and maternal characteristics: A pilot study in West Bengal, India. *Am. J. Clin. Nutr.*, 29(3):305–319.
94. Graves, P. L. (1978): Nutrition and infant behavior. A replication study of Katmanda Valley, Nepal. *Am. J. Clin. Nutr.*, 31(3):541–545.
95. Gross, M. D. (1975): Caffeine in the treatment of children with minimal brain dysfunction or hyperkinetic syndrome. *Psychosomatics*, 16(1):26–27.
96. Guy, W. (1976): *ECDEU Assessment Manual for Psychopharmacology* (Revised). DHEW Publication No. (ADM) 76-338, Rockville, Maryland.
98. Harley, J. P., Matthews, C. G., and Eichman, P. (1978): Synthetic food colors and hyperactivity in children: A double-blind challenge experiment. *Pediatrics*, 62(6):975–983.
99. Harley, J. P., Ray, R. S., Tomasi, L., Eichman, P. L., et al. (1978): Hyperkinesis and food additives: Testing the Feingold hypothesis. *Pediatrics*, 61(6):818–828.
100. Harner, I. C., and Lopp-Foiles, R. A. (1980): Effect of Feingold's K-P diet on a residential, mentally handicapped population. *J. Am. Diet. Assoc.*, 76(6):575–578.
101. Harrison, F. I. (1968): Relationship between home background, school success, and adolescent attitudes. *Merrill-Palmer Quarterly*, 14:331–344.
102. Helper, M., Wilcott, R., and Garfield, S. (1963): Effects of chlorpromazine on learning and related processes in emotionally disturbed children. *J. Consult. Psychol.*, 27:1–9.
103. Hersen, M., and Barlow, D. H. (1976): *Single Case Experimental Designs.* Pergamon Press, New York.
104. Hindle, R. C., and Priest, J. (1978): The management of hyperkinetic children: A trial of dietary therapy. *NZ Med. J.*, 88(616):43–45.
105. Hoorweg, J., and Stanfield, J. P. (1976): The effects of protein-energy malnutrition in early childhood on intelligence and motor abilities in later childhood and adolescence. *Dev. Med. Child Neurol.*, 18:330–350.
106. Howell, D. (1971): Significance of iron deficiencies. Consequences of mild deficiency in children. Extent and meaning of iron deficiency in the United States. *Summary Proceedings of Workshop of the Food and Nutrition Board.* National Academy of Sciences, Washington, D.C.
107. Huestis, R. D., Arnold, L. E., and Smeltzer, D. J. (1975): Caffeine versus methylphenidate and

d-amphetamine in minimal brain dysfunction: A double-blind comparison. *Am. J. Psychiatry*, 132(8):868–870.

108. Hunt, J. McV. (1961): *Intelligence and Experience*. Ronald Press, New York.
109. Hurwitz, I. (1976): Psychological testing in studies of malnutrition. In: *Malnutrition and Intellectual Development*, edited by J. D. Lloyd. Publishing Sciences Group, Littleton, Massachusetts.
110. Hutt, S., Jackson, P., Belshaw, A., and Higgins, G. (1968): Perceptual-motor behavior in relation to blood phenobarbitone levels: A preliminary report. *Dev. Med. Child Neurol.*, 10:626–632.
111. Institute of Food Technologists' Expert Panel on Food Safety and Nutrition and the Committee on Public Information. (1976): Diet and hyperactivity: Any connection? A scientific status summary. *Nutr. Rev.*, 34:151–158.
112. Interagency Collaborative Group on Hyperkinesis. (1975): First report of the preliminary findings and recommendations. HEW, Washington, D.C.
113. Jastak, J. F., and Jastak, S. (1978): *Wide Range Achievement Test Manual*. Jastak Associates, Wilmington, Delaware.
114. Kallen, D. J., Haddy, T. B., Narins, D., et al. (1972): Maternal correlates of iron deficiency anemia in infants. Paper presented at the IX International Nutrition Congress, Mexico City, September, 1972.
115. Kaufman, A. S. (1979): *Intelligent Testing with the WISC-R*. John Wiley & Sons, New York.
116. Kaufman, A. S., and Kaufman, N. L. (1977): *Clinical Evaluation of Young Children with the McCarthy Scales*. Grune & Stratton, New York.
117. Klein, R. E., Freeman, H. E., and Millett, R. (1973): Psychological test performance and indigenous conceptions of intelligence. *J. Psychol.*, 84:219–222.
118. Kupietz, S., Bialer, I., and Winsberg, B. C. (1972): A behavior rating scale for assessing improvement in behaviorally deviant children: A preliminary investigation. *Am. J. Psychiatry*, 128(11):1432–1436.
119. Langseth, L., and Dowd, J. (1978): Glucose tolerance and hyperkinesis. *Food Cosmet. Toxicol.*, 16:129–133.
120. Lasky, R. E., and Klein, R. E. (1980): Fixation of the standard and novelty preference in six-month old well and malnourished infants. *Merrill-Palmer Quarterly*, 26(2):171–178.
121. Leibel, R. L., Greenfield, D. B., and Pollitt, E. (1979): Iron deficiency: Behavior and brain biochemistry. In: *Nutrition: Pre- and Postnatal Development*, edited by M. Winick. Plenum Press, New York.
122. LeVine, R. A. (1970): Cross-cultural study in child psychology. In: *Carmichael's Manual of Child Psychology, Vol. 2*, third edition. John Wiley, New York.
123. Levy, F., Dumbrell, S., Hobbes, G., et al. (1978): Hyperkinesis and diet: A double-blind crossover trial with a tartrazine challenge. *Med. J. Aust.*, 1(2):61–64.
124. Levy, F., and Hobbes, G. (1978): Hyperkinesis and diet: A replication study. *Am. J. Psychiatry*, 135(12):1559–1562.
125. Lezak, M. (1976): *Neuropsychological Assessment*. Oxford University Press, New York.
126. Lick, J. R., and Katkin, E. S. (1976): Assessment of anxiety and fear. In: *Behavioral Assessment*, edited by M. Hersen and A. S. Bellack. Pergamon Press, New York.
127. Life Sciences Research Office, Federation of American Societies for Experimental Biology (1978): Evaluation of the health aspects of caffeine as a food ingredient. Bethesda, Maryland.
128. Linshaw, M. A., Harrison, H. L., Gruskin, A. B., et al. (1980): Hypochloremic alkalosis in infants associated with soy protein formula. *J. Pediatrics*, 96(4):635–640.
129. Lipton, M. A., Nemeroff, C. B., and Mailman, R. B. (1979): Hyperkinesis and food additives. In: *Nutrition and the Brain, Vol. 4*, edited by R. J. Wurtman and J. J. Wurtman. Raven Press, New York.
130. Lloyd-Still, J. D. (1976): Clinical studies on the effects of malnutrition during infancy on subsequent physical and intellectual development. In: *Malnutrition and Intellectual Development*, edited by J. D. Lloyd-Still. Publishing Sciences Group, Littleton, Massachusetts.
131. Logan, W., and Freeman, J. (1969): Pseudodegenerative disease due to diphenylhydantoin intoxication. *Arch. Neurol.*, 21:631–637.
132. Luria, A. R. (1980): *Higher Cortical Functions in Man;* 2nd edition, Basic Books, New York.
133. Mann, R. A. (1976): Assessment of behavioral excesses in children. In: *Behavioral Assessment*, edited by M. Hersen and A. S. Bellack. Pergamon Press, New York.
134. Mattes, J., and Gittelman-Klein, J. R. (1978): A crossover study of artificial food coloring in a hyperkinetic child. *Am. J. Psychiatry*, 135(8):987–988.

135. McGhee, P. E., and Crandall, V. (1968): Beliefs in internal-external control of reinforcement and academic performance. *Child Dev.*, 39:91–102.
136. McNair, D. M. (1973): Antianxiety drugs and human performance. *Arch. Gen. Psychiatry*, 29:611–617.
137. Meiers, R. L. (1973): Relative hypoglycemia in schizophrenia. In: *Orthomolecular Psychiatry: Treatment of Schizophrenia*, edited by D. Hawkins and L. Pauling. Freeman, San Francisco. pp. 452–462.
138. Millichap, J., and Johnson, F. (1974): Methylphenidate in hyperkinetic behavior: Relation of response to degree of activity and brain damage. In: *Clinical Use of Stimulant Drugs in Children*, edited by C. Conners. Excerpta Medica, Amsterdam.
139. Mirsky, A., and Kornetsky, C. (1964): On the dissimilar effects of drugs on the digit symbol substitution and continuous performance tests. A review and preliminary integration of behavioural and physiological evidence. *Psychopharmacologia*, 5:161–177.
140. Mitchell, S., and Shepherd, M. (1966): A comparative study of children's behaviour at home and at school. *Br. J. Educ. Psychol.*, 36:248–254.
141. Montgomery, L. E., and Finch, A. J. (1974): Validity of two measures of anxiety in children. *J. Abnorm. Child Psychol.*, 2:293–298.
142. Monckeburg, F. B. (1969): Malnutrition and mental behavior. *Nutr. Rev.*, 27:191–193.
143. Naatanea, R. (1975): The inverted relationship between activation and performance: A critical review. In: *Attention and Performance, Vol. 5*, edited by P. M. A. Rabbitt and S. Cornic. Academic Press, New York.
144. National Advisory Committee on Hyperkinesis and Food Additives. (1975): *Report to the Nutrition Foundation*. The Nutrition Foundation, New York.
145. Needleman, H. L. (1977): *Studies in Subclinical Lead Exposure*. Environmental Health Effects Research Series. PB-271649. Health Effects Research Laboratories, U.S. Environmental Protection Agency, Research Triangle Park, North Carolina.
146. Needleman, H. L., Gunnoe, C., Leviton, A., and Peresie, H. (1978): Neuropsychological dysfunction in children with "silent" lead exposure. *Paper presented at the American Pediatric Society Meeting*, April 27, 1978, New York.
147. Needleman, H. L., Gunnoe, C., Reed, M., Peresie, H., et al. (1979): Deficits in psychological and classroom performance of children with elevated dentine lead levels. *N. Engl. J. Med.*, 300:689–695.
148. Neil, J. F., Himmelhoch, J. M., Mallinger, A. G., Mallinger, J., and Hamin, I. (1978): Caffeinism complicating hypersomnic depressive episodes. *Comp. Psychiatry*, 19(4):377–385.
149. Newmark, C. S., Wheeler, D., Newmark, L., and Stabler, B. (1975): Test-induced anxiety with children. *J. Personal. Assessment*, 39:409–413.
150. Nowak, T. S., and Munro, H. N. (1977): Effects of protein-calorie malnutrition on biochemical aspects of brain development. In: *Nutrition and the brain, Vol. 2*, edited by R. J. Wurtman and J. J. Wurtman. Raven Press, New York.
151. Nowicki, S., and Roundtree, J. (1971): Correlates of locus of control in secondary school age students. *Dev. Psychol.*, 4:477–478.
152. Nowicki, S., and Strickland, B. R. (1973): A locus of control scale for children. *Journal of Consulting and Clinical Psychology*, 40(1):155–159.
153. O'Shea, J. A., and Porter, S. F. (1981): Double-blind study of children with hyperkinetic syndrome tested with multi-allergen extract sublingually. *J. Learn. Disabil.*, 14(4):189–191.
154. Palmer, S., Rapoport, J. L., and Quinn, P. O. (1975): Food additives and hyperactivity. *Clin. Pediatr.*, 14(10):956–959.
155. Piers, E. V. (1969): *Manual for the Piers-Harris Children's Self Concept Scale*. Counselor Recordings and Tests, Nashville, Tennessee.
156. Pollitt, E., Gersovitz, M. S., and Gargiulo, M. (1978): Educational benefits of the United States school feeding program: A critical review of the literature. *Am. J. Publ. Health*, 68(5):477–481.
157. Pollitt, E., and Leibel, R. L. (1976): Iron deficiency and behavior. *J. Pediatr.*, 88(3):372–381.
158. Pollitt, E., Leibel, R. L., and Greenfield, D. (1981): Brief fasting, stress and cognition in children. *Am. J. Clin. Nutr.*, 34(8):1526–1533.
159. Pollitt, E., Leibel, R., and Greenfield, D. (1983): Iron deficiency and cognitive test performance in preschool children. *Nutrition & Behavior (in press)*.
160. Pollitt, E., and Thomson, C. (1977): Protein-calorie malnutrition and behavior: A view from

psychology. In: *Nutrition and the Brain, Vol. 2*, edited by R. J. Wurtman and J. J. Wurtman. Raven Press, New York.

161. Pollitt, E., Viteri, F., Saco-Pollitt, C., and Leibel, R. (1980): Iron deficiency anemia and cognitive test performance in Guatemalan preschool children. *Paper presented at the Conference on Iron Deficiency, Brain Biochemistry, and Behavior*, The Woodlands, Texas, December 4–5, 1980.

162. Porrino, L., Rapoport, J., et al. (1983): Twenty-four hour activity in hyperactive children and controls. *Arch. Gen. Psychiatry (in press)*.

163. Prinz, R. J., Roberts, W. A., and Hantman, E. (1980): Dietary correlates of hyperactive behavior in children. *J. Consult. Clin. Psychol.*, 48(6):760–769.

164. Quay, H. C. (1979): Classification. In: *Psychopathological Disorders of Childhood*, 2nd edition, edited by H. C. Quay and J. S. Werry. John Wiley, New York.

165. Quinn, P., and Rapoport, J. (1975): One-year follow-up of hyperactive boys treated with imipramine or methylphenidate. *Am. J. Psychiatry*, 132:241–245.

166. Rapoport, J. L. (1979): Self-report measures. In: Appendix for *Guidelines for Evaluation of Psychoactive Agents in Infants and Children*, U.S. Government Printing Office, HEW Publication #79-3055, pp. 133–138.

166a. Rapoport, J., Abramson, A., Alexander, D., and Lott, I. (1971): Playroom observations of hyperactive children on medication. *J. Am. Acad. Child Psychiatry*, 10:524–534.

167. Rapoport, J., and Benoit, M. (1975): The relation of direct home observations to the clinic evaluation of hyperactive school age boys. *J. Child Psychol. Psychiatry*, 16:141–147.

168. Rapoport, J. L., Buchsbaum, M., Weingartner, H., Zahn, T., et al. (1980): Dextroamphetamine: Behavioral and cognitive effects in boys and adult males. *Arch. Gen. Psychiatry*, 37:933–943.

169. Rapoport, J., Buchsbaum, M., Zahn, T., Weingartner, H., et al. (1978): Dextroamphetamine: Cognitive and behavioral effects in normal prepubertal boys. *Science*, 199:560–563.

170. Rapoport, J. L., Elkins, R., Neims, A., Zahn, T., and Berg, C. J. (1981): Behavioral and autonomic effects of caffeine in normal boys. *Dev. Pharmacol.*, 3:74–82.

171. Rapoport, J. L., and Ferguson, B. (1981): Biological validation of the hyperkinetic syndrome. *Developmental Medicine and Child Neurology*, 23:667–682.

172. Rapoport, J. L., Jensvold, M., Elkins, R., Buchsbaum, M. S., et al. (1981): Behavioral and cognitive effects of caffeine in boys and adult males. *J. Nerv. Ment. Dis.*, 169:726–732.

173. Rapoport, J., Quinn, P., Bradbard, G., Riddle, D., and Brookes, E. (1974): Imipramine and methylphenidate treatment of hyperactive boys: A double blind comparison. *Arch. Gen. Psychiatry*, 30:789–793.

174. Rapp, D. J. (1978): Does diet affect hyperactivity? *J. Learn. Disabil.*, 11(6):383–389.

175. Reynolds, C. R., and Richmond, B. O. (1978): What I Think and Feel: A revised measure of children's manifest anxiety. *J. Abnorm. Child Psychol.*, 6(2):271–280.

176. Reynolds, C. R., and Richmond, B. O. (1979): Factor structure and construct validity of "What I Think and Feel": The Revised Children's Manifest Anxiety Scale. *J. Personal. Assess.*, 43(3):281–283.

177. Richardson, S. A. (1974): The background histories of school children severely malnourished in infancy. *Adv. Pediatrics*, 21:167–195.

178. Rie, E., and Rie, H. (1977): Recall, retention and Ritalin. *J. Consult. Clin. Psychol.*, 45:967–972.

179. Rose, T. L. (1978): The functional relationship between artificial food colors and hyperactivity. *J. Appl. Behav. Anal.*, 11(4):439–446.

180. Roy, S., and Arant, B. S. (1981): Metabolic alkalosis and chloride deficiency. *Pediatrics*, 67(3):423–429.

181. Rutter, M. (1980): Raised lead levels and impaired cognitive/behavioral functioning. A review of the evidence. *Dev. Med. Child Neurol. (Suppl.)*, 22(1):1–26.

182. Rutter, M., Tizard, J., and Whitmore, K. (1970): *Education, Health and Behavior*. Longmans Green, London.

183. Salzman, L. K. (1976): Allergy testing, psychological assessment, and dietary treatment of the hyperactive child syndrome. *Med. J. Austr.*, 2:248–251.

184. Sameroff, A., and Chandler, M. (1975): Reproductive risk and the continuum of caretaking casualty. In: *Review of Child Development Research*, edited by F. Horowitz. University of Chicago Press, Chicago.

185. Samter, M. (1973): Intolerance to aspirin. *Hosp. Pract.*, 12:85–90.

186. Satterfield, J. H. (1975): Neurophysiologic studies with hyperkinetic children. In: *The Hyperactive Child*, edited by D. P. Cantwell. Spectrum Publications, New York.
187. Satterfield, J. H., Cantwell, D. P., and Satterfield, B. T. (1974): Pathophysiology of the hyperactive child syndrome. *Arch. Gen. Psychiatry*, 21:839–844.
188. Sattler, J. M. (1974): *Assessment of Children's Intelligence*. W. B. Saunders, Philadelphia.
189. Schachar, R., Rutter, M., and Smith, A. (1981): The characteristics of children: Implications for syndrome definition. *J. Child Psychol. Psychiatry*, 22(4):375–392.
190. Schnackenberg, R. C. (1973): Caffeine as a substitute for schedule II stimulants in hyperactive children. *Am. J. Psychiatry*, 130(7):796–798.
191. Seone, N., and Latham, M. C. (1971): Nutritional anthropometry in the identification of malnutrition in childhood. *J. Trop. Environ. Child Health*, 17:198.
192. Shoemaker, W. J., and Bloom, F. E. (1977): Effect of undernutrition on brain morphology. In: *Nutrition and the Brain, Vol. 2*, edited by R. J. Wurtman and J. J. Wurtman. Raven Press, New York.
193. Silbergeld, E. K., and Anderson, S. M. (1982): Artificial food colors and childhood behavior disorders. *Bull. NY Acad. Med.*, 58(3):275–295.
194. Simopoulos, A. P., and Bartter, F. C. (1980): The metabolic consequences of chloride deficiency. *Nutr. Rev.*, 38(6):201–205.
195. Spielberger, C. D. (1973): *Preliminary manual for the State-Trait Anxiety Inventory for Children ("How I Feel Questionnaire")*. Consulting Psychologists Press, Palo Alto, California.
196. Sprague, R. L. (1972): Psychopharmacology and learning disorders. *J. Oper. Psychiatry*, 3:56–67.
197. Sprague, R. L. (1979): Performance tests for pediatric psychopharmacology studies. In: *FDA Guidelines for the Clinical Evaluation of Psychoactive Drugs in Infants and Children*. U.S. Government Printing Office, HEW(FDA) 79-3055.
198. Sprague, R. L., Barnes, K. R., and Werry, J. S. (1970): Methylphenidate and thioridazine: Learning, reaction time, activity, and classroom behavior in disturbed children. *Am. J. Orthopsychiatry*, 40:615–628.
199. Sprague, R. L., Cohen, M. N., and Eichlseder, W. (1977): Are there hyperactive children in Europe and the South Pacific? In: *The Hyperactive Child: Fact, Fiction, and Fantasy*, edited by R. Halliday. Symposium presented at the meeting of the American Psychological Association, San Francisco, August, 1977.
200. Sprague, R. L., and Sleator, E. K. (1973): Effects of psychopharmacologic agents on learning disorders. *Pediatr. Clin. North Am.*, 20:719–735.
201. Sprague, R. L., and Sleator, E. K. (1975): What is the proper dose of stimulant drugs in children? *Int. J. Mental Health*, 4:75–118.
202. Sprague, R. L., and Sleator, E. K. (1977): Methylphenidate in hyperkinetic children: Differences in dose effects on learning and social behavior. *Science*, 198:1, 274-1, 276.
203. Stein, Z., and Susser, M. (1975): The Dutch famine, 1944–45, and the reproductive process. I. Effects on six indices at birth. *Pediatr. Res.*, 9:70–76.
204. Stein, Z., Susser, M., Saenger, G., and Marolla, F. (1972): Nutrition and mental performance. *Science*, 178:708.
205. Stephens, M., and Delys, P. (1973): External control expectancies among disadvantaged children at preschool age. *Child Dev.*, 44(3):670–674.
206. Stine, J. S. (1976): Symptom alleviation in the hyperactive child by dietary modification: A report of two cases. *Am. J. Orthopsychiatry*, 46(4):637–645.
207. Stores, G. (1978): Antiepileptics (anticonvulsants). In: *Pediatric Psychopharmacology*, edited by J. S. Werry. Brunner/Mazel, New York.
208. Stores, G., Hart, J., and Piran, N. (1978): Attentiveness and related behaviour in boys and girls with epilepsy attending ordinary school. Cited in G. Stores, Antiepileptics. In: *Pediatric Psychopharmacology*, edited by J. S. Werry. Brunner/Mazel, New York.
209. Sulzer, J. L., Wesley, H. H., and Loenig, F. (1973): Nutrition and behavior in head start children: Results from the Tulane study. In: *Nutrition, Development and Social Behavior*, edited by D. J. Kallen. DHEW Publication No. (NIH) 73-242, Washington, D.C.
210. Sunderman, F. W., and Boerner, F. (1949): *Normal Values in Clinical Medicine*. W. B. Saunders, Philadelphia.
211. Swanson, J. M., and Kinsbourne, M. (1980): Food dyes impair performance of hyperactive children on a laboratory learning test. *Science*, 207:1485–1486.

212. Tchicaloff, M., and Gaillard, F. (1970): Quelques effects indesirables des medicaments anti-epileptiques sur les rendements intellectuals. *Rev. Neuropsychiatrie Infantile*, 18:599–602.
213. Trimble, M. (1979): The effect of anti-convulsant drugs on cognitive abilities. *Pharmacol. Thera.*, 4:677–685.
214. Trites, R. L., Blouin, A. G. A., Ferguson, H. B., and Lynch, G. (1981): The Conners' Teacher Rating Scale: An epidemiologic, inter-rater reliability and follow-up investigation. In: *Psychosocial Aspects of Drug Treatment for Hyperactivity*, edited by K. D. Gadow and J. Loney. American Association for the Advancement of Science, New York.
215. Trites, R. L., Dugas, E., Lynch, G., and Ferguson, H. B. (1979): Prevalence of hyperactivity. *J. Pediatr. Psychol.*, 4(2):179–188.
216. Tryphonas, H., and Trites, R. (1979): Food allergy in children with hyperactivity, learning disabilities and/or minimal brain dysfunction. *Ann. Allergy*, 42:22–27.
217. Vahlquist, B., Engsner, G., and Sjogren, I. (1971): Malnutrition and size of the cerebral ventricles. *Acta Paediatr. Scand.*, 60:533.
218. Wapner, I., Thurston, D., and Holowach, J. (1962): Phenobarbital: Its effect on learning in epileptic children. *JAMA*, 182:937.
219. Waterlow, J. C., and Scrimshaw, N. S. (1957): The concept of kwashiorkor from a public health point of view. *Bull. WHO*, 16:458.
220. Webb, T. E., and Oski, F. A. (1973): Iron deficiency anemia and scholastic achievement in young adolescents. *J. Pediatr.*, 82:827–830.
221. Weingartner, H., Langer, D., Grice, J., and Rapoport, J. L. (1982): Acquisition and retrieval of information in amphetamine treated hyperactive children. *Psychiatry Res.*, 6:21–29.
222. Weingartner, H., Rapoport, J. l., et al. (1980): Cognitive processes in normal and hyperactive children and their response to amphetamine treatment. *J. Abnorm. Psychol.*, 89(1):25–37.
223. Weiss, B., and Laties, V. G. (1962): Enhancement of human performance by caffeine and the amphetamines. *Pharmacol. Rev.*, 14:1–36.
224. Weiss, G., Minde, K., Douglas, V., Werry, J., and Sykes, D. (1971): Comparison of the effects of chlorpromazine, dextroamphetamine and methylphenidate on the behavior and intellectual functioning of hyperactive children. *Can. Med. Assoc. J.*, 104:20–25.
225. Weiss, G., Minde, K., Werry, J., Douglas, V., and Nemeth, E. (1971): Studies on the hyperactive child. *Arch. Gen. Psychiatry*, 24:409–414.
226. Weiss, G., Werry, J., Minde, K., Douglas, V., and Sykes, D. (1968): The effects of dextroamphetamine and chlorpromazine on behavior and intellectual functioning. *J. Child Psychol. Psychiatry*, 9:145–156.
227. Weiss, B., Williams, J. H., Margen, S., et al. (1980): Behavioral responses to artificial food colors. *Science*, 207:1487–1489.
228. Werner, E., Berman, J., and French, F. (1971): *The Children of Kauai: A Longitudinal Study from the Prenatal Period to Age Ten*. University of Hawaii Press, Honolulu.
229. Werner, E. E., Honzik, M. P., and Smith, R. S. (1968): Prediction of intelligence and achievement at ten years from twenty months pediatric and psychologic examinations. *Child Dev.*, 39:1063–1075.
230. Werner, E., and Smith, R. (1977): *Kauai's Children Come of Age*. University of Hawaii Press, Honolulu.
231. Werry, J. S. (1978): Measures in pediatric psychopharmacology. In: *Pediatric Psychopharmacology*, edited by J. S. Werry. Brunner/Mazel, New York.
232. Werry, J. S., and Aman, M. G. (1975): Methylphenidate and haloperidol in children: Effects on attention, memory, and activity. *Arch. Gen. Psychiatry*, 32:790–795.
233. Werry, J., Dowrick, P., Lampen, E., and Vamos, M. (1975): Imipramine in enuresis—psychological and physiological effects. *J. Child Psychol. Psychiatry*, 16:289–300.
234. Werry, J. S., and Hawthorne, D. (1976): Conners Teacher Questionnaire—norms and validity. *Austr. NZ J. Psychiatry*, 10:257–261.
235. Werry, J., and Sprague, R. (1974): Methylphenidate in children—effect of dosage. *Austr. NZ J. Psychiatry*, 8:9–19.
236. Werry, J. S., Sprague, R. L., and Cohen, M. N. (1975): Conners' Teacher Rating Scale for use in drug studies with children—an empirical study. *J. Abnorm. Child Psychol.*, 3(3):217–229.
237. Whalen, C. K., and Henker, B. (1976): Psychostimulants and children: A review and analysis. *Psychol. Bull.*, 83(6):1113–1130.
238. Whalen, C. K., and Henker, B. (1980): The social ecology of psychostimulant treatment: A model

for conceptual and empirical analysis. In: *Hyperactive Children: The Social Ecology of Identification and Treatment*, edited by C. K. Whalen and B. Henker. Academic Press, New York.

239. Wiener, J. M., and Jaffe, S. (1977): History of drug therapy in childhood disorders and adolescent psychiatric disorders. In: *Psychopharmacology in Childhood and Adolescence*, edited by J. M. Wiener. Basic Books, New York.

240. Willerman, L., Broman, S. H., and Fiedler, M. (1970): Infant development, preschool IQ, and social class. *Child Dev.*, 41:69–77.

241. Williams, J. I., Cram, D. M., Tausig, F. T., and Webster, E. (1978): Relative effects of drugs and diet on hyperactive behaviors: An experimental study. *Pediatrics*, 61(6):811–817.

242. Winer, B. J. (1962): *Statistical Principles in Experimental Design*, McGraw-Hill, New York.

243. Winick, M. (1976): *Malnutrition and Brain Development*. Oxford University Press, New York.

244. Wolf, S. M., Carr, A., Davis, D. C., et al. (1977): The value of phenobarbital in the child who has had a single febrile seizure: A controlled prospective study. *Pediatrics*, 59(3):378–385.

245. Wolf, S. M., and Forsythe, A. (1978): Behavior disturbance, phenobarbital, and febrile seizures. *Pediatrics*, 61(5):728–731.

246. Wong, G., and Cock, R. (1971): Long-term effects of haloperidol on severely emotionally disturbed children. *Austr. NZ J. Psychiatry*, 5:296–300.

247. Wurtman, J., and Wurtman, R. (1979): Drugs that enhance central serotonergic transmission diminish elective carbohydrate consumption by rats. *Life Sci.*, 24:895–904.

248. Wurtman, R. J., Hefti, F., and Melamed, E. (1981): Precursor control of neurotransmitter synthesis. *Pharmacol. Rev.*, 32(4):315–335.

248a. Wurtman, J. J., and Wurtman, R. J. (1982): Suppression of carbohydrate consumption as snacks and at mealtime by dl fenfluramine or tryptophan. In: *Anorectic Agents: Mechanisms of Actions and of Tolerance*, edited by S. Garranttini. Raven Press, New York.

248b. Wurtman, J. J., Wurtman, R. J., Growdon, J. H., Henry, P., Lipscomb, A., and Zeisel, S. (1981): Carbohydrate craving in obese people: suppression by treatments affecting serotoninergic transmission. *Int. J. Eating Disord.*, 1:2–11.

249. Yepes, L., Balka, E., Winsberg, B., and Bialer, I. (1977): Amitriptyline and methylphenidate treatment of behaviorally disordered children. *J. Child Psychol. Psychiatry*, 18:39–52.

250. Zentall, S. S., and Barack, R. S. (1979): Rating scales for hyperactivity: Concurrent validity, reliability, and decisions to label for the Conners and Davids Abbreviated Scales. *J. Abnorm. Child Psychol.*, 7(2):179–190.

GLOSSARY

Bayley Scales of Infant Development

This developmental scale is appropriate for assessing infants and young children between 2 months and 30 months of age. Separate mental and motor scales yield a Mental Developmental Index and Psychomotor Developmental Index. An accompanying Infant Behavior Record provides for ratings of the qualitative aspects of infant behavior.

Children's Manifest Anxiety Scale (CMAS)

This is a self-report scale, appropriate for use with children in grades 1 through 12, that measures anxiety as a trait.

Conners Abbreviated Parent–Teacher Questionnaire (PTQ)

This is a shortened, 10-item version of Conners' earlier rating scale for measuring hyperactivity.

Conners Parent Questionnaire (PQ)

This is a 93-item scale for measuring hyperactivity through the use of parent's ratings. Factor analytic studies have suggested several basic factors or dimensions: conduct disorder, anxiety, impulsivity, immaturity, psychosomatic complaints, obsessionality, antisocial problems.

Conners Teacher Questionnaire (TQ)

This is a scale used for obtaining teacher's ratings of hyperactivity. Both a 39-item and a shorter, 28-item version are available. Factors underlying the items include conduct problems, inattention, anxiety, hyperactivity, and sociability.

Continuous Performance Test (CPT)

This is a laboratory task that requires monitoring of either visual or auditory stimuli and sustained vigilance. The subject's task is to detect certain target stimuli while monitoring an ongoing series of stimuli.

Davids' Rating Scale for Hyperkinesis

This is a rating scale for hyperactivity, consisting of seven items: hyperactivity, short attention span, behavioral variability, impulsiveness, instability, explosiveness, and poor school work.

Global Clinical Impressions Scale

This is a 7-point scale on which a parent, physician, or other observer rates the degree and general direction (improved, unchanged, or worse) of behavioral changes. The specific nature of behavioral changes is not indicated.

Gray Oral Reading Test

This test measures fluency and accuracy of oral reading. Comprehension questions follow each of 13 reading passages and give an indication of the reader's understanding at a concrete level. Difficulty ranges from an early first grade to a college level.

Halstead-Reitan Neuropsychological Test Battery

This is a comprehensive neuropsychological test battery for use with adults and older adolescents. Individual test scores and an overall impairment index can be calculated.

Halstead-Reitan Neuropsychological Test Battery for Children

This is an adaptation of the Halstead-Reitan adult test battery, appropriate for children, ages 9 to 15 years of age. It consists of simplified versions of the individual tests included in the adult battery.

Illinois Test of Psycholinguistic Abilities (ITPA)

This test consists of 12 subtests originally intended to measure various specific psycholinguistic abilities. Its psychometric characteristics, validity as a measure of linguistic functions, and educational significance have, however, been questioned and criticized.

Intellectual Achievement Responsibility Questionnaire

This self-report measure, appropriate for children in grades 3 through 12, measures locus of control for successes and failures related to the academic setting.

Iowa Tests of Basic Skills

These achievement tests, designed for administration to groups, measure basic skills related to the school curriculum across grades kindergarten through grade 14. Skills such as vocabulary, reading comprehension, spelling, mathematical concepts, mathematical problem-solving, and computations are tested.

Matching Familiar Figures Test

This test requires a subject to select from among several variants a picture that precisely matches a standard picture. It provides a measure of cognitive impulsivity.

McCarthy Scales of Children's Abilities

These scales, designed for children, ages 2½ to 8½ years, assess both intellectual and motor development. The scales yield separate scores for verbal ability, short-term memory, numerical ability, perceptual performance, motor coordination, lateral dominance, and overall cognitive competence.

Metropolitan Achievement Tests

These tests are norm- and criterion-referenced measures of academic achievements that cover grades kindergarten through 12. Individual tests are available for estimating instructional levels in reading, mathematics, language, social studies, and science.

Nowicki and Strickland Locus of Control Scale

This is a self-report scale for measuring locus of control, appropriate for children beyond the second grade.

Peabody Individual Achievement Test (PIAT)

This individually administered achievement test, designed for use with kindergarten through 12th grade students, tests reading recognition, reading comprehension, spelling, mathematics, and general information.

Peabody Picture Vocabulary Test (PPVT)

This test primarily measures receptive vocabulary. The subject must identify which of four pictures matches a stimulus word read by the examiner. The PPVT was standardized on children, ages 2½ to 18 years. Its recent (1979) revision—the PPVT-R—was standardized for ages 2½ through 40 years.

Piers-Harris Self-Concept Scale (The Way I Feel About Myself)

This is a self-report, norm-based measure of self-concept, appropriate for children from grades 4 through 12.

Porteus Mazes Test

This is a nonlanguage test of mental ability. The subject's task is to trace his way through paper and pencil mazes. Impulsive darting into blind alleys is penalized, while planning and foresight result in a higher score.

Raven's Progressive Matrices

This nonverbal test of reasoning and problem-solving requires the subject to choose from among four to eight pictured inserts the one that will complete a visuospatial pattern. Items range from the concrete and simple to the complex and abstract. Various versions, which differ in difficulty level, provide tests that are appropriate for children, ages 5 years through adult ages.

Reitan-Indiana Neuropsychological Test Battery for Children

This represents a modification of the tests of the Halstead-Reitan battery for adults, for children, ages 5 to 8 years.

Stanford Achievement Tests

This is a group-administered achievement battery for grades 1 through 9, which assesses reading comprehension, language skills, mathematical skills, science concepts, social science inquiry skills, and auditory skills.

Stanford-Binet Intelligence Scale

This is an individually administered, age-based measure of general cognitive functioning, appropriate for ages 2 years through adult. Test scores include an Intelligence Quotient (IQ) and a Mental Age.

State-Trait Anxiety Inventory for Children (STAIC)

This is a self-report measure of anxiety for use with elementary school children that consists of separate scales for assessing anxiety as a trait (a stable aspect of personality functioning) and anxiety as a state (one that fluctuates with changes in the social situation).

Stephens-Delys Reinforcement Contingency Interview

This is a standard interview for assessing generalized life expectancies (or "locus of control"), useful for children, ages 4 to 10 years.

Wechsler Adult Intelligence Scale (WAIS)

The WAIS is an individually administered, general intelligence test for adolescents and adults, ages 16 to over 75 years. It contains six verbal and five performance subtests, which yield standard scores, which are summed and translated into Verbal, Performance, and Full-Scale IQ scores. This test, originally standardized in 1955, has recently (1981) been updated and restandardized (WAIS-R).

Wechsler Intelligence Scale for Children (WISC)

This widely used intelligence scale for children, ages 6 to 16 years, contains six verbal and six performance subtests, which yield standard scores, which are summed and converted into a Verbal IQ, Performance IQ, and Full-Scale IQ. In addition to its use as a global measure of intelligence, it has been widely used as part of neuropsychological test batteries to provide information concerning patterns of abilities and deficits. It is being replaced by the 1974 revision (WISC-R).

Wechsler Intelligence for Children-Revised (WISC-R)

The WISC-R, published in 1974, represents a revision of the WISC. It has retained the basic format of the WISC and was standardized for use with children, ages 5 to 15 years.

Wechsler Preschool and Primary Scale of Intelligence (WPPSI)

The WPPSI provides a general measure of intelligence in children, ages 4 to 6½ years. It contains five verbal and five performance subtests and one alternate subtest, which yield standard subtest scores, a Verbal IQ, a Performance IQ, and a Full-Scale IQ.

Werry-Weiss-Peters Activity Rating Scale

This is an experimental scale for measuring hyperactivity.

Wide Range Achievement Test (WRAT)

This is an individually administered achievement test designed for ages five through adult. Skills measured are word recognition (reading), spelling, and mathematical computation.

Nutrition and the Brain, Vol. 6 edited by
R. J. Wurtman and J. J. Wurtman.
Raven Press, New York © 1983.

Problems and Processes Underlying the Control of Food Selection and Nutrient Intake

John E. Blundell

Department of Psychology, The University of Leeds, Leeds LS 2 9JT, U.K.

I. INTRODUCTION

More than 40 years ago it was noted that "the ability of animals and humans to make dietary selections which are conducive to normal growth and reproduction has not received much attention in modern nutritional studies" (150). Considering the importance attached to such a capacity, the issue has not received a commensurate degree of attention from researchers during the intervening period. Indeed, two reviewers (100,133) particularly lamented the lack of investigation of mechanisms underlying the phenomenon of food selection. However, in recent years, overtaking the slowly accumulating body of data, certain theoretical propositions have been put forward that have provoked the interest of researchers. Moreover, there has recently been a sharp increase in the publication of experimental reports on food selection. There are clear signs that within the study of food intake, we are beginning a period in which attention will be focused not solely on total caloric intake and regulation of body weight but will be directed to an examination of the mechanisms influencing the choice of specific nutritional commodities. Accordingly, it is now appropriate to describe recent theoretical developments, to assemble recently acquired experimental evidence, to examine critically the techniques and methods being used in such experiments, and to appraise the implications—academic and clinical—of the phenomenon of food selection. This chapter will incorporate studies on food selection by animals and man.

In laboratories, experimental animals are usually maintained on single-composite balanced diets designed to provide a nutritional input optimal for biological functioning. Consequently, most animals are not permitted to display any potential capacity to select particular dietary items. Any test of this capacity must involve a deliberately designed experiment. However, in the wild, many animals have the opportunity to consume a variety of edible materials, and the variability of the pattern of intake often suggests that a capacity for selection is being demonstrated. However, it is clear that the mere observation that a variable array of foods is being consumed alone does not imply the articulation of a power to select a diet purposefully. Such variability could arise capriciously for reasons unrelated to internal physiological events or to qualities inherent in the food materials. Accordingly, it is first necessary to ascertain that the selection is systematic and rational before undertaking the investigation of the mechanisms responsible. This theoretical point has methodological implications, since in laboratory experiments the simultaneous presentation of different diets and the consumption of some of each by an experimental animal does not automatically mean that a physiological process of nutrient selection is operating, even though the animal may possess some capacity for selection.

It is clear that under natural conditions the problems of selecting appropriate food material are not equally intense for all species. Indeed the tasks confronting herbivores, carnivores, and omnivores are quite different. In general herbivores spend a large amount of time feeding on material of low caloric density and low nutritional quality. In some ways the nutrient quality of food is more important to herbivores than to carnivores and insectivores because plants often lack essential dietary components, and only by careful selection of plant species can a herbivore obtain a balanced intake (95). One example is the moose living on the shores of Lake Superior that feeds on deciduous leaves from the forest, which have a high energy yield, and on aquatic plants, which contain sodium (15). Since the moose needs both energy and sodium it must eat a mixed diet. Moreover, many animals are anatomically specialized, for example, as browsers (eating from bushes, shrubs, or trees) or grazers (eating from the ground); consequently the type of food eaten and the place from which it can be procured are often severely limited. Carnivores typically consume all their essential nutrients from a single source, the nutrients having maintained the life of the prey. Although carnivores feed on high-density material of good nutritional quality, they are often as limited as herbivores in the varieties of food that they are capable of consuming. This feature of feeding behavior has been characterized by referring to animals as either specialists or generalists (157). Although all animals must overcome environmental obstacles in the procurement of food, selecting superior items and avoiding inferior or contaminated material, it is omnivores who face the most severe problems of nutrient selection. By definition omnivores eat a wide range of foods among which no single item contains all of the essential materials for optimal biological functioning. Consequently, to maximize its chances of survival, an omnivore must select foods containing essential materials appropriate to its internal physiological requirements, a feature that exemplifies the strength and the weakness in development of omnivores. In one respect the capability of eating a wide variety of materials is useful, since it allows omnivores to colonize new habitats. Whereas the loss of a single food source may be fatal to a particular herbivore or carnivore, for omnivores it presents simply an obstacle that can be overcome. On the other hand this capability demands specialized mechanisms to harmonize physiological information in the internal milieu with nutritional information in the external environment. These mechanisms clearly involve physiological processes for accurate monitoring of the internal need state; perceptual capacities to identify the characteristics of food materials located in the environment; and a mechanism to link the biochemical features of ingested food with the consumed structural form. The freedom afforded by an omnivorous life style can be juxtaposed with the complexity and vulnerability of the mechanisms developed to deal with this mode of living. Two prominent examples of omnivores are the rat, which has been the target of most animal research, and man. How well do these species select appropriate foods and what are the mechanisms involved?

It is obvious that dietary self-selection involves the gathering and consumption of all the elements of what is usually considered to be a balanced diet, including essential vitamins, minerals, and salts, together with the macronutrients—protein, carbohydrate, and fat. Current interest is focused particularly on this last group of materials; thus this chapter will be concerned only with control of the selection of macronutrients, and especially with protein and carbohydrates. General mechanisms involved in the control of total caloric intake and body weight have been recently reviewed (e.g., refs. 83,116) and will not be dealt with here. Attention will be directed to the question of internal validity, that is, to an understanding of the mechanisms (or causes) underlying food selection, and to the issue of external validity—the extent to which the methodology adopted in laboratory investigations permits an extrapolation of the findings to more natural circumstances.

II. TRANSLATION OF NEEDS INTO BEHAVIOR

Nothing is more important to animals than that they approach features of the environment that are beneficial and avoid those elements that are dangerous. A prerequisite for accomplishing this is the development of brain mechanisms to reflect positive and negative experiences (e.g., ref. 175). In this exercise the two major tasks of managing the internal and the external environments (71) merge into a single task. Consequently, animals in a state of internal need (which may be defined as the departure from optimal value of any essential item) must be able to recognize and approach the environmental features that will rectify the need. In much of the traditional literature on dietary self-selection it was assumed that animals have a need for all basic dietary items (macronutrients, vitamins, and minerals). Experiments sought to determine how well animals could satisfy their needs when allowed to select their intake from a "cafeteria" array of dietary materials. Since animals will normally sample from most items in a presented series, this alone, as noted above, does not indicate the existence of purposeful selection. Accordingly, some criterion must be set to judge the adequacy of the selection. This is usually rate of growth, reproductive capacity, or longevity (survival time)—parameters believed to reflect a biological advantage. Alternatively, Lát (100) has reported the use of "unspecific excitability level of the brain," measured indirectly by monitoring some aspect of behavioral activity, as an index for assessing qualitative and quantitative differences in selection capacity. Although omnivores such as the rat can grow and survive when allowed to self-select their dietary intake, experimental results show great variability. For example, in the classic early study of Kon (94) some animals failed to ingest a particular form of protein (casein), failed to grow properly, and subsequently died. Similar results were obtained in later experiments (e.g., refs. 142,164).

An alternative strategy used in traditional studies involves the experimental manipulation of a need by withdrawing an essential element from the diet, by removal of an endocrine gland, or by imposing certain physiological demands, e.g., pregnancy, on the animal. The dependent variable then becomes the capacity of the animal to adjust its selected intake to cope with the new demand. The outcome of these traditional approaches is far from satisfactory, for, as Lát noted in his 1967 review, "different methods of studying SSDC (self-selection of dietary components) lead to contradictory results" (100). Clearly, if different experimental strategies lead to discrepant observations, the search for mechanisms underlying the translation of needs into behavior is problematic, and implies that methodological issues are of paramount importance.

A. What Is Diet Selection?

The essence of dietary selection in experimental studies is to present animals with the possibility of making choices among dietary items offered simultaneously (not sequentially). When faced with an array of foods in the laboratory, animals choose more from some than from others. Research is concerned with the nature of the mechanisms underlying this proven phenomenon.

Researchers have used a number of techniques to measure the extent of an animal's (usually a rat's) capacity to select from a range of dietary items:

(a) Certain studies have forced rats to choose from up to 15 substances including pure protein (casein), carbohydrate (sucrose) and fat (olive oil), sodium as sodium chloride, potassium as potassium chloride, calcium as calcium lactate, magnesium as magnesium chloride, phosphorus in dibasic sodium phosphate, vitamin B complex in baker's yeast, vitamin D in cod liver oil, and vitamin E in wheat germ oil. In certain experiments the various vitamin components in baker's yeast have been presented separately.

(b) More frequently experimenters have employed a more limited set of choices in which separate containers of pure macronutrients have been presented alongside a container of a mixture of vitamins and minerals.

(c) A third strategy includes presentation of macronutrients in combination with vitamins and minerals to reduce the number of choices facing experimental animals. For example, in one study animals were offered separate containers of carbohydrate (glucose), fat (corn oil and tallow), and protein (casein plus methionine), each of which was supplemented with a basal mixture of minerals and vitamins (155). In some studies only proteins and carbohydrates were supplemented by minerals and vitamins (e.g., ref. 88).

(d) An alternative technique is the use of composite diets, which are frequently employed when only two macronutrients (e.g., protein and carbohydrate) are under investigation. A now-traditional procedure is to construct two isocaloric diets containing minerals and vitamins, and the same amount of the nutrient not being tested. The diets are prepared so that one contains large amounts of the test nutrient (for example, 45% protein or 70% carbohydrate) and the other diet contains very small amounts of the nutrient (5% protein or 25% carbohydrate). Fat is varied between the diets to keep them isocaloric (e.g., refs. 119,188). In certain cases composite diets may be entirely free of carbohydrate (the protein fraction) or protein (the carbohydrate fraction), and presented in combination with a single food containing all dietary elements (control diet), e.g., ref. 49.

In other forms of nutritional experiments animals may be presented with unbalanced diets that may contain, for example, an excess or deficit of amino acids. Such studies have been used to determine mechanisms of protein regulation. However, it is only those studies that offer animals *choices* between nutritionally different diets that can be referred to as self-selection experiments. When confronted with containers of foods that are nutritionally different animals adjust their consumption from the various sources. It is equally clear that humans modulate their food intake from nutritionally different food items. Although the practical problems of investigating this phenomenon are more severe in humans than in animals, methods have been developed to track consumption of at least macronutrients. For example, the use of a vending machine to dispense isocaloric, high-carbohydrate or high-protein snacks allowed the identification of individuals predisposed to selecting one set or the other (190). Consequently, in both animals and humans, experimental techniques exist for monitoring the self-selection of nutritionally different foods. What mechanisms regulate this phenomenon and what are the methodological problems that confront its investigation?

B. Learning or Physiology?

It appears that processes of food selection depend heavily on mechanisms of learning. That is, the omnivores profit by experience. In learning about food materials it is necessary to monitor and store information about the taste and texture of food items, their frequency of occurrence, their location, and other factors including their total concentrations of key nutrients and their nutrient densities. To be useful, all of this information must be matched against conditions in the internal environment. The classic studies in this area concern thiamine. Initially, it was demonstrated that thiamine-deficient rats could make appropriate dietary choices to alleviate the vitamin deficiency (82). Given a choice of three foods, one supplemented with B vitamins, rats deficient in vitamin B quickly came to choose the enriched food. Whereas thiamine-deficient animals strongly preferred the thiamine-enriched choice, control animals did not. Subsequently, it was shown that thiamine-deficient rats display an inclination to sample new foods at well-spaced intervals. The spacing allows time for the emergence of the metabolic consequences of consuming the food. If a vitamin-B-deficient animal samples a thiamine-rich diet it apparently is able to associate the diet's beneficial effects with its perceived sensory properties (for review, see ref. 158). The animal behaves in the most logical way to overcome the problem faced by the metabolic deficiency, and this strategy provides an opportunity of gaining the information that can lead to a solution. This general paradigm can account for deficiency learning (learning to overcome the lack of a particular item), poison avoidance (learning to avoid a diet that has produced illness), and specific appetites (learning to select essential dietary components).

This paradigm involves the particular sequence of behavioral acts carried out by an animal together with the synthesis of sensory and metabolic information. It can account in large part for the adaptability displayed by omnivores. However, this type of process, usually referred to as learning, is often set against an alternative so-called physiological process in which an internal sensor mechanism detects the elements of a dietary input and guides the animal's actions accordingly. However, even in this type of system the animal must always relate the reading of the sensor mechanism to certain external features associated with the food material—its taste, texture, or location. This association can also be called learning. Consequently the distinction between learning and physiology is false. All rational selection of dietary materials involves the process of relating the physiological consequences of eating a food to its external properties. It therefore seems appropriate to avoid confrontations between psychological (learning) and physiological explanations for selection, and instead to direct attention to identifying the mechanisms which couple a food's metabolic effects to its sensory properties.

C. Statement of Problem

Much of the research that has been carried out on nutrient selection would be referred to as normal science (96) and has been concerned with the solving of puzzles and with the gradual accumulation of knowledge from small amounts of information. This is the most common form of progress in basic science (97). In contrast, only a small portion of research could be called "extraordinary science," which is concerned with the testing of theories. Although a certain theoretical picture has developed from the normal-science approach, in recent years one clearly stated theory has emerged from biochemical and behavioral experiments. This theory arose initially as a proposal of the relationship between the effects of foods modifying plasma amino acid levels and the synthesis of neurotransmitters in the brain (see refs. 63,64 for reviews). The resulting changes in release of the neurotransmitters are thought to be involved in the mechanisms controlling food choice, particularly the selection of dietary protein and carbohydrate (65,191). This theory, which incorporates a mechanism of nutrient selection, is limited in that it is not concerned with the selection of fats, vitamins, or minerals, nor with deficiency learning or poison avoidance. However, the theory embodies proposals for the control of specific appetites for protein and carbohydrate and has prompted the use of pharmacological and neurochemical tools to study this process. This chapter will present a critical review of such theoretical approaches in the light of the conceptual issues set out above and in relation to methodological factors involved in research on nutrient selection. The review will examine processes and problems in the control of food selection.

III. MACRONUTRIENT SELECTION: MAJOR ISSUES

At the present stage of research, the field may be divided into three interrelated issues:

(a) Are macronutrient intakes (particularly protein and carbohydrate) independently regulated?

(b) If regulation exists, what is the nature of the regulatory mechanism? If there is no strict regulation, what processes control the intakes of protein and carbohydrate?

(c) Can protein and carbohydrate intakes be experimentally manipulated as predicted from our understanding of the regulatory mechanisms?

A. Are Protein and Carbohydrate Intakes Regulated?

Mechanisms underlying food selection clearly depend on the regulation of macronutrients. If protein and carbohydrate are not regulated, then maintaining adequate supplies of these items cannot be attributed to food selection. In turn, the issue is related to the question of whether or not total food intake is precisely controlled and whether this serves to regulate some ulterior parameter such as body weight.

For many animals, including man, once the period of rapid growth has occurred the body size remains fairly constant over a period of time. This observation has led some theorists to suppose that the size of the body or some feature correlated with body size is actively regulated. In turn, one suggestion is that constancy is maintained by reference to a "set point" embodied in physiological mechanisms that ultimately control energy intake and expenditure (e.g., refs. 92,127). Other theorists have argued that bodily features (total body energy, body fat, or body weight) are not actively regulated about set values but that apparent constancy is maintained by a natural balance between intake and output (34,73). Moreover, it is known that stability within a controlled system can be maintained by regulatory factors without the inclusion of a set point; accordingly, the term "settling point" may give a more appropriate description of the working of such a system (54,182). Incorporated in the idea that body weight "settles" but is not "set" is the concept that food intake is not precisely controlled but may be stabilized by an *interaction* between factors in the internal and external domains. The notion of a set point is an integral part of mathematical control theory but the set point may not have a physiological counterpart (145). This does not mean that the system does not possess regulatory properties. The system will display purposeful activity (drive) and will seek to maintain bodily constituents around preferred values, but this tendency is mitigated by circumstances in the external environment.

In the short term, if total food intake is subject to regulatory influences but not precisely controlled, what happens to the selected intakes of protein and carbohydrate? Most research has been devoted to the problem of protein regulation. To what extent do omnivores exert control over the intake of protein? For some years the possibility has been recognized that dietary proteins and plasma amino acids play a role in the control of total food intake (123). Generally, animals decrease their food intake when fed diets in which the protein content is very low, very high, or deficient in an indispensable amino acid, or in which the protein intake pattern is grossly different from that needed to supply the animal's amino acid requirements (for reviews see refs. 80,81).

This suppression of food intake has been attributed to alterations in free amino acids in body fluids that provide signals monitored by the brain (154). However, it is perhaps more feasible that amino acids should be involved in the control of protein rather than total food intake. First, it has been demonstrated that rats allowed to select from a protein-containing but energy-free diet or a protein-free but otherwise complete diet tended to adjust intakes over a few days in the direction appropriate to maintain a fairly constant protein intake (33). This presumably would occur most effectively when feeding is not heavily influenced by energy need, extremes of palatability, or other environmental demands such as selection habits. Second, when weanling rats self-selected their intake from two diets varying in protein content (quantity, quality, or density), although absolute intake of protein (casein) varied, the rats were observed to maintain a constant value of the protein energy percent—the amount of protein relative to total calories consumed (128). This finding was in agreement with a previous study also carried out on young (30-day-old) rats (49). Here rats choosing from a protein or carbohydrate diet selected a constant proportion of protein to carbohydrate when the nature of the protein diet was experimentally manipulated. In a similar choice experiment in which rats (60 days old) were allowed to select from a protein-free diet or from two diets varying in protein concentration (at various stages of the experiment) a constant absolute intake of protein was observed (161). However, the protein also remained a constant percentage of the total calories suggesting that, in some way, the nonprotein portion of the intake (a mixture of sucrose, dextrose, dextrin, minerals, vitamins, celluflour, vegetable shortening, and corn oil) was being adjusted to protein intake. These findings have been interpreted as evidence for the separate identity of mechanisms controlling protein and total energy intake. On the basis of the rat's ability to increase pure protein intake when the source was experimentally diluted, Rozin (156) had earlier concluded that protein intake could be separately regulated.

However, if protein intake is independently controlled, it is not clear what internal parameter is maintained as a result of this management. Certainly, the quantity of protein selected does not appear to be closely related to requirements for growth or weight gain (4,49), parameters that had earlier been considered criterion indices for the rational control of food selection. Moreover, it is noticeable that there is not total agreement among the results of the above experiments; some report constancy of absolute protein values, others a constancy of protein intake relative to total, whereas others show only approximations to maintenance of stable protein intake. This variability may be a function of the degree of imprecision in the underlying mechanism (or mechanisms), or it could depend on technical and procedural differences of the experiments including the nature of the protein offered (e.g., casein vs. cottonseed flour), the percentage of protein in the diet (pure, 100%, or some lower fraction), or textural features (solid, liquid, or gel) that affect the sensory properties and the acceptability of the diet. Although it is clear that protein is regulated metabolically through the balance of body nitrogen, the evidence suggests that there is some behavioral control of protein intake. This evidence does not reveal the reason for this control or the mechanism involved. Indeed the variability of the above findings (control of absolute or relative protein intake) suggests that the mechanism guiding behavioral control of protein intake may not be aimed at preserving protein intake at a particular set value but rather to keep intake within upper and lower limits. Provided that an animal eats enough protein to satisfy minimal requirements for growth and tissue repair, and avoids excessive overload of amino acids, the mechanism for behavioral control could operate over a fairly broad range. Small errors in behavior control could be compensated for by metabolic regulation. Two further points can be mentioned here. First, the rather precise control noted in some experiments could arise when the behavioral mechanism acts to maintain protein intake at the previously "educated" level for that particular group of rats. Naturally this learned level of intake need not be the same for all animals. Second, in a self-selection design the avoidance of very low or very high protein intakes could be managed by mechanisms for "poison avoidance" (e.g., ref. 158). Of course this mechanism requires a constant set of environmental circumstances to operate effectively. Accordingly, some mechanism for the behavioral control of protein, under circumstances permitting selection, is required that operates within the quantitative middle ranges of intake and that could act in the short term to cope with shifting environmental circumstances.

B. Mechanisms Controlling Macronutrient Intake

For the control of total food intake theoretical approaches have embodied a variety of levels of explanation and have emphasized different types of structures and events in the physiological system. For example, the central focus of Young's theory has been the sensory impact of food (194), whereas certain neural theories have emphasized the integrative capacity of brain structures, particularly the hypothalamus (79,170) or monoamine pathways (19,83,86). Other approaches have given priority to peripheral physiological systems (66), gastrointestinal structures such as the stomach (55), or peripherally acting hormones such as cholecystokinin (168). Conceptions emphasizing the monitoring of physiological parameters have included the traditional thermostatic (40), lipostatic (93), and aminostatic (123) theories, together with a more recent postulation of energy flow (39). In summary, it can be noted that theoretical attempts have favored almost every aspect of the total physiological system, some hypotheses covering the interaction between central and peripheral events (e.g., refs. 129,135), and some constructed on the interplay between internal and external factors (e.g., ref. 151) or between physiological variables and psychological constructs (20). Very few approaches have attended to food choice or nutrient selection.

In the opinion of the author the weakness of many of the theoretical statements described above resides in the consideration of food intake as a unitary variable. Feeding behavior is a complex and adaptable activity that is articulated in a pattern of behavioral actions that can be regarded as "behavioral flux" (29). The search for a single regulatory principle for food intake has frequently overlooked the behavioral complexity of feeding and has tended to simplify the nature of the underlying mechanism. The characterization of this mechanism could be more realistically described by including processes of nutrient selection.

As noted in the previous section, when animals are given a choice of diets, they can maintain fairly constant absolute or proportional intakes of protein. This does not prove that some constituent is being monitored—such stability could arise from external qualities of the diets—but it constitutes *prima facie* evidence for the existence of control. What is the nature of the control? Schonfeld and Hamilton (161) have suggested that "mechanisms controlling protein intake could include (a) a monitor of the absolute amount of protein ingested with adjustment to a value that varies with age and sex; (b) an adjustment of caloric intake such that protein remains a fixed percentage of total calories ingested; (c) a sensing of concentration (and other properties) of protein sources to elicit behaviors that would maintain a constant input of protein or protect against an imbalance of blood amino acids; and (d) an adjustment of behavior to drastic changes in availability and quality of protein sources, perhaps by means of conditioned aversions or preferences."

It has already been recognized (see previous section) that in the long term the main task of such a mechanism should be to control intakes over moderate ranges and not at extreme values. However, in the short term (i.e., meal-to-meal regulation) the mechanism may act to ensure that a meal high in one nutrient (e.g., protein) will be followed by a meal high in the other (e.g. carbohydrate). In general terms this mechanism must possess:

(a) a means of reflecting the protein content of the diet in some metabolized internal variable;

(b) a process whereby the level of this variable is detected or interpreted by the brain;

(c) a way of associating this brain information with perceptual characteristics of the consumed diet, and of maintaining a memory for this;

(d) some means of initiating and guiding behavior toward an appropriate diet (in the laboratory this would consist of a constraint over an animal's choice of an available sample, but under natural circumstances it may require the initiation of a search process to locate and then sample a particular type of food).

Of course, in considering a scheme such as this to account for purposeful and selective behavior by an animal it must be remembered that animals (not least the rat) can cope to some extent with nonpreferred protein intakes by adjustments of the many enzymes responsible for degrading amino acids (6,172).

At the base of most conceptualizations of the control of protein intake is the proposal that the protein content of the diet (identified as dietary amino acids) is reflected in the profile of blood plasma amino acids (step a above). In turn, it is argued that some rational relationship should exist between the plasma amino acid profile and the pattern of amino acids in the brain (e.g., ref. 140). Brain lesion studies (113,114) have been interpreted as suggesting that a receptor system for the growth-limiting amino acid may exist in the prepyriform cortex or the medial amygdala. The nature of this receptor system is not known. More recently, other researchers have suggested that branched-chain amino acids (leucine, isoleucine, valine) may serve as the signal of protein intake that is detected by the brain. The site or mechanism of the brain's interpretation of this central amino acid signal is not known.

An alternative view has arisen from research at the University of Toronto and at MIT. The major unique element of this view is that the amino acid profile in the brain contains precursors of neurotransmitters; consequently, the protein content of the diet can be represented, via plasma and brain amino acid patterns, in brain neurochemical activity. This process dispenses with the need for specialized chemoreceptors to detect amino acids.

A number of dietary constituents can affect central metabolism in this way. All neurotransmitters whose syntheses are known to be influenced by precursor availability are produced from compounds that must be obtained in whole or in part from the diet (see ref. 191 for review). Tryptophan, like threonine, cannot be synthesized at all by mammalian cells and is truly an essential amino acid. Tyrosine is formed in the liver and in the brain from phenylalanine, but phenylalanine is itself an essential amino acid. Choline, like tyrosine, can be formed in liver and brain but the major portion of choline in the blood normally derives from dietary lecithin. With regard to food selection, the important precursors are tryptophan and tyrosine, and of these the most cohesive body of evidence exists for the synthesis of brain serotonin from tryptophan. The details of this process have been presented by Fernstrom and Wurtman (61–63). Crucial features include the competition between plasma tryptophan and other large neutral amino acids (leucine, isoleucine, valine, phenylalanine, threonine, and methionine) for the transport system of the blood–brain barrier, and the influence of insulin on brain serotonin synthesis. It follows that entry of circulating tryptophan into the brain can be facilitated by raising plasma tryptophan or by lowering plasma levels of other large neutral amino acids. Insulin has little effect on plasma tryptophan levels but does lower plasma levels of other large neutral amino acids (LNAA), thereby increasing the plasma tryptophan ratio. The maintenance of plasma tryptophan is brought about by an increase in the amount of tryptophan bound to albumin (at the expense of nonesterified fatty acids), which makes up for the fall in plasma free tryptophan. Therefore, the effect of any meal on the plasma tryptophan ratio will depend on the contribution of amino acids in the diet and the postprandial secretion of insulin. A high carbohydrate meal—causing a substantial release of insulin—will cause the plasma tryptophan ratio to rise whereas a high protein meal will cause it to fall. Since the plasma tryptophan ratio is related to brain serotonin synthesis, it has been argued that serotonin-releasing brain neurons can function as variable ratio sensors that respond to the protein content of the diet. Consequently, in this hypothesis nutrient selection is related to plasma and brain tryptophan and ultimately to the neurotransmitter serotonin.

Studies have also been carried out to examine plasma amino acid patterns in relation to protein intake in rats self-selecting from a choice of diets (5,9,10). After weanling rats had stabilized their selection of food from diets varying only in the quantity of protein (amino acid manipulations altered the quality of the protein), blood was taken, and the plasma amino acid composition was related to the proportion of protein to energy consumed. The most striking relationship—irrespective of the amino acid content of the proteins fed—was the inverse correlation between protein intake and plasma tryptophan ratio. Ashley and Anderson (10) suggested that this plasma tryptophan to LNAA ratio triggered a brain serotoninergic mechanism dealing mainly with the control of protein intake.

There is a good deal of evidence showing that experimental manipulations of serotonin exert strong effects on total food intake (for reviews see refs. 19,21) and on various aspects of the behavioral patterns of feeding (26,27,101). Since most of the studies have used only single-composite diets it is conceivable that under such circumstances rats may adjust total intake as their only available means of altering protein (or carbohydrate) intake.

Despite the arguments set out above, it should be considered that any relationship existing between dietary manipulation, brain neurotransmitters, and feeding behavior is probably complex and will be very difficult to investigate. Some dietary-induced increases or decreases in whole brain tryptophan and serotonin do not appear to be readily linked to eating behavior. This is necessarily true since a 24-hr period of food deprivation has been shown to increase brain tryptophan concentration (53) and to increase sertonin synthesis (141) in a manner similar to the administration of certain diets. Indeed, it has been shown that food restriction will significantly decrease protein intake and the ratio of protein to total energy (120). The reason why deprivation and feeding may, under certain circumstances, show apparently similar effects on serotonin metabolism yet opposite effects on eating is almost certainly because the procedures differentially influence other amine systems involved in feeding, and these changes must be considered together with the modification of serotonin systems. For example, Fig. 1 illustrates one way in which

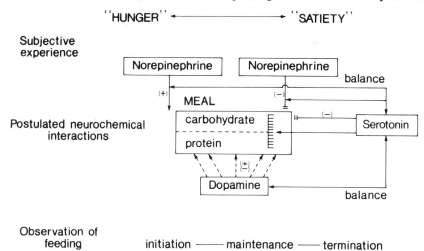

FIG. 1. Working conceptualization of the way in which neurotransmitter systems may interact to control food intake. This model implies that these neurotransmitters (and others) act conjointly to organize the expression of feeding behavior—certain systems initiate consumption, others bring an episode of eating to a halt or adjust the selection of macronutrients, whereas others alter the rate of eating. It follows that manipulation of any of these systems will influence consumption but that the characteristics of the adjustment will depend on the particular neurotransmitter chiefly involved.

various neurotransmitter systems may influence total food intake and selection by acting upon various aspects—initiation, maintenance, termination, and choice of eating behavior (22,30). Ultimately, elucidation of the neurochemical links between diet and eating behavior will probably require the simultaneous monitoring of alterations in several brain amines and other neurotransmitters as well. Moreover, the feedback effect from neurotransmitter synthesis to feeding behavior may involve qualitative rather than quantitative adustments in food intake. One qualitative aspect of food intake is nutrient selection, and the following section will examine the results of recent experimental manipulations—mainly pharmacological, neurochemical, and hormonal—of the selection of nutrients and the implications of these findings for theories of nutrient intake and for the methodology of studies on feeding.

IV. STRUCTURE OF SELF-SELECTION EXPERIMENTS

Most of the experimental investigations of nutrient intake to be considered here have used a self-selection design in which animals (usually rats) have been allowed to eat from two or more foods. Clearly the designs of such investigations may vary in a number of experimental parameters, each of which could potentially influence the outcome. Experiments are constructed with the understanding that rats will select from particular diets on the basis of the nutrient content, but it is clear that selection may be influenced heavily by the number of choices offered, differences in taste and texture of the diets, location of the foods, concentration of nutrients, physical structure of the diets, temperature, housing conditions, and length of habituation to the experimental regimen. Interestingly, in a comparison of seven studies judged to produce favorable outcomes and seven regarded as unfavorable, Lát (100) found that conditions such as those mentioned above were not critical to the outcome. This did not mean that the conditions were ineffective. However, Lát's judgments of favorable or unfavorable were based on the rate of growth, one of the criteria traditionally used to assess the adequacy of diet selection. However, in many studies on the *mechanisms* of nutrient intake the experiments are brief and often no attempt is made to evaluate the long-term effect of consumption on rate of growth or longevity. Accordingly, the interpretation of diet selection in *short-term studies* is not straightforward, and adjustments in the pattern of selection cannot be assumed to have arisen because of the nutrient content of the diet. Moreover, it seems likely that peripheral variables would exert a disproportionately great influence in studies involving brief data-collection periods, particularly when some further strong experimental manipulation is operating. For these reasons *brief* experiments on nutrient intake using the self-selection design should be subjected to critical examination. Some variables most likely to influence selection are considered below.

A. Sensory Characteristics of Diets

It is obvious that the sensory impact of a food influences the preference, or liking, for that diet. The acceptability, or initial willingness to consume, is only one way in which sensory factors (particularly taste) can modulate intake. Sensory data can be used in the following ways:

(a) *Trigger:* To induce early or anticipatory responses to consumption such as the cephalic phase of insulin release (144).

(b) *Cue (signal):* Essential element of associative processes such as those involved in taste-aversion conditioning (e.g., refs. 72,146), and more generally in the conditioning of appetite (acceptance) and satiation (rejection) (35,171). Sensory cues have been demonstrated to be operative in animal and human studies (37).

(c) *Reward:* Taste qualities alone can be used as reinforcers to increase the probability of occurrence of responses occurring immediately before. Saccharine, a nonnutritive sweetener, is widely used as a reinforcer in operant learning situations.

(d) *Pleasure:* Difficult concept to deal with in the context of animal experiments but may be regarded as an internal state that mediates in the expression of a preference. In human experiments subjectively experienced liking for a food may be evaluated by rating scales or other devices (e.g., ref. 32). In animal studies such a state may only be inferred, or may be defined operationally by an animal's willingness to begin eating or to continue eating (*see* f, *below*).

(e) *Identifier (label):* Taste may be used to inform about some aspect of the content of a diet, such as its protein or carbohydrate value, not necessarily related to the capacity of the diet to bring about satiation. Identifying characteristics may be either innate, such as sweetness, or acquired.

(f) *Releaser:* Qualities of the diet give rise to oral responses of acceptance or rejection (78). The basic pattern is innate but use of conditioning techniques allows these responses to be separated from other internal responses such as insulin release (18).

It follows that the influence on consumption contributed by taste cannot be considered a unitary effect. This sensory dimension can affect the initiation, maintenance, or termination of consumption in a variety of ways.

B. Structural Form of Diet

Obviously, the structural characteristic of a diet—its texture—is one aspect, along with taste, of its sensory properties. Texture is considered here as a separate factor although the two dimensions of taste and texture will certainly act conjointly to determine a food's acceptability. Generally speaking, diets may be presented as liquids, gels (semisolids), or solids. In the solid form foods may occur as powders, granules, chips, or blocks. In these forms it is possible to obtain good control over the nutritional content of the diets (cf situation used to induce dietary obesity in which a variety of human foods of uncontrolled nutritional value is presented to the rat, e.g., refs. 89,163). Not surprisingly rats do not find all of these dietary forms equally acceptable; though given the choice between eating a nonpreferred food or nothing rats will normally eat. Powders appear to be least preferred and are difficult for rats to consume; they may be regarded as slightly aversive. Granules are more readily accepted, and blocks of food are probably most preferred because of the rat's natural tendency to grasp food materials with its forepaws and to nibble. Gels are accepted by rats but may be low in nutrient concentration, owing to their inclusion of nonnutritional agar or of similar substance to bind the elements together. Is it possible that the same diet presented in different physical forms (in a self-selection design) will affect nutrient intake? In a test of this possibility, McArthur and Blundell (121) presented rats with a choice of isocaloric 5 and 45% protein diets (see Table 1). The diets were available in three textures. In one diet a granular form of casein was used (ANRC), whereas a second diet included a powdery form of casein (BDH). An addition of agar converted the BDH diet into a gel form. Groups of rats were allowed to feed freely from these diets for 21 days. Figure 2 illustrates that during this period the structure of the diets not only influenced the body weight of the rats but also affected total food consumed, absolute protein intakes, and protein energy percent. This experiment incorporated an important control for evaporation sustained by gel diets. In this study gel lost weight linearly at the rate of 0.31 g/hr. With daily measurements this factor makes a considerable difference to the calculated consumption of gel.

These data illustrate that rats will vary nutrient intake according to the form of the diet and are an example of the type of interaction referred to in section II.A.

Apart from these dietary forms rats are sometimes obliged to consume all of their nutrients as liquids. Indeed, Rozin (156) used a liquid cafeteria in which the three major macronutrients—protein, fat, and carbohydrate—were all presented sepa-

TABLE 1. *Composition of the experimental diets and calculation of caloric density*

	Nutrient composition (g/100)		Caloric density (kJ/g)[a]	
	5% Protein	45% Protein	5% Protein	45% Protein
Cornstarch	80.70	40.70	13.48	6.80
Casein	5.00	45.00	0.83	7.51
Corn oil	10.00	10.00	3.77	3.77
Vitamin mix[b]	0.50	0.50	—	—
Mineral mix[c]	3.80	3.80	—	—
Total caloric density			18.08	18.08

[a]Based on the Atwater factors of cornstarch (16.7), casein (16.7), and corn oil (37.7 kJ/g).

[b]The vitamin mixture was composed of: vitamin D_3 (4,000,000 IU/g) (0.4%), vitamin A (5,000,000 IU/g) (3.2%), vitamin E (250 IU/g) (48.0%), thiamin (0.8%), riboflavin (1.6%), niacinamide (10.0%), DL-pantothenic acid (80% Ca salt) (3.0%), folic acid (2.0%), vitamin B_{12} (relative potency of 1 mg vitamin B_{12}/kg) (2.4%), pyrodoxine (1.2%), vitamin K (22.5% menadione) (2.0%), nonnutritive fiber (925.4 g/kg of mixture) (Labsure Animal Foods, Poole, Dorset).

[c]The mineral mixture was prepared according to the procedure described previously (Musten et al., ref. 128).

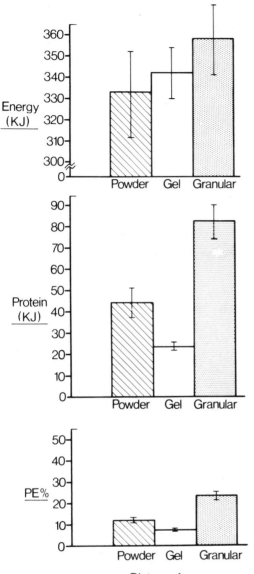

FIG. 2. Effect of the form of the diet (powder, granular, gel) on intake of total calories, protein, and PE%. The diets have significant effects on protein intake [$F(2,21) = 20.4$, $p < 0.01$] and PE% [$F(2,21) = 24.4$, $p < 0.01$]. KJ, kilojoules. PE% = protein consumed (KJ) as percentage of total energy.

rately as fluids. In certain self-selection experiments (see ref. 100) a mixed array of solid and liquid dietary commodities was presented. Here, basic preferences based on texture are likely to bias short-term consumption. Moreover, even when all nutrients are presented as liquids, textural differences will be apparent depending on the nature of the fluid, whether aqueous or oily. Consequently, sensory preferences may again interfere with the selection of nutrients. Even with very careful control of diet composition and structure it is unlikely that diets can be produced with absolutely equal levels of acceptability. Moreover, when rats are offered liquid diets, even with additional water present, there exists the possibility of confounding food ingestion with drinking behavior. Under these circumstances there seems to be no way of judging the extent to which animals are consuming a particular fluid in the interests of osmoregulation or the regulation of nutrients or calories. Consequently, the amount of fluid consumed (usually a dependent variable) may not be a good indicator of the amount of nutrient required. Of course, if rats are to learn an association between nutrient contents and diets, then the diets must be discriminable on the basis of sensory qualities—smell, taste, or texture—or according to the place where they are located (or some cue such as color or pattern of food dish acting as an identifier). Since the positions of diets are normally randomized in self-selection tests and visual coding is rarely used, the diets must be sensorily different to permit rational selection to occur. The problem is how to create discriminable diets without introducing a sensory preference. In addition to the way in which structural features of the diet point out methodological issues pertinent to the design of experiments, more fundamental problems concerning the theoretical basis of selection are raised *(see below)*.

C. Nutrient Composition of Diets

When the purpose of experiments was to establish whether or not animals could self-select a balanced diet capable of supporting growth it was sufficient to present a complete array of all essential dietary elements—macronutrients, minerals, vitamins, and salts. However, in experimental manipulations of the selection process in which only one dietary factor may be the dependent variable, it is essential that animals maintain an adequate supply of all elements apart from the critical factor being allowed to vary. Consequently, the vast topic of nutrient compositions can be reduced to two fundamental issues:

    (a) Should macronutrients be used in a pure form or as part of a composite diet?
    (b) How many choices should be available?

In assessing the effects of manipulations on individual macronutrients, the presentation of individual dishes containing fats, proteins, and carbohydrates obviously affords a clear separation of the measurable elements (usually a vitamin-salt supplement is supplied). However, the individual nutrients differ in smell, taste, and texture as well as in caloric density. When there is large variation in caloric density, rats may consume a diet for calories rather than for specific nutrients. Intake may, therefore, be unduly biased by a variety of uncontrolled variables. On the other hand, composite diets containing different proportions of macronutrients can be made isocaloric and attempts made to minimize differences in sensory qualities. In the preparation of composite diets each choice usually contains a complete range of vitamins and minerals. However, one problem arises immediately, for it has been demonstrated that the nature of the mineral mixture can significantly influence the amount of protein consumed (108). In addition, it should be noted that mineral oil, when used as a noncaloric constituent to equate diets for textural qualities (e.g., ref. 136), impairs the digestion of sucrose and starch, produces diarrhea, and leads to the expulsion of fat-soluble vitamins.

Manipulation of the proportions of macronutrients of composite diets has two implications. First, researchers are forced to disclose the particular macronutrient under investigation; second, they are faced with the question of how many choices to present to the animals. (For researchers using separate purified macronutrients the choice of number is made automatically and simultaneous observations can be made of all three components). The choice facing researchers is not merely one of technical neatness, for the experimental designs differentiate between the inductive and deductive approaches.

In using composite diets a two-choice paradigm has become established. However, a problem arises because with two choices and three macronutrients the adjustment of one factor must result in the alteration of another if the diets are to remain isocaloric. For example, if two diets vary in protein content (say 20 vs. 40%) and if fat content is held constant, then the proportion of carbohydrate must also vary. Therefore, a low-protein diet will also be a high-carbohydrate diet and vice versa. Alternatively, a low-protein, isocaloric diet could be achieved by adjustments in the proportions of both the other commodities. To maintain diets isocaloric and to vary protein inclusion while holding each of the other two macronutrients constant in turn will obviously require four choices, not two. However, it is likely that the introduction of this experimental maneuver would only serve to complicate outcomes, for such macronutrient adjustments cannot be carried out with impunity; each alteration changes the sensory qualities of the diet. Without undermining methodological rigor, perhaps it should be admitted that food consumption will always be based on some balance between macronutrient content and sensory characteristics. There may be circumstances in which animals will compromise macronutrient intake to maintain intake of a food preferred for its taste, texture, or ease of consumption. A massive undertaking would be required to test this hypothesis and to provide complete control over the sensory dimension while manipulating macronutrient values.

D. Ecological Validity and Preparedness

One of the major reasons for examining the structure of self-selection experiments is to evaluate external validity, that is, the capacity of experiments to be representative of natural circumstances. In the laboratory, rats are required to lick liquid foods from a drinkometer, scrape or bite pieces from a gel block, lick up powdered food from a dish, pull blocks from a hopper, and recognize varying concentrations of nutrients presented separately or in combination. Thinking teleologically, one can ask whether or not the biological system was designed to cope equally well with all of these tasks. This raises the issue of "preparedness" (166,167), a concept that arose out of a consideration of mechanisms of learning and of the tasks that animals are obliged to learn in laboratories. A dimension of preparedness was suggested by means of which each species, according to biological endowments and evolutionary history, would be prepared, unprepared, or contraprepared to acquire certain skills or to solve particular problems. This concept can be applied to the self-selection of nutrients. For example, how well are rats conceptually equipped to consume all of their nutrients in liquid form? First, it is known that a liquid diet causes malabsorption of nutrients through diarrhea, and, given alternative sources of food, rats would presumably strive to alleviate this condition by choosing solid food. Second, the rat's physiological system has not developed to accommodate the possibility of meeting all proteins, carbohydrates, and fats as fluids. Consequently, the regulatory system may not function optimally when dealing with the rate of intake, gastric filling, and intestinal absorption associated with this form of diet.

Criticisms may be raised also against the use of powdered food. The act of licking up finely milled materials without use of the forepaws is a very unusual eating posture for the rat. Consumption of powders tends to be lower than other forms of food; one reason may be the difficulty of making the appropriate motor movements and the problems of ingesting a very dry material. If rats are unprepared or contraprepared to consume a particular form of food then the problems of overcoming this disadvantage may interfere with the monitoring of nutrient content or with the development of associations between nutrient content and sensory characteristics.

The use of purified and separate sources of nutrients may also be questioned, since the rat's system would not be expected to deal with such isolated and concentrated forms of nutrients. Studies of pure stimuli out of context may not explain what happens in real life. With composite diets, artificially produced, problems exist in the blending of nutrient content, texture, and taste. It may be presumed that rats are not naturally prepared to form associations between all possible combinations of nutrient density and the taste (or texture) of a diet. Moreover, the capacity of rats to perform place learning experiments suggests that the common precaution of randomly adjusting the position of food containers in self-selection experiments may fail to capitalize on the rat's ability to recognize a food according to its usual location, and may serve to restrict the rat's repertoire for obtaining information about the nature of the food it eats.

Self-selection experiments are tests of an organism's adaptability. In turn, adaptability represents the capacity to use informational cues to make appropriate behavioral actions. Some cues are more important than others (carry more information) and have a greater probability of being associated with a veridical outcome. The notion of probabilistic functionalism (43) can be applied to the selection of foods. Designs that compromise the preparedness of rats to display their abilities may be expected to distort the outcomes of experiments. Even if animals possess the capacity to regulate macronutrient intake, their capacity to demonstrate this may be distorted by arbitrary choice of experimental parameters. Differences in results from different laboratories should be expected, and we should not be surprised by this. The real question is to decide whether these differences are due to idiosyncratic selection of variables or to the absence of a precise regulatory system.

V. EXPERIMENTAL MANIPULATIONS OF NUTRIENT INTAKE

A. Drug Treatments

Drugs have been widely used in the study of food intake, and agents exist that give rise to hypo- or hyperphagia, or to both effects depending on experimental circumstances (e.g., 24). The most common effect is a suppression of intake.

1. Pharmacology of Anorexia

This field of study has been characterized by four predominant experimental features:

(a) Presentation of a single food. Traditionally rats (or other small animals) have been allowed access to only a single diet. In most cases this is a composite diet containing a balanced range of nutrients. However, exceptions to this rule make it clear that not only is one food considered sufficient to investigate drug effects but also that for certain researchers all foods may be considered equal. Table 2 illustrates the wide range of foods that have been presented to rats as alternatives to rodent laboratory chow. Clearly these foods differ greatly in macronutrient content and in sensory characteristics. The suppression of intake by drugs therefore represents a severe and global inhibition, particularly since drug effects are often considered significant only when they produce a 50% reduction in intake (ED_{50}).

(b) Single variable measured. The use of a single diet is often coupled with the use of one dependent variable—total amount of food eaten, usually expressed in grams rather than calories. Accordingly, the pharmacology of anorexia is primarily concerned with the mass of consumed material rather than with its nutritional or metabolic qualities.

TABLE 2. *Various test foods used in evaluating the effects of chemical agents on food consumption*

Food	Investigators
Beef broth	Abdallah and White (1970)
Carrots	Zelger and Carlini (1980)
Potatoes	Cross et al. (1977)
Spaghetti	Wynn and Redgrave (1979)
Meal worms	Broekamp et al. (1974)
Condensed milk	Numerous investigators
Dog food	Watson and Cox (1976)
Breakfast cereal	Edwards and Ritter (1981)

(c) Food deprivation and feeding regimens. In most experiments with drugs as the independent variable rats are subjected to lengthy periods of food deprivation (16 to 48 hr) prior to the test period. Alternatively, the animals may be placed on cyclic feeding regimens in which food is available for only a few hours per day.

(d) Short food tests. Experiments with anorectic drugs typically use brief measurement periods of 1 or 2 hr.

There are good reasons for believing that these procedures are not optimally effective for producing precise information about drug action or for shedding light on the processes controlling food intake. First, a simple measure of the weight of food consumed in a discrete interval of time may conceal information about the manner in which pharmacological treatment inhibited food consumption. For example, an animal may fail to eat because of the nonspecific disruption of any controlled sequential behavior by competing or interfering activities. Second, although brief periods of eating following long periods of deprivation are typical of drug experiments, they are not typical of animal behavior and are not usually encountered in natural rat feeding repertoires. Consequently, it is possible that drugs are being evaluated under highly abnormal circumstances. Certain researchers (47,84) have specifically drawn attention to the need to construct experimental analogues of the natural environment to discover the nature of the systems governing natural feeding. Third, it is known that food deprivation can modify brain neurotransmitter levels. Consequently, agents administered to severely deprived animals may be intervening in atypical brain metabolism.

In summary, the combined use of severe deprivation periods and short food tests represents a procedure that may be highly insensitive to certain pharmacological effects, may create circumstances for abnormal animal behavior, and may modify drug action in an unknown way by altering brain chemistry. In addition, the normal use of one single food prevents the disclosure of any information about nutrient preferences or food selection. Most of these defects can be overcome by using free-feeding animals, allowed access to a choice of diets, and monitoring the pattern of nutrient selection in addition to various meal parameters such as meal number, meal size, and intermeal intervals together with ratios between these values. In addition, continuous sampling procedures can be used to describe changes in the microstructure of feeding events (e.g., 180,181). Such recordings provide an indication of an animal's rate of consumption and elucidate mechanisms controlling the onset, maintenance, and termination of eating episodes (26). These methodological issues are important for, in observing the effect of a drug on nutrient selection, it is necessary to establish whether some adjustment has been made to a control mechanism or whether the result has come about because of some arbitrary selection of experimental parameters. However, one possible problem with using free-feeding animals is that amino acid blood levels (dependent on the time since the animal's last meal) may not be similar in all animals at the start of the period of data collection.

Interestingly, in his 1967 review, Lát drew attention to the necessity of obtaining "continuous data" by means of automatic recording techniques to refine the analysis of self-selection. This idea was subsequently taken up by Leung and Rogers (114) to observe the effects on eating patterns of feeding an imbalanced diet. More recently a complete system (Fig. 3) has been developed for the continuous monitoring of nutrient selection, meal parameters, and intrameal events together with behavioral episodes that precede and follow episodes of eating (29). This system involves the on-line recording and computer analysis of intake from two different diets and the continuous video recording of the rat's behavior. It is, therefore, possible to relate nutrient selection to other qualitative features of a rat's feeding repertoire. In this way the mechanisms controlling nutrient selection can be investigated simultaneously with mechanisms involved in total food intake and in the expression of activities intimately associated with the feeding cycle. Central to this analysis is the identification of a feeding cycle in addition to a "meal." This feeding cycle includes three elements: first an appetitive phase of activity following a period of rest and before the occurrence of eating. Second, a feeding phase that includes all the activities occurring during the period of a traditionally defined meal, and leading up to, third, the period of sustained rest.

Analysis of the characteristics of the feeding cycle reveals a number of interesting features. First, once the rats have awakened from the period of sleep they rarely rest during the course of the feeding cycle until the onset of the next long episode of sleep. The feeding cycle is a very active period characterized by considerable locomotor activity and a great deal of grooming. Indeed, grooming is the most frequently displayed behavior during the period of wakefulness, and is particularly

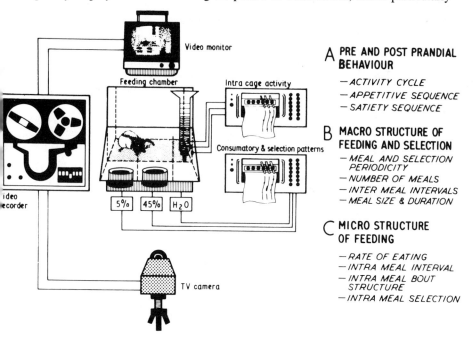

FIG. 3. General plan of the technique for the continuous monitoring of diet selection, meal patterns, and associated behaviors.

dominant during the appetitive phase (before the onset of eating) and during the satiety phase (following the cessation of eating and prior to sleep).

During the meal itself the rats in this study showed between 20 and 30 (average = 27.9) changes in behavior. Accordingly, the meal phase of the feeding cycle is a particularly active episode during which rats change frequently from one behavior to another.

Table 3 illustrates the patterns observed at each of the four meals chosen for analysis. These data show that the basic pattern of behavior shown in the "average" feeding cycle is preserved in the profiles of individual meals. It is noticeable that resting and drinking seldom occur during the appetitive phase. However, whereas rats show considerable drinking during the meal, resting rarely takes place in this phase. The dominance of grooming is again evident, particularly during the appetitive and satiety phases.

With regard to food consumption, it is clear that the rats spend more time eating from the low-protein source. However, since approximately equal amounts are eaten from each cup over the course of 24 hr, it follows that the high-protein diet must be eaten more rapidly.

The consistency with which various behaviors are represented in the phases of the feeding cycles, and the relationship between periods of sleep and of waking activities, suggests the existence of a firm structure to these patterns of activity. In addition, these data indicate that a behavior such as feeding is not an isolated event but is related to phases of activity that precede and follow a meal, and that within

TABLE 3. *Structure of feeding cycles at various times during the day*

	Behaviors (sec)	First meal	Second meal	Third meal	First meal after longest IMI
	Premeal IMI[a] rest	327.3	1,619.3	3,656.5	20,015.0
Appetitive phase	General activity	88.5	106.5	67.0	81.0
	Grooming	368.0	362.0	314.0	141.0
	Drinking	0.0	15.0	0.0	0.0
	Resting	6.0	0.0	0.0	1.5
Feeding phase	Low protein (5%)	197.0	422.0	341.0	411.0
	High protein (45%)	38.0	131.0	96.0	54.0
	General activity	108.0	86.0	90.0	40.0
	Grooming	416.0	475.0	606.0	269.0
	Drinking	17.0	37.0	34.0	3.0
	Resting	3.0	0.0	13.5	0.0
Satiety phase	General activity	27.0	92.0	44.0	62.0
	Grooming	242.0	470.0	187.0	624.0
	Drinking	6.0	29.0	12.0	33.0
	Resting	17.0	53.0	32.0	27.0
	Postmeal IMI rest	1,348.5	2,858.5	1,670.3	1,966.0

[a]IMI = intermeal interval.

the meal there is some rational relationship between episodes of eating, activity, and grooming. It may be presumed that these relationships are functional and play some role in the overall physiological economy of the animal. Accordingly, this behavioral structure provides an appropriate base on which to study the effects of pharmacological agents. Two points follow from this enterprise. First, any agent that interferes with the natural assembly of episodes of behavior during a feeding cycle may hinder the expression of eating; this would happen by an alteration of the basic behavioral pattern of which eating is a part. Second, because eating is intimately related to other behaviors, any drug-induced alteration in feeding is likely to produce some adjustment in the behaviors to which it is linked. Consequently, "specific" effects on eating should not be expected.

The use of a double-dissociation design involving two anorectic drugs (amphetamine and fenfluramine) with contrasting pharmacological profiles has revealed differences in nutrient selection patterns, differences in the profile of meal structure, and differences in the cycles of feeding and rest, which form a major part of a rat's behavioral repertoire (29). This is illustrated in Table 4, which shows that, during the feeding phase, amphetamine and fenfluramine have quite distinctive effects on consumption of high and low protein diets. These adjustments in diet intake can be related to other behavioral changes in the feeding cycle. However, most pharmacological experiments on nutrient selection have used less extensive experimental designs.

TABLE 4. *Effects of amphetamine and fenfluramine on diet selection and on the structure of behavior within the feeding cycle*

Behaviors	Saline	Amphetamine (1.0 mg/kg)	Saline	Fenfluramine (4.0 mg/kg)
Premeal IMI[a] rest	327.3	1,090.0	1,619.3	1,382.7
General activity	88.5 (4.5)	81.8 (6.5)	106.5 (6.5)	120.0 (5.8)
Grooming	368.0 (2.3)	385.5 (5.5)	362.0 (5.5)	320.0 (3.3)
Drinking	0.0	0.0	10.5 (0.8)	6.8 (0.5)
Resting	6.0 (0.3)	0.0	0.0	49.5 (1.5)
Low protein	197.0 (5.0)	335.3 (9.3)	422.0 (5.0)	403.0 (4.3)
High protein	38.0 (3.8)	72.8 (5.0)	131.0 (4.3)	231.0 (5.3)
General activity	108.0 (12.3)	615.8 (39.0)	86.0 (9.8)	132.0 (10.7)
Grooming	416.0 (10.3)	1,138.5 (37.8)	475.0 (13.8)	204.0 (6.3)
Drinking	17.0 (2.0)	62.3 (5.5)	37.0 (2.8)	10.0 (1.0)
Resting	3.0 (0.3)	0.0	0.0	0.0
General activity	27.0 (2.5)	3.5 (1.3)	92.0 (7.3)	103.0 (3.7)
Grooming	242.0 (4.8)	296.0 (4.3)	470.0 (10.0)	158.0 (3.0)
Drinking	6.0 (0.3)	0.0	29.0 (2.0)	30.0 (1.3)
Resting	17.0 (1.0)	7.0 (1.3)	53.0 (2.5)	52.0 (1.7)
Postmeal IMI rest	1,348.5	2,516.3	2,858.5	8,454.0

[a]IMI = intermeal interval.

2. *Serotoninergic Modulations of Nutrient Intake*

The first experiments in which anorectic drugs were used to modify nutrient intake were reported in 1977 (187) and were directly related to the proposed role for serotonin in protein selection. The purpose of the experiments was to separate the effects of drugs on total caloric intake from their effects on the consumption of a particular nutrient. In the major study male weanling rats (21 to 48 days old) were placed on an 8-hr cyclic feeding regimen and during the feeding period allowed to select food from two isocaloric diets containing 5 or 45% protein. The rats were injected with one of two drugs known to act on serotonin metabolism. Fenfluramine reduces serotonin levels in the brain with little effect on catecholamines (57) and increases the turnover rate of serotonin (51). This drug appears to act by releasing and blocking the reuptake of serotonin (69). Fluoxetine also exerts an effect on serotonin metabolism (68) and is a more specific inhibitor of the serotonin membrane pump than chlorimipramine (67). Fluoxetine, like fenfluramine, causes a powerful depression of food intake (26,77). With fenfluramine no adjustments were observed during the first hour after injection, but during the following 3 hr "fenfluramine-treated animals selectively decreased their consumption of the low-protein diet and increased their consumption of the high-protein food so that total caloric intake was depressed while protein intake was spared" (187). This action was generally in keeping with fluctuations of the plasma levels of fenfluramine (25). Like fenfluramine, fluoxetine suppressed food intake but spared protein consumption, thereby increasing the proportion of calories consumed as protein. On the other hand, amphetamine—a drug with little known action on serotonin-mediated neurotransmission—was reported to reduce food consumption but failed to alter the proportion of total calories consumed as protein. The action of serotoninergic drugs was characterized as a protein-sparing effect.

These first studies were carried out on young rats subjected to food deprivation prior to testing. To investigate the robustness of the findings, Blundell and McArthur (28) administered fenfluramine to adult rats maintained on a deprivation regimen or allowed to feed freely. For deprived animals the data were broadly in keeping with the findings of Wurtman and Wurtman (187); fenfluramine gave rise to an increase in the proportion of protein in the total food consumed (protein-sparing effect). However, under free feeding conditions the protein-sparing effect of fenfluramine was not apparent. It has since been revealed that food deprivation significantly decreases protein intake and the ratio of protein to total energy consumed in both adult and weanling rats (120). The alteration of this baseline should be considered in evaluating the effects of drugs on nutrient intake.

A further difference between the two sets of experiments is the nature of the food available for consumption: powder versus gel. In a previous section (IV.B.) it was reported that this variable can exert a significant effect on the absolute amount of protein consumed and on the proportion of proteins to total calories (protein energy percent). Figure 4 illustrates that sensory characteristics can also modify the action of fenfluramine. Under free-feeding conditions fenfluramine reduces protein

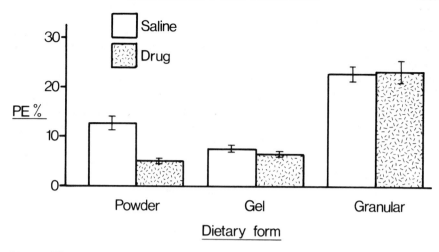

FIG. 4. Effect of fenfluramine on PE% of three diets varying in form (powder, granular, gel). In the 0 to 4 hr measurement period the drug produced a marked suppression of protein intake (relative to total energy intake) in the powder diet. Drug × diet interaction is significant [$F_{(2,20)}$ = 5.6, $p < 0.05$].

energy percent for the powder diet (cf. ref. 28) but leaves unaltered this parameter with the gel and granular diets. Clearly taste and textural qualities may influence a drug's effect on nutrient intake—at least in short-term tests. This factor may have had some bearing on the outcome of a further recent experiment in which fenfluramine was administered to rats offered a choice of pure separate portions of protein (casein), carbohydrate (corn starch and dextrin), and fat (vegetable fat and safflower oil) (132). In one experiment in which the fat ration contained more calories than the other two nutrient rations, fenfluramine reduced protein and fat intakes and tended to spare carbohydrate. When all diets were made isocaloric, fat intake was again severely depressed with a relative and weak sparing of protein and carbohydrate.

The overall picture is somewhat complicated. Different studies involving differences in the age of animals, sensory characteristics of diets, concentration of nutrients, number of choices, feeding regimens, and test intervals have produced widely varying results. According to these data the protein-sparing effect of fenfluramine can be observed but is not a particularly robust phenomenon.

If animals are given diets containing differing proportions of two nutrients and if the treatment selectively alters their intake of one of the diets, it may not be clear which of the nutrients the animal is choosing or avoiding. For example, if a treatment causes rats to consume less of diet A (high-carbohydrate, low-protein) than diet B (low-carbohydrate, high-protein), it can be said to be exerting either a "protein-sparing" or a "carbohydrate-suppressing" effect. A decision about which action is primary and which secondary requires the use of different types of test diets in which only one of the nutrients in question is varied. In experiments (188) on the effect of serotoninergic drugs on carbohydrate intake, rats were allowed to consume from two isocaloric, isoprotein diets containing either 25% or 75% dextrin. Following administration of fenfluramine or MK212, a drug reported to exert a serotonin-like effect at the central synapses (46), rats specifically decreased their consumption of the high (75%)-carbohydrate diet and consumed relatively more of the low-carbohydrate diet. Consequently, the absolute intake of carbohydrate was reduced together with the proportion of total food represented by carbohydrate. The role of serotonin may be to control the proportion of carbohydrate to protein consumed rather than absolute amounts. [The depression of fat intake by fenfluramine noted above (132) was not observed in these experiments as the preferred low-carbohydrate diet contained substantially more fat than the high-carbohydrate diet. Thus it remains uncertain whether fenfluramine has an effect on fat intake.]

3. Catecholaminergic Manipulations

In self-selection experiments using amphetamine it has been reported that this drug has no selective action on nutrient intake (187), produces a protein suppressive effect (28), and decreases fat consumption (90). However, it is well known that amphetamine has an action on both major catecholamines—dopamine and noradrenaline (e.g., ref. 76). Using the more specific α-adrenergic agonist, clonidine, it was reported that low doses (25 to 50 mg/kg), which may selectively affect presynaptic α_2 receptors, increase food consumption and selectively enhance preference for protein (119). This suggests that noradrenergic neurons may participate in mechanisms controlling the selection of proteins so that lowered noradrenergic activity leads to an increase in protein intake. One puzzling feature of this study was the observation that yohimbine, a drug thought to block presynaptic α-receptors, brought about a massive increase in food intake and a much larger increase in protein than did clonidine. Obviously, synaptic pharmacology will have to be very carefully controlled to allow an unambiguous interpretation of these data.

In addition, other evidence hinders the interpretation of the effect of clonidine. In a preliminary study using similar doses of clonidine and a variety of diets, the drug actually increased a carbohydrate preference in a manner similar to that produced by insulin (60). There is no doubt that clonidine is a potent pharmacological tool, but calibrating the dose to ensure an action at specific neuronal sites is clearly a problem in the absence of biochemical data. The opposing effects observed in the above-mentioned studies could arise because of differing actions of clonidine at noradrenergic synapses or because of other factors associated with diet design, test interval, or pretreatment conditions. In the absence of knowledge about the stability of these findings the development of a theoretical framework is hazardous.

4. Other Treatments

It has been known for some years that insulin increases the intake of dextrose when it is supplied in liquid form along with a normal diet (147). More recently, it has been shown that rats offered separate pure macronutrients markedly increase caloric intake following insulin administration, this being entirely a function of raised carbohydrate (cornstarch and dextrin) consumption (91).

However, although these actions of insulin illustrate that animals will selectively adjust their dietary intake the mechanism is not clear. Although the findings are in keeping with the actions of insulin on glucose metabolism, neither blood glucose levels nor levels of amino acids in blood were measured in these studies. Moreover, it is not clear whether the animal's dietary pattern was adjusted to regulate total caloric intake or the intake of specific nutrients.

Other effects are also not easy to interpret. For example, morphine produces a general but short-lasting suppression of the intake of all three macronutrients with a longer lasting inhibition of protein and carbohydrate (118). On the other hand, naloxone, the opiate antagonist, appears to exert a suppression of fat intake but spares protein (117). Since opiate agonists and antagonists display varied effects on total intake depending on the dose and deprivation conditions (160), it is not easy to embrace these findings within possible mechanisms for the control of total intake or nutrient selection.

5. Conclusions

Drugs can produce dramatic effects on the intake of specific nutrients. These effects appear to vary with a variety of experimental factors. However, there is a lack of information about the effect of these drugs on receptor systems dealing with sensory information from the diets and on effector mechanisms to deal with the consumption of various structural forms of diet. Moreover, the diffuse actions of drugs on many tissues in the body and sites within the brain suggests a cautious interpretation of pharmacological manipulations of food selection.

B. Brain Treatments

Direct manipulations of the brain have not been widely used in investigations of nutrient selection but techniques include the use of neurotoxins, direct microinjections of chemicals, and electrode-induced brain lesions.

1. Neurochemical Alterations

Investigations of the role of serotonin in the regulation of protein intake have used the self-selection procedure to monitor food choices following the chronic lowering of brain serotonin levels by synthesis blockers, neurotoxins, and specific lesions of clusters of cell bodies of serotonin neurons. All of these treatments have been shown to produce effects on total food intake or body weight, but the evidence for a serotonin control mechanism is equivocal (see ref. 21). Rats were allowed to select food from two isocaloric powder diets containing 15 or 55% casein. Fat content was held constant and carbohydrate (cornstarch) allowed to vary (11). Systemic injections of p-chlorophenylalanine, an inhibitor of serotonin synthesis, reduced brain levels of serotonin and 5-hydroxyindoleacetic acid (5-HIAA) and also reduced the proportion of protein consumed. Intraventricular injections of the serotonin neurotoxin 5,7-dihydroxytryptamine (13), and radio frequency lesions of dorsal and medial raphé nuclei both decreased whole brain levels of serotonin and reduced protein energy percent. These results are quite in keeping with some earlier data on the effects of pharmacological adjustments of serotonin (187), and taken together strengthen the belief that serotonin neurons have a function in the control of protein intake. However, two qualifying features should be considered. First, although these treatments might produce a long-lasting depletion of brain serotonin (whose levels were not measured directly), their effects on protein intake decreased with time. Second, these alterations in protein selection are in the opposite direction to that predicted by some previous post hoc correlations of dietary selection and plasma tryptophan-to-natural amino acid ratios (9,10).

2. Direct Intracranial Injections

Balanced amino acid mixtures injected into the dorsolateral perifornical hypothalamus inhibit feeding (137), whereas similar mixtures injected at a wide variety of sites cause an aversion when paired with odorized foods (38). These experiments suggest only that the monitoring of protein ingestion is involved in the control of food intake. The vast majority of studies on the neurochemistry of feeding have examined the role of noradrenergic systems, probably because this transmitter is relatively easy to measure and to manipulate. Critical sites where its direct injection produces maximum effects are the paraventricular nucleus and the perifornical hypothalamic area, which receive projections from the dorsal and ventral central tegmental tracts, respectively (86,105,106). It is well established that paraventricular injections of noradrenaline stimulate eating, and this effect has been linked to carbohydrate metabolism (104). Using a self-selection paradigm and various sets of diets, noradrenergic stimulation of the paraventricular nucleus was found in a preliminary study to increase the elective consumption of carbohydrate, independently of the sweetness of the diet (173). Interestingly, amphetamine injected into the perifornical zone decreased preference for protein (Leibowitz, *personal communication*), an effect similar to that seen with peripheral injections (28). These experiments, although not conclusive, raise the possibility that chemosensitive sites in the hypothalamic region may be linked to mechanisms for nutrient selection.

3. Brain Lesions

Lesions of the prepyriform cortex and medial amygdala (114) prevent the normal decrease in food intake in response to imbalanced amino acid diets. Lesions of the ventromedial hypothalamus, well known to produce hyperphagia and obesity, failed to alter consumption of the imbalanced diet. However, in self-selection experiments there is disagreement about the effects of ventromedial hypothalamic lesions. Neuringer and Mayer (131) reported that lesioned animals failed to maintain sufficient protein to maintain weight. More recently, lesioned animals offered a choice of 10% or 60% protein (casein) diets overate and gained weight by consuming more of the low-protein diet while maintaining normal levels of protein intake (7). However, in another study ventromedial hypothalamic lesions increased fat intake, had no effect on carbohydrate intake, and decreased protein intake (88a). It was argued that protein intake remained intact in these medial lesioned rats, and does not appear to be affected by lesions of the lateral hypothalamus (176). However, rats with lesions of the dorsomedial nucleus of the hypothalamus show an interesting pattern of selection (17). When offered three diets high in fat, protein, or carbohydrate, lesioned rats displayed a much-reduced intake of the high protein diet, but maintained overall consumption of all three macronutrients in proportions equivalent to those of control rats.

What can be deduced from these lesion experiments? The studies with deficient or imbalanced amino acid diets suggest the involvement of an extra-hypothalamic site. The dissociation of "energy" and "protein" intake following medial hypothalamic lesions implies that their consumption may be under the control of separate mechanisms in different brain sites. Increased intake of energy, but ot protein, may be related to changes in peripheral metabolism (66) unrelated to plasma profiles of amino acids. However, most of the experiments quoted above were inductive (data gathering) rather than deductive (theory testing). Taken together they eliminate certain possibilities but do not greatly elucidate mechanisms for the control of macronutrient intake.

C. Hormonal Manipulations

There is ample evidence that modulation of sex hormones in male and female rats gives rise to changes in total food intake and body weight (e.g., refs. 130,177). Most research has been carried out on female animals and has almost invariably been based on the use of single balanced diets. Four experimental strategies have been widely used:

1. Measurement of variability over the estrus cycle
2. Ovariectomy
3. Ovariectomy plus estrogen replacement
4. Pregnancy

All of these models have been used in conjunction with the self-selection technique, the major purpose of most of these four strategies being the identification of alterations in nutrient selection that may account for the observed changes in food intake and body weight. This field illustrates clearly the problems that characterize the experimental modification of nutrient intake: wide variety in the structure and composition of diets, considerable variability in the baseline intake of nutrients, and almost no agreement between the outcomes of different studies.

A summary of the researches is presented in Table 5. There is agreement that during pregnancy food intake and body weight invariably increase, but less agreement about changes in food selection. It has been variously reported that proportions of nutrients chosen remain constant (165), that only fat intake increases (174), that

TABLE 5. *Summary of experiments on female sex hormone manipulations and nutrient self-selection by rats*

Authors	Diet	Manipulation	Outcome
Richter and Barelare (1938)	Olive oil, sucrose, casein, salt	Pregnancy	Increased olive oil, casein, NaCl
Scott et al. (1948)	Vegetable oil, sucrose, casein, salt mix, vitamins (pills)	Pregnancy	Proportions of nutrients constant
Tribe (1955)	Seven foods: maize starch, glucose, margarine, yeast, casein, salt mix, cod liver oil	Pregnancy	Depressed total caloric intake
Leshner et al. (1972)	Three isocaloric diets Control: 22% protein Protein: 45% protein Carbohydrate: 0% protein	Pregnancy	Increased protein intake
		Estrus	No change in nutrient selection
Leshner and Collier (1973)	Three isocaloric diets Control Protein 90%, carbohydrate 0% Protein 0%, carbohydrate 90%	Ovariectomy	Increased protein intake and protein %
Wurtman and Baum (1980)	Isocaloric 5 and 45% protein diets (40% carbohydrate; fat varies)	Estrus	Decreased carbohydrate, protein stable ∴ increased PE%
		Ovariectomy	No change in nutrient intake (Tables 1 and 2)
		Ovariectomy plus estradiol benzoate	Decrease in low protein intake ∴ PE% increased
	Isocaloric isoprotein 25% and 70% carbohydrate diets		Decreased carbohydrate intake
Kanarek and Beck (1980)	Three diets: casein (+ salts and minerals), carbohydrate (cornstarch, dextrin + salt and minerals), vegetable oil	Ovariectomy	No change in selection patterns
Geiselman et al. (1981)	Olive oil, sucrose, casein, neutral bulk (+ salts)	Estrus	Increased carbohydrate, decreased fat
		Ovariectomy	Increased fat, decreased carbohydrate

protein consumption increases but not carbohydrate (111), and that oil (fat), casein, and salt intakes increase (149).

When selective nutrient intake has been measured over the stages of the estrous cycle, measurements on the day of ovulation (as determined by vaginal smears) show no change in the pattern of nutrient selection (111), a decrease in carbohydrate and fat intakes, and an increase in protein energy percent (186), or an increase in carbohydrate and decrease in fat (74). One interesting feature of these studies is the decrease in fat intake at estrous observed in two out of three cases. In the third study (111), fat intake was kept constant as a fixed proportion of each diet.

After ovariectomy the pattern of selection shows no change (88,186—by inspection of Tables 1 and 2), an increase in protein and protein energy percent (109), or an increase in fat and decrease in carbohydrate (74). Where estradiol benzoate has been administered to ovariectomized animals it has been reported to lower intake of a low-protein diet and raise protein energy percent (186), an effect also attributed to ovariectomy itself (109).

What can explain the lack of agreement between the outcomes of these studies? One possibility is the composition of the diets offered, which vary widely in number of choices; nutrient density and purity; constancy of key elements; and combinations of tastes, favors, and textures. For example, some studies have used pure substances such as olive oil, sucrose, and casein as specific representatives of fats, carbohydrates, and proteins (74,149). This array contains a mixture of tastes and textures. Obviously other types of pure nutrients could have been chosen. An alternative series of separated nutrients has been constructed around a protein ration (casein plus salts and minerals), carbohydrate ration (cornstarch, dextrin, plus salts and minerals), and vegetable oil (88). Other composite diets have manipulated protein and carbohydrate while allowing fat to vary (186) or adjusted protein and carbohydrate while keeping fat constant (111). The diets have been presented as powders, gels, aqueous solutions, or oils. This sensory dimension creates variability in preferences both within and between studies. Coupled with the extensive range of nutrient inclusion behind this sensory field, rats in different studies are confronted with nutritional puzzles of varying difficulty. These differences lead to varying profiles of baseline nutrient intakes before the application of hormonal adjustments. For example, with composite diets rats selected 8% protein (111) or about 25% (186). Using pure nutrients Kanarek and Beck (88) reported intakes of 35%, 34%, and 31% for protein, carbohydrate, and fat, respectively, whereas intakes of 16%, 35%, and 49% were observed elsewhere (74). Faced with discrepancies in every aspect of experimental procedure and in the results, the present reviewer is unable to discern any clear principle linking fluctuations in estrogen levels with patterns of nutrient intake. It seems certain that in this area of research the variability in the results of experiments has been brought about by the great variability in the experimental parameters manipulated. (These discrepancies may to some extent be resolved by determining whether baseline nutrient intake is compatible with normal growth and development. For example, the level of protein (8%) selected by the rats in the study of Leshner et al. is considerably lower than the amount needed to sustain normal growth, raising doubts about its significance. Baseline measurements should be carried out for several weeks to ensure that the experimental diets allow the animal to consume nutrients in proportions needed for its age, sex, and physiological condition (for example, pregnant or lactating) before experimental manipulations to alter nutrient selection are begun. Moreover, if possible, the elective caloric intake of control animals should be determined using a composite food such as chow, and this intake compared with that observed when animals are given the pure nutrients.)

D. Circadian Rhythms in Nutrient Selection

Any theory linking neurotransmitter activity with nutrient selection would be markedly strengthened if it could be demonstrated that the daily oscillation of neurotransmitter level in the brain was synchronized with the daily rhythm of nutrient intake. Circadian variation in protein intake has been reported in at least two studies. Rats given a choice of two powder diets containing either 60% or 0% protein showed clear differences in total food intake and the type of diet selected during the light and dark periods (87). Although consumption of the high-protein diet remained fairly constant over 24 hr, rats ate much more of the protein-free diet during the dark period. Naturally, this uneven pattern of consumption leads to fluctuations in the proportion of calories consumed as protein with maximum PE% occurring during the second portion of the light period. However, when rats were allowed to eat from diets containing 55% or 0% protein and obliged to perform the operant response of bar pressing to obtain pellets of food, a different pattern of selection was observed (102). PE% varied from a peak of 38.3% during the first 4 hr of daytime to a low of 22.9% during the first hours of darkness. In a further study using different animals and expressing the data as intake for each 6-hr period the profile shown in Fig. 5 was observed (103). When the pattern obtained by Johnson et al. (87) is superimposed on this profile there appears to be little concordance between the two studies. What factors could have given rise to this discrepancy? Variables to do with diet construction and acquisition appear most likely. Although there is little difference between the proportions of nutrients in the diets, one study used powdered food whereas the other used small pellets, and whereas the powder was licked and lapped from a Fallon eatometer, the pellets were collected one by one from a trough after the depression of a lever. Differences in the animals' preferences for type of food and mode of acquisition could account for the observed differences. If so, this demonstrates that sensory and sensorimotor factors probably contribute as much as metabolic factors to the displayed pattern of intake.

E. Other Variables

In addition to the experimental manipulations described in previous sections, a number of other variables have been shown to influence the pattern of nutrient intake.

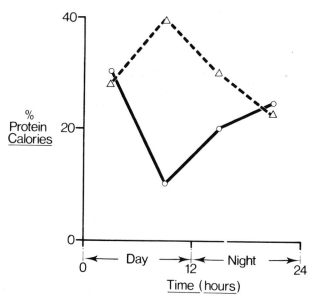

FIG. 5. Circadian rhythms in protein selection taken from the diagram in ref. 103 (o) and computed from data reported by Johnson et al. (87) (Δ).

(a) *Water restriction.* Relative to rats allowed water *ad libitum*, rats subjected to water rationing showed a decreased preference for a nutritious high-protein diet and gradually developed a preference for an isocaloric high-carbohydrate diet (134). In a similar study using two isocaloric powder diets rats were restricted to 6 ml of water per day for 8 days (50). During this period rats increased the proportion of food taken from the low-protein diet. This adjustment is highly adaptive, since protein releases half as much water of metabolism as carbohydrate because water is required for excretion of the nitrogenous products of protein. The crucial stimulus leading to carbohydrate preference appears to be a dry mouth, since understandable shifts in preferences were also seen in desalivate rats (50). Accordingly, any treatments—pharmacological, neurological, or hormonal—that lead to changes in water balance or to a dry mouth may bias the pattern of nutrient intake.

(b) *Food restriction.* Using purified separate dietary components, a number of studies have shown that total starvation or food restriction leads to an increase in fat intake (8,122,162). Following 5 days of starvation after baseline intakes of 65% carbohydrate, 21% protein, and 13.5% fat, Piquard et al. (143) observed a compensatory increase in fat and carbohydrate intakes over 23 days. Interestingly, with rats allowed to feed for only 1 hr per day, McDonald et al. (122) noted a decrease in protein intake. A similar effect has been observed in weanling and adult rats offered a choice of 5 and 45% composite protein diets (120).

(c) *Activity.* Rats selecting from two composite diets containing 0 to 46% protein were kept in home cages or allowed access to activity wheels (49). Interestingly, the active rats ate less food than the inactive group but consumed a higher proportion of carbohydrate (17.5% protein versus 19.9% for the inactive group). In a later study (112) rats made hypoactive by the administration of thiouracil reduced carbohydrate intake but maintained normal levels of protein. These studies were interpreted as showing that the patterns of nutrient intake reflect intermediate metabolism and are related to animals' energy requirements.

(d) *Housing*. In a comparison of rats living in groups of 12 or in single cages and fed separate diets of sucrose, salt, casein, and vegetable oil (122), the grouped animals adapted more readily to the self-selection regimen. Indeed, half of the individually housed rats refused to eat casein and did not gain weight. In response to a combined schedule of restricted feeding (1 hr daily) and 5 hr of daily cold stress, the grouped rats ate more of all components than the individually housed animals. Little can be discerned about nutrient preferences, since animals had access to food for only 1 hr every day, and, as the data show, the animals were probably eating in response to immediate energy demands.

(e) *Cold*. In a more systematic study of self-selection at low temperatures, rats were kept for 33 days at ambient temperatures of 2° or 22°C (110). Protein intake was maintained but rats ate an increased absolute amount of carbohydrate (thereby leading to a reduction in PE%). A similar increased intake of a carbohydrate diet has been observed in mice (56).

The effect of these systematic experimental treatments on apparent nutrient preferences can be added to knowledge of the actions of additional variables such as age (e.g., ref. 139), artificial alteration of taste (50), adjustment of the amino acid content of protein (e.g., ref. 183), and type of protein offered (see section D).

VI. IMPLICATIONS

The previous sections have illustrated the wide range of circumstances in which an animal's selection of nutrients, within a self-selection experiment, is responsive to experimental manipulations. Indeed, inspection reveals that fewer than 5% of treatments fail to modify the pattern of selection. Variables that give rise to alterations in macronutrient intake include *inter alia* age, time of day, physical activity, ambient temperature, a wide variety of drugs, reproductive hormones, metabolic manipulations, food or water restriction, housing, brain lesions, and neurochemical interventions, as well as direct adjustments of the sensory or nutritional components of the foods offered. This may indicate only that the phenomenon is labile. However, the lack of accord, frequently encountered, between the results of similar treatments is puzzling and there appears to be no single theme that can unify the widely divergent observations. Outcomes appear to depend on a variety of mechanisms. But it remains possible that there exists a single dominant principle governing nutrient selection whose expression may be masked, overcome, suppressed, or blocked by the operation of collateral mechanisms. This issue will be taken up later.

A. Homeostasis, Adaptability, and Interactions

For more than 50 years the dominant principle governing studies on food intake has been the notion of homeostasis—the idea that organisms eat, and display other behaviors, to maintain stability within the internal environment and, by implication, stability of body mass. Many internal metabolic processes are devoted to maintaining physiological equilibrium, but since eating is a form of behavior this led to the conceptualization of a "behavioral regulation" of internal state (e.g., ref. 148). However, the way in which behavior is used as an expression of an internal need may be questioned. It is obvious that the internal environment must be protected— from overloading, underloading, and contamination—and behavioral strategies have developed to cope with this problem. But there is a difference between maintaining fixed values of certain parameters of the internal environment and defending tolerated limits of these parameters. In other words, the internal environment is, in certain aspects, robust and may withstand fluctuations in levels and rates of reaction without sustaining catastrophic consequences.

Clearly, homeostatic considerations are important influences on the behavior of all mammals, but the major characteristics of omnivore feeding behavior are its adaptability and selectivity. The strength of the omnivore feeding style is the capacity to adjust to meet the requirements of changing environmental circumstances. In other words, feeding behavior is flexible, and this flexibility is critical to the biological success of omnivores. This principle is illustrated in Fig. 6, in which food intake, of which nutrient selection is a fundamental part, is seen as the outcome of an interaction between internal and external constraints. Indeed, rather than viewing feeding behavior solely as the expression of an internal need state it may be profitable to consider feeding as an activity that bridges the internal and external environments. The especially intimate relationship of food as part of the external environment that subsequently becomes incorporated into the internal environment means that feeding can be considered more as a *transaction* than an interaction.

From this perspective it became impossible to disengage feeding from either the internal or the external environment. Just as the nature of eating is influenced by the levels of various internal parameters, so it is modulated by a variety of external conditions. Accordingly, feeding, including the selection of nutrients, does not automatically follow invariable rules set by the internal system. Under certain circumstances, regulation can be offset, overcome, or modulated by external conditions or demands (e.g., refs. 47,48). Indeed, certain concepts commonly used in biorhythm research may be usefully considered to apply to feeding patterns. Internal or endogenous constraints may be "entrained" by the equivalents of zeitgebers to produce a profile of nutrient selection. If it were possible to suspend all of the external agents, then it would be possible to evaluate completely the characteristics of the endogenous rules. In practice this can never be achieved. Consequently, mechanisms governing food selection should be sought not only in the internal environment but also in the interactional processes that give rise to the observed structure of feeding behavior.

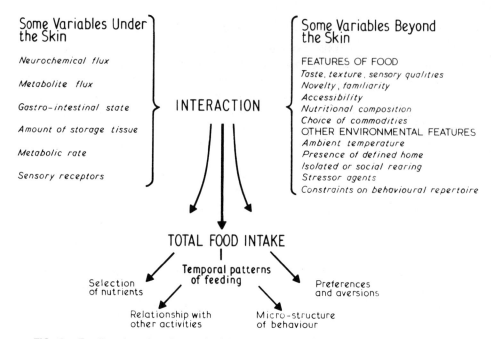

FIG. 6. Feeding viewed as the result of the interaction between two domains of events. Variables in the internal and external environments have been demonstrated to exert effects on total food intake and on qualitative aspects of feeding behavior. Consequently, the rules governing feeding ultimately reside in the interactional processes that bridge these two domains.

B. Design Problems

A number of factors bearing on the design of self-selection experiments have been discussed in section D. However, it became clear in considering experimental manipulations that the proper interpretation of the effects of certain treatments could be made only by reference to the experimental design. Different designs, independent of the experimentally manipulated variable, produced different outcomes. This situation existed when Lát wrote his review (100); it still exists now, and it will probably get worse. It will undoubtedly hinder the development of a coherent theory. These issues seem particularly important.

(a) *Pure nutrients versus composite foods.* Studies that use one or the other of these techniques differ on a bewildering range of factors including number of choices, nutrient density, freedom available for extremes of selection (e.g., with three pure nutrients an animal can choose not to eat a particular nutrient, whereas with two composite diets the animal must eat the proportion contained in the diets), freedom to modify intake according to the circadian rhythm (e.g., to eat fat at night but not during the day), range of tastes and textures within the array, and differences between the pure and composite foods (e.g., pure foods may have more intense sensory characteristics than mixtures). These variables compromise a proper understanding of both the *sensory* and *metabolic* aspects of nutrient selection. Mechanisms apparently revealed by research on one type of material founder when compared with results using an alternative dietary array. It is unlikely that researchers will agree to dispense with one particular procedure. However, it would be extremely productive if some studies could test the effect of variables against both pure substances and composite foods. In that case a discrepancy between the results would have to be resolved by the researcher rather than by some third party (a reviewer of the field), attempting a *post hoc* comprehension of events.

(b) *Choice of nutrient.* There is a good deal of conformity in the elements chosen to represent a particular class of nutrient. Carbohydrates usually appear as sucrose, cornstarch, or dextrin, fats as some sort of vegetable oil, and protein as casein. Although low carbohydrate intakes are recorded with sucrose and dextrose as the source of carbohydrate (100), the critical choice appears to be the particular protein used. For years it has been known that rats do not appear to enjoy eating pure casein and a number of experiments have reported abstinence, sometimes resulting in death (94,142,165). Casein additions to composite diets are likely to detract from the acceptability of the food. Other sources of protein, for example, beef protein, are more readily consumed by rats (P. Leathwood, *personal communication*), and the importance of this element of diet construction should be further explored.

(c) *Baselines.* It is a matter of logic that experimentally induced changes in nutrient intake are always related to the departure from a natural level. It is also true that some levels may be defended more vigorously than others. For example, a rat eating 10% protein may be less prepared to reduce intake (and more prepared to increase it) than a rat eating a diet, 35% of which is protein. Accordingly, the baseline intake or "educated level" arrived at after some period of familiarization with the diets can mitigate or enhance the apparent effect of an experimental treatment.

(d) *Discrimination and preference.* Ideally, an investigation of the metabolic effects of nutrients would measure some internal variable (or a behavioral variable covarying with the internal one) when one nutrient in the dietary array was adjusted while others were left untouched. Unfortunately, a manipulation of this type does not simply exert metabolic consequences since the dietary adjustment would alter the sensory characteristics of the food and hence its discriminability, acceptability, or palatability. If rats (and humans) are to choose between certain offered diets then these diets must be discriminable from one another on the basis of taste, smell, or texture or according to the place where they are normally found. Gross differences in palatability can obviously bias a choice. But attempts to smother natural tastes by contaminating foods with quinine or saccharine (or some other adulterant) may decrease discriminability to the extent that rats fail to distinguish one from the other according to their tastes. An optimal situation would be one in which foods were equally preferred but highly discriminable, since presumably "learning" which diet to eat in response to metabolic requirements is made easier by being able to tell one food from another. This problem is difficult to resolve since in many cases equating preferences would detract from discriminability while improving discriminability would probably tend to create unequal preferences.

(e) *Diet dilution and adulteration.* The observation that macronutrient intakes can be independently manipulated, albeit often in an unpredictable manner, and the belief that they are separately regulated have implications for experiments that do not employ self-selection designs. If experimental animals are treated in such a way as to provoke an adjustment in the intake of a particular nutrient while being offered a single diet, then the proportion of the nutrient in that diet is critical. For it follows that an animal may over- or undereat the entire food simply to control the intake of one item. If this possibility is taken seriously it offers alternative interpretations for thousands of experiments in which single diets have been fed and measures of intake have been expressed as total grams or calories consumed. An example of research where revision may be needed is work on ventromedial hypothalamic hyperphagia. The findings of Anderson et al. (7) (see section V), if interpreted literally, imply that on those occasions on which hypothalamically lesioned animals overeat a single diet, the rats are attempting to maximize intake of nonprotein energy. To accomplish this the animals must also overeat the protein fraction. Another example would be the many situations in which experimental animals are induced to overeat by being offered a high-fat diet. It is usually acknowledged that overeating occurs because of an improved sensory acceptability of the diet, i.e., it becomes more palatable. However, it follows that if fat is added to a composite food and nothing is removed then the percentage of other macronutrients diminishes. Consequently a high-fat diet may carry a reduced proportion of protein and to maintain a continuing constant level of protein intake animals must overeat the whole food. In this way, adulterations of diet, whether with the intention of "diluting" or "concentrating" calories, introduce the operation of metabolic mechanisms unrelated to the control of total bulk consumed.

C. What Makes a Good Experiment?

Given the number of problems listed above it may be questioned whether or not it is possible to control for sufficient of the confounding variables to design a good experiment. One first step is the recognition that diets that differ in nutritional composition will probably differ in sensory characteristics. These sensory differences may lead to one diet being consumed more than others on account of its sensory rather than nutritional value. How can this be controlled? The palatability of diets can be tested in short-term preference tests by offering rats an array of samples. If after initial investigation one diet is initially consumed by all animals, this would suggest that the food contained some intrinsic factor making it more preferred. Where diets are of similar consistency and texture small amounts of nonnutritious sweetening could be added to the less preferred diets to raise them to a similar preference level. This precaution, or some similar manipulation, should ensure that at the outset of the experiment all choices facing the animal are equally acceptable. Subsequent disproportionate consumption of particular diets could then be attributed to their metabolic, rather than sensory, qualities.

The choice of nutritional parameters including the inclusion of particular concentrations of macronutrients is more problematical. Clearly the establishment of equal preferences will be more difficult where diets vary greatly in texture and the most extreme case will be that in which the array contains both solids and liquids. The use of pure substances may compromise the dimension of sensory acceptability. In the case of composite diets the proportion of macronutrients included should always allow the animals' baseline intake to remain within physiologically accepted values. Obviously, if the choice of parameters means, for example, that rats consume very large amounts of protein then any further experimental manipulation may make it difficult to increase protein intake owing to a ceiling effect. The stricture must be that the overall proportions of macronutrients consumed should be such as to allow for increases or decreases following experimental treatment.

Even if composite diets are equally preferred the choice of nutrient proportions is critical and may influence the overall amounts of particular macronutrients consumed. For example, it has been demonstrated for mice that the replacement of carbohydrate by fat (in diets in which the other major component was protein) lowered the overall percentage of the protein self-selected from the choices of the composite diets (45). This means that in experiments focusing on protein intake and protein regulation the source of nonprotein energy in the diet is an important factor.

All of these comments illustrate that a single experiment cannot provide a definitive statement about the effects of an experimental manipulation. Adjusting the parameters may alter the outcome. This is understandable for we are dealing with biological systems that have evolved because of their robustness. However, it also means that this is a field in which the "one-off" crucial experiment is unlikely to play a role. The elucidation of mechanisms will probably come about through the carrying out of a series of experiments during which the same treatment can be applied to a set of situations in which particular parameters are systematically varied. Knowledge of mechanisms of self-selection will yield only to long-term research programs rather than brief and limited experimental thrusts.

D. Idiographic and Nomothetic Approaches

These terms are used in other fields of science to connote an interest in individual characteristics or in the "general responses" of groups of animals. The terms represent the distinction between "individual differences and general rules." Naturally the study of self-selection of nutrients has sought to establish general principles through which the levels of particular nutrients are regulated and according to which animals adjust their elective consumption. Although the bulk of experiments have been mounted in the attempt to elucidate general rules the literature abounds with mention of exceptions and with references to individual differences. Leaving aside the individual differences in survival when young rats are offered a choice of foods (e.g., refs. 94,174), other less dramatic cases occur. For example, Pilgrim and Patton (142), following studies on the self-selection of purified components, observed that "Animals show a wide variability in their choices of the components of a diet. Even though all of the essentials may be present, not all of the rats eat them. Even two series of animals similar in their genetic and physiological background, and tested under the same conditions do not exhibit the same patterns of selection." The authors go on to assert that the experiments "demonstrate the necessity for determining the patterns of choice of dietary components by the *individuals* of any given group of rats before the effect of a variable... can be properly evaluated" (my italics). Considerable interanimal variation is also the experience of the present writer. Experiments in which rats have been allowed to select from the composite diets varying in protein inclusion have revealed stable daily intakes varying from 9% to 37% protein. Indeed, rats have frequently been encountered whose daily protein intake has been less than that commonly accepted as a minimum for the maintenance of normal growth.

Considering interactions between components of a diet, Lát (100) has observed not only interanimal differences but also the existence of distinct subgroups. According to Lát, underlying biochemical factors were responsible for determining two basic patterns designated as a "glucogenic" and "gluconeogenic type" depending on the relative proportions of fat, carbohydrate, and protein regularly consumed together with certain salts and vitamins. These profiles suggest the operation of differing modes of regulation of nutrients in different animals and the existence of such patterns should be encompassed by any theoretical account of mechanisms of regulation.

In contrast with the wide variability between individual rats and between subgroups, patterns of food intake are remarkably stable in any one animal. Consequently, it appears that voluntary self-selection of nutrients by animals is characterized by pronounced *inter*subject variability and notable *intra*subject stability. The search for general rules of nutrient regulation, particularly in experiments that involve the introduction of a potent manipulative treatment, may well founder on the infrastructure of individual variability. Certainly this variability between individuals, between groups, and between laboratories will contribute to the lack of concordance of experimental outcomes.

E. Theories of Food Intake

It has been stressed repeatedly in this chapter and by other authors that research on nutrient selection should have implications for theories of food intake. At the present time theoretical formulations of feeding have restricted scope and deliberately do not attempt to embrace the great variety of factors known to influence intake. For example, although food consumption is modified by the novelty, familiarity, and safety of food, its ease of acquisition and consumption, taste, texture, and discriminability, together with a host of metabolic and physiological variables— and although feeding is articulated through a variety of complex and sophisticated actions, most theories attempt only to explain abrupt quantitative shifts in intake through a few critical brain zones or neurochemical pathways. The focus of such theories is the definition of the critical integrative or command loci. The model has been the multifactorial dual-center theory (3,170) in which specialized zones within the hypothalamus are deemed to control the initiation and cessation of episodes of eating. In turn, certain theoretical approaches have identified these critical areas as long-term or short-term regulators, each subject to influences such as the familiarity/ novelty of food or circadian oscillators (e.g., ref. 135). Acknowledgment of the multiple inputs controlling food intake has also been expressed in the two-profile statement (129), which envisages feeding as the ultimate outcome of a peripheral and central profile of neurotransmitters, hormones, enzymes, and meabolites.

A number of more recent attempts have been made to fit together various pieces of the neural jigsaw puzzle believed to articulate the brain's control over food intake. For example, Morley (126) has attempted to work out, in terms of facilitatory and inhibitory actions, the roles for all neurotransmitters and hormones that have been shown to influence consumption. This enterprise suffers from two defects. First, all brain processing is explained by reference to either an increase or a decrease in a single outcome variable—total food intake—often measured during a brief period. Second, all influences are channelled through the lateral or ventromedial regions of the hypothalamus, a restriction that illustrates the legacy of dual-center thinking. A more diffuse brain control system is likely, and researchers are now being advised to seek answers within broad functional networks of limbic–forebrain relationships (125). One step in this direction has been embodied in a summary model that has retained the idea of feeding and satiety neurons but embraced this concept within a framework of aminergic pathways known to influence food intake in the short or long term (83). This model draws largely on evidence from microinjection experiments that have identified sensitive zones in the paraventricular and perifornical zones of the hypothalamus receiving inputs from ascending monoaminergic pathways (see refs. 105,106). In turn, data from knife-cut studies (e.g., ref. 75) and from experiments using specific neurotoxins (e.g., ref. 2) have been used to illustrate how particular neurotransmitter pathways converge on critical zones in the hypothalamus to adjust consumption. A later version of the model (86) incorporates a specific action for noradrenaline, adrenaline, dopamine, and serotonin. This type of spatial model provides one way of arranging a complex body of data around a core of anatomical evidence. However, at this stage the model can only account for adjustments in the total amount of food eaten.

How can data on food selection be incorporated into conceptualizations for the control of food intake? Clearly, if some anatomical map were to be drawn up it should include some role for the prepyriform cortex and medial amygdala where lesions adjust the response to imbalanced diets (see section V.B.3) as well as hypothalamic areas. Regarding neurochemical mechanisms, evidence in the literature is not unanimous in support of any specific system (see section V.A.4). However, influential but inconclusive evidence exists for serotonin and, to a lesser extent, for noradrenaline. The anatomical distribution of such aminergic projections that could bias food selection has not been investigated, but it remains possible that the neuronal systems incorporated into the models mentioned above could be the ones to direct organisms to the consumption of certain macronutrients rather than others. A simple model based on an interaction between neurotransmitter systems and embodying a process for the selection of nutritional commodities has already been presented (Fig. 2). This type of conceptualization draws attention to the structure of behavior and gives importance to temporal as well as spatial aspects of feeding control. The selection of foods represents a structural characteristic of feeding behavior and entails the appropriate ordering of sequences of actions. Accordingly, a temporal model of feeding can readily incorporate a process to guide the selection of nutrients. One possible arrangement is set out in Fig. 7. This approach is suggested as a heuristic device to demonstrate how moment-to-moment adjustments in preferences and selection may be related to the operation of particular neurotransmitters and how these may be inserted into the sequential flow of actions making up feeding behavior. The capacity to select foods means that animals stop eating one commodity and begin consuming another; that is, the process entails changes in behavior. If these changes are determined, at least in part, by underlying activity in neurochemical systems, then the arrangement in Fig. 7 shows how the interdigitation may occur. The selection of nutrients must be related not only to the overall control of caloric intake, but also to the periodic nature of feeding behavior and to the way in which episodes of eating are intimately embraced by a behavioral flux comprising, for the rat, episodes of grooming, activity, sedation, and sleep.

Over the years, the way in which theories of food intake have been constructed has made it difficult to assimilate data on food selection. On the other hand, theoretical statements for the regulation of macronutrient ingestion have been formulated through experimental strategies not easily blended with techniques for investigating food consumption. The two approaches must merge. The conceptualization in Fig. 7 provides a provisional statement for the way in which a comprehensive theory could develop.

F. Clinical Applications

The bulk of the experimental work discussed in this chapter has been carried out on animals, but a clear articulation of processes underlying food selection has implications for man. "The construction of animal models for human behaviour can be a seductive pastime or a serious scientific enterprise. Valid models may increase our understanding of animal and man, but invalid ones lead to theoretical confusion and their practial application may have undesirable social consequences." This was how Beach (14) has described the value of animal models for understanding human sexuality. In making comparisons across species two principles should be kept in mind. First, meaningful comparisons are based not on formal characteristics of behavior, but on its causal mechanisms and functional outcomes. It is true that rats select their intake from a variety of available macronutrients; humans also choose foods varying in the protein, carbohydrate, and fat content. Rats also select according to the sensory qualities of dietary commodities; so apparently do humans. But considered at the level of descriptive phenomenology, neither set of facts helps us to understand the other. Only comparative study can discover whether similar causes are involved and similar functions served.

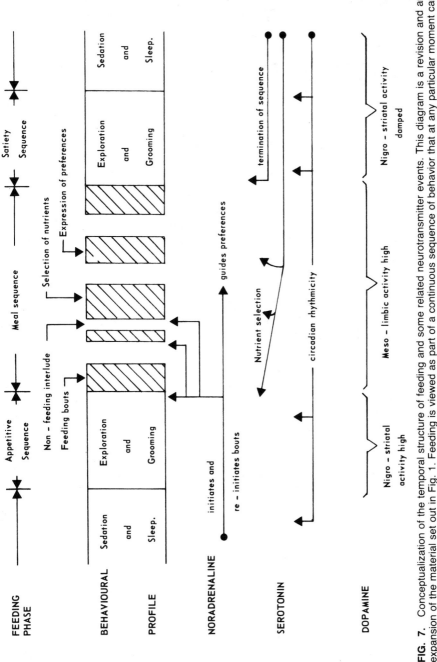

FIG. 7. Conceptualization of the temporal structure of feeding and some related neurotransmitter events. This diagram is a revision and an expansion of the material set out in Fig. 1. Feeding is viewed as part of a continuous sequence of behavior that at any particular moment can be related to the state of activity in a number of different neurotransmitter systems. The conjoint and harmonious action of these systems allows for the expression of feeding behavior. Consequently, the description of one aspect of food intake such as the selection of a particular macronutrient is complex and may require the specification of the level of activity in all of the systems set out in the diagram.

The second principle is that the validity of interspecific (cross-species) generalization cannot exceed the reliability of intraspecific analysis. "Significant comparison of a particular type of behavior in two different species is impossible unless and until the behavior has been adequately analysed in each species by itself. Only after independent, intraspecific analysis is achieved can we properly interpret the nature and degree of interspecific similarities and differences" (14). Accordingly, comparisons of food selection behavior in rats and humans will remain scientifically weak until both phenomena have been examined by similar analytical procedures and according to similar theoretical principles.

It is known that humans display clear preferences and aversions for particular foods. Aversions have attracted most interest because of the manner in which they could be established according to theoretical principles derived from animal studies. In two surveys (70,115), a total of 1213 subjects were asked to report relationships between food aversions and the occurrence of illness. In one study, gastrointestinal illness was associated with acquisition of aversions in 87% of subjects, and in the other survey more than 95% of the aversions appeared to have been established by means of orthodox conditioning mechanisms. Moreover, Logue et al. (115) reported that approximately 29% of the aversions generalized to foods that tasted and smelled similarly to the food that had been paired with the illness.

Although this chapter has been largely concerned with metabolic processes capable of mediating short-term oscillations in food selection, it is clear that in man long-standing preferences and aversions may interfere with the articulation of moment to moment choices. Although taste-aversion conditioning has not been examined in humans with the same intensity as the animal studies, the phenomenon appears to be real and is in accord with principles of biological adaptability. The existence of these and other (cognitive and economic) restrictions on human food selection means that the study of metabolic and neurochemical processes governing macronutrient selection in humans will be inherently more difficult than in animal studies.

However, certain reports have provided *prima facie* evidence for the modulation of human food preferences by hormones or neurotransmitters. For example, the hormonal fluctuations underlying the menstrual cycle have been related to changes in some sensory thresholds (107,193), and for the taste modality there appears to be a depression of the liking for sweet substances between ovulation and the premenstrual phase (185). However, the reduction in the perceived pleasantness of sucrose solutions (alliesthesia) that occurs following a glucose load (44) occurs more slowly at the time of ovulation than at other phases of the cycle (185). If these shifts are important in determining the consumption of sweet foods and the onset of satiety, then these data indicate that a greater quantity of sweet commodities may be consumed at the time of ovulation. This may explain why weight gains of the order of 1% have been reported at midcycle in women (159). However, this argument should be considered alongside the observation that a craving for sweet foods has been reported to occur during periods of premenstrual tension (169). These pieces of evidence need not be in conflict for there is clearly a difference between the active seeking of a sweet food (craving) and the tendency for a slow decline in preference for sweet commodities (alliesthesia). These differences are reflected in the processes of hunger and satiation (20,32). The adjustments in these processes at different times of the menstrual cycle may indicate the existence of separate mechanisms related to differing biological requirements for sweet materials. Of course, this may be related to macronutrient intake only if it is accepted that the sweet taste is normally associated with particular nutrient composition of foods.

There is also evidence that certain commonly administered psychoactive drugs exert effects on food preferences. Although all the major classes of drugs including neuroleptics, benzodiazepines, and antidepressants produce changes in appetite, total food intake, and body weight (22), the antidepressant drugs appear to give rise to selective preferences. For example, depressed patients on maintenance therapy with amitriptyline (Elavil) showed an excessive weight gain that subsided when the amitriptyline was stopped. The patients on amitriptyline complained of weight gain and also displayed a craving for foods rich in carbohydrate (138). Interestingly, in a participant observer study of two schizophrenic patients on imipramine treatment, kept in isolation for 3 weeks, the author reported that these patients "seemed to have an endless appetite for tea, sugar, bread and potatoes but not much else," while one patient "refused chicken, lamb chops, pork chops, steak, stew, liver and even mince" (124). It is tempting to suggest that these particular drug treatments may have influenced mechanisms responsible for specific appetites and for the control of carbohydrate and protein intake.

These reports suggest that pharmacological treatments may alter food preferences in unexpected ways when carried out for the alleviation of a psychological disorder. This capacity may be an unhelpful or even distressing adjunctive action of drug treatment. However, it may be questioned whether drugs could be used deliberately to bring about desired changes in food preferences. Although the data from animal studies are not in total agreement (see section V.A.), the most coherent body of knowledge exists for pharmacological manipulations of the neurotransmitter serotonin. Using amphetamine and fenfluramine as a drug pair, in a manner similar to that used in animal experiments, it was reported that amphetamine produced a marked suppression of protein consumption whereas fenfluramine exerted a greater suppression of carbohydrate intake (31). Similar directional effects were observed on a food preference questionnaire, and it was noticeable that the subjective preferences were a more sensitive indicator of the presence of an active drug than actual behavior. This controlled study that examined subjective experiences and consumption across the course of a single meal shows that drugs may produce subtle but understandable adjustments to food selection in keeping with their presumed action on neurotransmitters. The study also revealed that strong changes brought about in subjective preferences for protein and carbohydrate are translated into a weaker effect on the actual consumption of these macronutrients. The reasons for this disparity are not obvious, but the phenomenon should be considered if drugs are to be used for the deliberate suppression or enhancement of macronutrient intake. Indeed, it has been argued that drugs such as fenfluramine, which enhance activity at serotoninergic synapses, could be used in the treatment of eating disorders to suppress appetite selectively for carbohydrate (188). In a test of this hypothesis a group of subjects prone to snack on high-carbohydrate foods were treated separately with tryptophan and fenfluramine (189). The treatment period for each compound was 5 days, and during this time fenfluramine significantly reduced the number of carbohydrate foods taken in snacks. Tryptophan gave rise to a weaker effect. Since a predilection for carbohydrates is often noted in overweight individuals, the use of fenfluramine alone, or together with tryptophan, could be useful in controlling this tendency. Accordingly, the extension of food selection mechanisms into the clinical arena assumes an importance related to hormonal fluctuations, the capricious or incidental effects of prescribed psychoactive drugs, and the deliberate, rational intention to adjust neurochemistry to provoke a desired change in preference and consumption.

G. Human Feeding: Physiology and Cognition

It is, of course, a truism to remark that human feeding is dependent on both physiological and environmental variables and may be viewed profitably as an interaction (see section II.A.). Indeed, many people would argue that human food habits are dominated by ethnic, racial, cultural, sociopolitical, and economic factors that collectively overwhelm any basic biological dispositions—in certain cases, for example, political hunger strikers, to the point of death. But in certain stable subpopulations where elective intake is not unduly hindered by religious or economic constraints it may be possible to detect the effective operation of physiological factors (see previous section). Moreover, Rozin (157) has drawn attention to three examples—carbohydrate metabolism in Eskimos, phenylthiocarbamide tasting, and lactase deficiency—where biological variables make a clear contribution to regional feeding habits. Between the committed activist who refuses all food for political reasons and the Yoruba tribesman who avoids milk because of lactase deficiency it is necessary to develop a framework to comprehend the interplay between biological variables and the mental processes that together determine human feeding practices.

1. Conceptual Coherence

In addition to considering the extent to which nutrient selection depends on neurotransmitter activity, and on the learned associations between metabolic events and behavior, one further domain of information has to be recognized. This domain involves the "sociology of knowledge" (16) and seeks to understand the way in which our "everyday" understanding of events arises and gives credibility to the world. One basic assumption is that every society contains a fabric of shared meanings that serve particular functions for individuals, allowing their actions to be consistent with those of others. Accordingly, a study of biological mechanisms underlying the selection of nutrients needs to take account of the sociology of knowledge since an individual's life is lived within boundaries of awareness and consciousness set by the social system. Reynolds (146a) has referred to this culturally defined knowledge entering the mind to give "contours" to the world, thus making sense of physiological functioning.

Food selection is not only an aspect of behavior, it is also a social action, and it can be argued that biological functioning (including changes in levels of hormones, neurotransmitters, etc.) achieves harmony with social actions through the mediating process of conceptual thought. Coherence is attained by way of cognitive structuring. Consistent with this supposition is the evidence that cognitive factors, concerning a person's belief about the strength of a need (preference) or about the power of a food to satisfy a need, can overcome objectively defined indices in the control of food consumption (184). The intervention of these cognitive factors—giving meaning to actions—may be one reason why drug-induced changes in nutrient preferences (see section VI.D.) are not inevitably converted into mutually consistent behavior. In other words, the necessity to have *reasons* for selecting one macronutrient rather than another may overcome or adjust any biological disposition to select based on fluctuating levels of hormones or neurotransmitters. In experiments on human *behavior*, biological manipulations should not be expected to induce unequivocal responses. Food selection is not a localized physicochemical parameter such as a glandular secretion or enzyme concentration, but involves the whole organism and occurs in the public world. Accordingly, it seems profitable to view man, and his selective capacity, simultaneously as a biological organism and as a social, intellectual being.

2. Uncoupling of Response Systems

The concept of uncoupling or disengagement is most widely known in the field of emotional arousal. For example, Lacey (98) has argued that electrocortical, autonomic, and behavioral indices of arousal are imperfectly coupled systems. In a study of subjectively felt fear in parachute jumpers, training and experience led to a dissociation of perceived avoidance (fear) and a physiological index of fear such as heart rate (59). Lang (99) has construed emotional behavior as verbal–cognitive, motor, and physiological events interacting through interoceptive and exteroceptive channels. These systems differ in sensitivity and in subtlety of response and can, therefore, be uncoupled. In simple terms this means that our thoughts, our behavioral actions, and our physiological variables do not appear always to act in synchrony. Food selection can be similarly conceived to consist of subjectively embedded preferences, actual selection behavior, and underlying physiological/neurochemical mechanisms. Indeed, in studies of food intake uncoupling has been demonstrated between cognitive and metabolic variables (184), subjective sensations and behavior (153), and physiological and behavioral measures (85). The obvious conceptualizing power of humans together with the known dissociation between biological, behavioral, and mental events means that research on biological mechanisms of human nutrient selection will have to be framed within meaningful boundaries. Paradigms used in animal experiments and in the typical clinical trials in man will be inadequate to detect the operation of biological factors obscured by desynchrony. Uncoupling does not mean that biological processes (hormones/neurotransmitters) are unrelated to nutrient selection, but it suggests that the classic cause–effect sequence may not always be found.

VII. CODETTA: FOOD SELECTION AS A BIOPSYCHOLOGICAL PROBLEM

Study of the self-selection of macronutrients can be regarded as a classic biopsychological problem. Not only does it require an examination of physiological processes and neurotransmitter mechanisms but it also demands a fastidious approach to the dismantling of variables in the behavioral domain. The task is made more difficult by the obvious fact that when manipulations are made to the system by drugs, brain lesions, removal of glands, hormonal treatments, and dietary adjustments many aspects of the system are disturbed simultaneously. In such a complex fabric of biological and psychological variables, experimentation is faced with severe methodological problems and theory development is difficult.

Considering the number of variables that can affect the self-selection of nutrients, a general consensus among the data would be unlikely and indeed is not apparent. Even certain clear contradictory findings may be observed, for example, following the manipulation of ovarian hormones (see section V.C.) or the drug clonidine (see section V.A.4.) or associated with circadian rhythms (see section V.D.). It may be questioned whether, out of this dense network of data, it is possible to extract a basic regulatory principle that governs nutrient selection. One possibility is that a direct metabolic–behavior link to control the amount of nutrient (particularly protein) does not exist. Under such circumstances approximate control of intake could be accounted for in two ways: first, by the action of avoidance mechanisms to cope with deficits and surfeits of a macronutrient such as protein, and second by the expression of the "variety" effect, which in rats manifests itself as the tendency to change from one food to another from meal to meal, thus ensuring some degree of variability in dietary intake.

However, although extremes of lack or excess can be accounted for, it is plausible that a more subtle mechanism has evolved to adjust nutrient selection within upper and lower boundaries. Evidence suggests that the neurotransmitter serotonin may be involved in this mechanism. Serotonin is synthesized from an essential amino acid and levels in the brain fluctuate in keeping with nutrient inflow (see section III.B.), although it is likely that a certain amount of buffering occurs. However, because of its dependence on a dietary amino acid, serotonin is usually perceived as exerting a "modulatory" influence on behavioral activities such as sleep and sex. This modulatory action could also apply to self-selection behavior, in which case a serotoninergic mechanism would work jointly with avoidance learning and behavioral change to keep protein intake within manageable limits. A group of mechanisms acting in this way would allow a flexible expression of behavior incorporating the selection of nutrients.

It is clear that any theoretical statement about the selection of nutrients must account for the widely observed range of individual variability. Individual experimental animals and humans display markedly discrepant idiosyncratic preferences and aversions for certain nutrients. The reasons for these peculiar patterns are not always obvious, but their existence in man invites the development of techniques to treat such anomalous, and possibly harmful, intakes.

In the view of the present author the further refinement of theory will depend on the clarification and resolution of certain methodological problems confronting experimenters. Foremost among these is reaching an agreement about the basic paradigm in those studies using a causal strategy. The continued use of separate purified nutrients and composite diets will inevitably lead to a proliferation of conflicting experimental reports. However, one further concern limits almost every one of the experiments in this research field. In experimental language, behavioral self-selection of nutrients means voluntary consumption in the presence of unlimited amounts of the food items. Almost nothing is known of the searching or foraging strategies that may be invoked when animals are obliged to seek *specific* nutritional commodities not immediately accessible. Indeed the various influences on elective consumption of nutrients, reviewed above, could be significantly adjusted by the economic cost involved in finding food instead of simply eating it. Such problems will remain unsolved for a considerable time to come.

ACKNOWLEDGMENTS

Part of this chapter was prepared while the author was Johananoff International Fellow in Advanced Biomedical Research at the Istituto di Ricerche Farmacologiche Mario Negri in Milan. I am grateful to Professors Silvio Garattini and Alfredo Leonardi for their support. I am also grateful to Bob McArthur for collaboration on research related to the topic of the review and for discussion of methodological problems. I thank Miranda Hughes for critical comments on the text and Mavis Walton for help with the preparation of the manuscript.

REFERENCES

1. Abdallah, A. H., and White, H. D. (1970): Comparative study of the anorexic activity of phen-inolamine, *d*-amphetamine and fenfluramine in different species. *Arch. Int. Pharmacodyn. Ther.*, 188:271–283.
2. Ahlskog, J. E., and Hoebel, B. G. (1973): Overeating and obesity from damage to a noradrenergic system in the brain. *Science*, 182:166–169.
3. Anand, B. K., and Brobeck, J. R. (1951): Localisation of a "feeding centre" in the hypothalamus of the rat. *Proc. Soc. Exp. Biol. Med.*, 77:323–324.
4. Anderson, G. H. (1977): Regulation of protein intake by plasma amino acids. *Adv. Nutr. Res.*, 1:145–166.
5. Anderson, G. H., and Ashley, D. V. M. (1974): Correlation of the plasma tyrosine to phenylalanine ratio with energy intake in self-selecting weanling rats. *Life Sci.*, 21:1227–1234.
6. Anderson, G. H., Benevenga, N. J., and Harper, A. E. (1968): Associations among food and protein intake, serine dehydratase and plasma amino acids. *Am. J. Physiol.*, 214:1008–1013.
7. Anderson, G. H., Leprohon, C., Chambers, J. W., and Coscina, D. V. (1979): Intact regulation of protein intake during the development of hypothalamic or genetic obesity in rats. *Physiol. Behav.*, 23:751–755.

8. Andik, I., Donohoffer, S., Moring, I., and Szentes, J. (1951): The effect of starvation on food intake and selection. *Acta Physiol. Acad. Sci. Hung.*, 2:363–368.

9. Ashley, D. V. M., and Anderson, G. H. (1975): Food intake regulation in the weanling rat: Effects of the most limiting essential amino acids of gluten, casein and zein on the self-selection of protein and energy. *J. Nutr.*, 105:1405–1411.

10. Ashley, D. V. M., and Anderson, G. H. (1975): Correlation between the plasma tryptophan to neutral amino acid ratio and protein intake in the self-selecting weanling rat. *J. Nutr.*, 105:1412–1421.

11. Ashley, D. V. M., Coscina, D. V., and Anderson, G. H. (1979): Selective decrease in protein intake following brain serotonin depletion. *Life Sci.*, 24:973–984.

12. Barker, L. M., Best, M. R., and Domjan, M. (1977): *Learning Mechanisms in Food Selection.* Baylor University Press.

13. Baumgarten, H. G., Bjorklund, A., Lachenmeyer, L., and Nobin, A. (1973): Long-lasting selective depletion of brain serotonin by 5,6-dihydroxytryptamine. *Acta Physiol. Scand. (Suppl.)*, 391:2–19.

14. Beach, F. A. (1979): Animal models for human sexuality. In: *Sex, Hormones and Behaviour.* Ciba Foundation Symposium 62 (new series), pp. 113–132. Excerpta Medica, Amsterdam.

15. Belovsky, G. E. (1978): Diet optimization in a generalist herbivore: The moose. *Theoret. Pop. Biol.*, 14:105–134.

16. Berger, P. L., and Luckmann, T. (1967): *The Social Construction of Reality.* Penguin, Harmondsworth.

17. Bernadis, L. L., and Bellinger, L. L. (1981): Dorsomedial hypothalamic hypophagia: Self-selection of diets and macronutrients, efficiency of food utilization, "stress and eating," response to high protein diet and circulating substrate concentrations. *Appetite*, 2:103–113.

18. Berridge, K., Grill, H. J., and Norgren, R. (1981): Relation of consummatory responses and pre-absorptive insulin release to palatability and learned taste aversions. *J. Comp. Physiol. Psychol.*, 95:363–382.

19. Blundell, J. E. (1977): Is there a role for serotonin (5-hydroxytryptamine) in feeding? *Int. J. Obes.*, 1:15–42.

20. Blundell, J. E. (1979): Hunger, appetite and satiety—constructs in search of identities. In: *Nutrition and Lifestyles*, edited by M. Turner, pp. 21–42. Applied Science Pub., London.

21. Blundell, J. E. (1979): Serotonin and feeding. In: *Serotonin in Health and Disease, Vol. 5, Clinical Applications*, edited by W. B. Essman, pp. 403–450. Spectrum, New York.

22. Blundell, J. E. (1980): Pharmacological adjustment of the mechanisms underlying feeding and obesity. In: *Obesity*, edited by A. J. Stunkard, pp. 182–207. W. B. Saunders, Philadelphia.

23. Blundell, J. E. (1981): Deep and surface structures: A qualitative approach to feeding. In: *The Body Weight Regulatory System: Normal and Disturbed Mechanisms*, edited by L. A. Cioffi, W. P. T. James, and T. Van-Itallie, pp. 73–82. Raven Press, New York.

24. Blundell, J. E. (1981): Biogrammar of feeding: Pharmacological manipulations and their interpretations. In: *Progress in Theory and Psychopharmacology*, edited by S. J. Cooper, pp. 233–276. Academic Press, London.

25. Blundell, J. E., Campbell, D. B., Leshem, M. B., and Tozer, R. (1975): Comparison of the time course of the anorexic effects of amphetamine and fenfluramine with drug levels in blood. *J. Pharm. Pharmacol.*, 27:187–192.

26. Blundell, J. E., and Latham, C. J. (1978): Pharmacological manipulation of feeding behaviour: Possible influences of serotonin and dopamine on food intake. In: *Central Mechanisms of Anorectic Drugs*, edited by S. Garattini and R. Samanin, pp. 83–109. Raven Press, New York.

27. Blundell, J. E., and Latham, C. J. (1979): Serotonergic influences on food intake: Effect of 5-hydroxytryptophan on parameters of feeding behaviour in deprived and free-feeding rats. *Pharmacol. Biochem. Behav.*, 11:431–437.

28. Blundell, J. E., and McArthur, R. A. (1979): Investigation of food consumption using a dietary self-selection procedure: Effects of pharmacological manipulation and feeding schedules. *Br. J. Pharmacol.*, 67:436P–438P.

29. Blundell, J. E., and McArthur, R. A. (1981): Behavioural flux and feeding: Continuous monitoring of food intake and food selection and the video-recording of appetitive and satiety sequences for the analysis of drug action. In: *Anorectic Agents, Mechanisms of Action and of Tolerance*, edited by S. Garattini, pp. 19–43. Raven Press, New York.

30. Blundell, J. E., and Rogers, P. J. (1978): Pharmacological approaches to the understanding of obesity. *Psychiatr. Clin. N. Am.*, 1:629–650.
31. Blundell, J. E., and Rogers, P. J. (1980): Effects of anorexic drugs on food intake, food selection and preferences, hunger motivation and subjective experiences. *Appetite*, 1:151–165.
32. Blundell, J. E., and Rogers, P. J. (1980): Fame e appetito—una prospettiva biopsicologica. In: *Obesita*, edited by M. Cairella and A. Jacobelli, pp. 99–119. Societa Editrice Universo, Roma.
33. Booth, D. A. (1974): Acquired sensory preference for protein in diabetic and normal rats. *Physiol. Psychol.*, 2:344–348.
34. Booth, D. A. (1976): Approaches to feeding control. In: *Appetite and Food Intake*, edited by T. Silverstone. Abakon, Berlin.
35. Booth, D. A. (1977): Satiety and appetite are conditioned reactions. *Psychosom. Med.*, 39:76–81.
36. Booth, D. A. (1978): *Hunger Models. Computable Theory of Feeding Control.* Academic Press, London.
37. Booth, D. A., Lee, M., and McAleavey, C. (1976): Acquired sensory control of satiation in man. *Br. J. Psychol.*, 67:137–147.
38. Booth, D. A., and Stribling, D. (1978): Neurochemistry of appetite mechanisms. *Proc. Nutr. Soc.*, 37:181–191.
39. Booth, D. A., Toates, F. M., and Platt, S. V. (1976): Control system for hunger and its implications in animals and man. In: *Hunger: Basic Mechanisms and Clinical Implications*, edited by D. Novin, W. Wyrwicka, and G. Bray, pp. 127–143. Raven Press, New York.
40. Brobeck, J. R. (1960): Food and temperature. *Recent Prog. Horm. Res.*, 16:439–459.
41. Brobeck, J. R. (1981): Models for analysing energy balance in body weight regulation. In: *The Body Weight Regulatory System: Normal and Disturbed Mechanisms*, edited by L. A. Cioffi, P. James, and E. Van-Itallie, pp. 1–9. Raven Press, New York.
42. Broekkamp, C. L. E., Honig, W. M. M., Pavli, A. I., and Van Rossum, J. M. (1974): Pharmacological suppression of eating behaviour in relation to diencephalic noradrenergic receptors. *Life Sci.*, 14:473–481.
43. Brunswik, E. (1950): *The Conceptual Framework of Psychology.* University of Chicago Press, Chicago.
44. Cabanac, M., and Duclaux, R. (1970): Specificity of internal signals in producing satiety for taste stimuli. *Nature*, 227:966.
45. Chee, K. M., Romsos, D. R., and Bergen, W. G. (1981): Effects of dietary fat on protein intake regulation in young obese and lean mice. *J. Nutr.*, 111:668–677.
46. Climchmidt, G. V., McGuffin, J. .C., Pflueger, A. B., Tevaro, J. A. (1978): A 5-hydroxytryptamine-like mode of action for *p*-chloro-2-(l-piperarinyl)-pyrazine (MK-212). *Br. J. Pharmacol.*, 52:579–589.
47. Collier, G., Hirsch, E., and Hamlin, P. H. (1972): The ecological determinants of reinforcement in the rat. *Physiol. Behav.*, 9:705–716.
48. Collier, G., Hirsch, E., and Kanarek, R. (1977): The operant revisited. In: *Handbook of Operant Behaviour*, edited by W. K. Honig and J. E. R. Staddon. Prentice-Hall, New Jersey.
49. Collier, G., Leshner, A. I., and Squibb, R. L. (1969): Dietary self-selection in active and non-active rats. *Physiol. Behav.*, 4:79–82.
50. Corey, D. T., Walton, A., and Wiener, N. I. (1978): Development of carbohydrate preference during water rationing: A specific hunger? *Physiol. Behav.*, 20:547–552.
51. Costa, E., Groppetti, A., and Revuelta, A. (1971): Action of fenfluramine on monoamine stores of rat tissues. *Br. J. Pharmacol.*, 41:57–64.
52. Cross, P. E., Dickinson, R. P. Halliwell, G., and Kemp, E. G. (1977): Substituted trifluoromethylphenyl piperazines as anorectic agents. *Eur. J. Med. Chem.*, 12:173–176.
53. Curzon, G., Joseph, M. H., and Knott, P. J. (1972): Effects of immobilization and food deprivation on rat brain tryptophan metabolism. *J. Neurochem.*, 19:1967–1974.
54. Davis, J. D., and Wirtshafter, D. (1978): Set points or settling points for body weight? A reply to Mrosovsky and Pawley. *Behav. Biol.*, 24:405–411.
55. Deutsch, J. A. (1978): The stomach in food satiation and the regulation of appetite. *Prog. Neurobiol.*, 10:135–153.
56. Donhoffer, S., and Vonotsky, J. (1947): The effect of enviornmental temperature on food selection. *Am. J. Physiol.* 150:329–333.
57. Duhault, J., and Verdavainne, C. (1967): Modification du taux de serotonine cerebrale chez le

rat par les trifluoromethyl-phenyl-2-ethyl-amino-propane. *Arch. Int. Pharmacodyn. Ther.* 170:276–283.

58. Edwards, G. L., and Ritter, R. C. (1981): Ablation of the area postrema causes exaggerated consumption of preferred foods in the rat. *Brain Res.*, 216:265–276.

59. Epstein, S., and Fenz, W. D. (1965): Steepness of approach and avoidance gradients in humans as a function of experience: Theory and experiment. *J. Exp. Psychol.*, 70:1–12.

60. Fahrbach, S. E., Tretter, J. R., Aravich, P. F., McCabe, J., and Leibowitz, S. F. (1980): Increased carbohydrate preference in the rat after injection of 2-deoxy-d-glucose and clonidine. In: *Proceedings of the Society for Neuroscience 10th Annual Meeting, Cincinnati, Nov. 9–14*, p. 784, Abstracts, Vol.6.

61. Fernstrom, J. D., and Wurtman, R. J. (1971): Brain serotonin content: Physiological dependence on plasma tryptophan levels. *Science*, 173:149–152.

62. Fernstrom, J D., and Wurtman, R. J. (1971): Brain serotonin content: Increase following injection of carbohydrate diet. *Science*, 174:1023–1025.

63. Fernstrom J. D., and Wurtman, R. J. (1972): Brain sorotonin content: Physiological regulation by plasma neutral amino acids. *Science*, 178:414–416.

64. Fernstrom, J. D., and Wurtman R. J. (1973): Control of brain 5-HT content by dietary carbohydrates. In: *Serotonin and Behaviour*, edited by J. Barchas and E. Usdin, pp. 121–128. Academic Press, New York.

65. Fernstrom, J. D., and Wurtman, R. J. (1974): Nutrition and the brain. *Sci. Am.*, 230:84–91.

66. Friedman, M., and Stricker, E. (1976): The physiological psychology of hunger: A physiological perspective. *Psychol. Rev.*, 83:409–437.

67. Fuller, R. W., Perry, K. W., Snoddy, H. D., and Molloy, B. B. (1974): Comparison of the specificity of 3-(p-trifluoromethylphenoxy)-N-methyl-3-phenylpropanolamine and chlorimipramine as amine uptake inhibitors in mice. *Eur. J. Phramacol.*, 28:223–236.

68. Fuller, R. W., and Wong, D. T. (1977): Inhibition of serotonin reuptake. *Fed. Proc.*, 36:2154–2158.

69. Garattini, S., and Samanin, R. (1976): Anorectic drugs and neurotransmitters. In: *Food Intake and Appetite*, edited by T. Silverstone, pp. 82–108. Dahlem Konferenzen, Berlin.

70. Garb, J L., and Stunkard, A. J. (1974): Taste aversions in man. *Am. J. Psychiatry*, 131:1204–1207.

71. Garcia, J., Hankins, W. G., and Rusiniak, K. W. (1974): Behavioural regulation of the milieu interne in man and rat. *Science*, 185:824–831.

72. Garcia, J., and Koelling, R. A. (1966): Relation of cue to consequence in avoidance learning. *Psychon. Sci.*, 4:123–124.

73. Garrow, J. S. (1978): *Energy Balance and Obesity in Man.* North Holland, Amsterdam.

74. Geiselman, P. J., Martin, J. E., Vanderweele, D. A., and Novin, D. (1981): Dietary self-selection in cycling and neonatally ovariectomized rats. *Appetite*, 2:87–101.

75. Gold, R. M., Jones, A. P., and Sawchenko, P. E. (1977): Paraventricular area: Critical focus of a longitudinal neurocircuitry mediating food intake. *Physiol. Behav.*, 18:1111–1119.

76. Goodman, L. S., and Gilman A. (1970): *The Pharmacological Basis of Therapeutics.* 4th edition. Macmillan, New York.

77. Goudie, A. J., Thornton, E. W., and Wheeler, T. J. (1976): Effects of Lilly 110140, a specific inhibitor of serotonin uptake, on food intake and on 5-hydroxytryptophan-induced anorexia. Evidence for serotonergic inhibition of feeding. *J. Pharm. Pharmacol.*, 28:318–320.

78. Grill, H. J., and Norgren, R. (1978): Chronically decerebrate rats demonstrate satiation but not bait shyness. *Science*, 201:267–269.

79. Grossman, S. P. (1976): Neuroanatomy of food and water intake. In: *Hunger: Basic Mechanisms and Clinical Implications*, edited by D. Novin, W. Wyrwicka, and G. Bray, pp. 51–59. Raven Press, New York.

80. Harper, A. E. (1967): Effects of dietary protein content and amino acid pattern on food intake and preference. In: *Handbook of Physiology, Vol. 6: Alimentary Canal*, edited by C. F. Code. American Physiological Society, Washington.

81. Harper, A. E. (1976): Protein and amino acids in the regulaton of food intake. In: *Hunger: Basic Mechanisms and Clinical Implications*, edited by D. Novin, W. Wyrwicka, and G. Bray, pp. 103–113. Raven Press, New York.

82. Harris, J. L., Clay, J., Hargreaves, I. J., and Ward, A. (1933): Appetite and choice of diet. The

ability of the vitamin-B deficient rat to discriminate between diets containing and lacking the vitamin. *Proc. Roy. Soc. Lond.* [Biol.], 113:161–190.

83. Hernandez, L., and Hoebel, B. G. (1980): Basic mechanisms of feeding and weight regulation. In: *Obesity*, edited by A. J. Stunkard, pp. 25–47. W. B. Saunders, Philadelphia.

84. Hirsch, E. and Collier, G. (1974): The ecological determinants of reinforcement in the guinea pig. *Physiol. Behav.*, 12:239–249.

85. Hodgson, R. J., and Greene, J. B. (1980): The saliva priming effect, eating speed and the measurement of hunger. *Behav. Res. Ther.*, 18:243–247.

86. Hoebel, B. G., and Leibowitz S. F. (1981): Brain monoamines in the modulation of self-stimulation, feeding, and body weight. In: *Brain, Behaviour and Bodily Disease*, edited by H. A. Weiner, M. A. Hofer, and A. J. Stunkard, pp. 103–142. Raven Press, New York.

87. Johnson, D. J., Li, E. T. S., Coscina, D. V., and Anderson, G. H. (1979): Different diurnal rhythms of protein and non-protein energy intake by rats. *Physiol. Behav.*, 22:777–780.

88. Kanarek, R. B., and Beck, J. M. (1980): Role of gonadal hormones in diet selection and food utilization in female rats. *Physiol. Behav.*, 24:381–386.

88a. Kanarek, R. B., Feldman, P. G., and Hanes, C. (1981): Pattern of dietary self-selection in VMH-lesioned rats. *Physiol. Behav.*, 27:337–343.

89. Kanarek, R. B., and Hirsch, E. (1977): Dietary-induced overeating in experimental animals. *Fed. Proc.*, 36:154–158.

90. Kanarek, R. B., Ho, L., and Meade, R. G. (1981): Amphetamine selectively decreases fat consumption in rats. *Pharmacol. Biochem. Behav. (In press)*.

91. Kanarek, R. B., Marks-Kaufman, R., and Lipeles, B. J. (1980): Increased carbohydrate intake as a function of insulin administration in rats. *Physiol. Behav.*, 25:779–782.

92. Keesey, R. E. (1978): Set points and body weight regulation. *Psychiatr. Clin. N. Am.*, 1:523–543.

93. Kennedy, G. C. (1953): The role of depot fat in the hypothalamic control of food intake in the rat. *Proc. R. Soc. Lond.*, 140:578–592.

94. Kon, S. (1931): The self-selection of food constituents by the rat. *Biochem. J.*, 25:473–481.

95. Krebs, J. R., and Davies, N. B. (1981): *An Introduction to Behavioural Ecology.* Blackwell, Oxford.

96. Kuhn, T. S. (1962): *The Structure of Scientific Revolution.* Chicago University Press, Chicago.

97. Kuhn, T. S. (1970): Logic of Discovery or Psychology of Research. In: *Criticism and the Growth of Knowledge*, edited by I. Lakatos and A. Musgrave. Cambridge University Press, London.

98. Lacey, J. I. (1967): Somatic response patterning and stress: Some revisions of activation theory. In: *Psychological Stress*, edited by Appley and Trumbell, Appleton-Century-Crofts, New York.

99. Lang, P. J. (1971): Application of psychophysical methods to the study of psychotherapy and behaviour modification. In: *Handbook of Psychotherapy and Behavioural Change—An empirical analysis*, edited by A. E. Bergin and S. L. Garfield, pp. 75–125. John Wiley, New York.

100. Lát, J. (1967): Self-selection of dietary components. In: *Handbook of Physiology, Vol. 1: Alimentary Canal*, edited by F. Code. American Physiology Society, Washington, D.C.

101. Latham, C. J., and Blundell, J. E. (1979): Evidence for the effect of tryptophan on the pattern of food consumption in free feeding and food deprived rats. *Life Sci.*, 24:1971–1978.

102. Leathwood, P., and Arimanana, L. (1980): Patterns of food intake in rats offered a choice of high and low protein diets. In: *Proceedings of the Seventh International Conference on the Physiology of Food and Fluid Intake* ("IUPS"), Warsaw, July 7–10, 1980.

103. Leathwood, P. D., and Ashley, D. V. M. (1981): Nutrients as regulators of food choice. In: *The Body Weight Regulatory System: Normal and Disturbed Mechanisms*, edited by L. A. Cioffi, P. James and E. Van-Itallie, pp. 263–269. Raven Press, New York.

104. Leibowitz, S. F. (1980): Neurochemical systems of the hypothalamus—control of feeding and drinking behaviour and water-electrolyte excretion. In: *Handbook of the Hypothalamus, Vol. 3*, pp. 299–437. Marcel Dekker, New York.

105. Leibowitz, S. F., and Brown, L. L. (1980): Histochemical and pharmacological analysis of noradrenergic projections to the paraventricular hypothalamus in relation to feeding stimulation. *Brain Res.*, 201:289–314.

106. Leibowitz, S. F., and Brown, L. L. (1980): Histochemical and pharmacological analysis of catecholaminergic projections to the perifornical hypothalamus in relation to feeding inhibition. *Brain Res.*, 201:315–345.

107. Le Magnen, J. (1950): Nouvelles donnes sur le phénomène de l'exaltolide. *Comptes Rendues H. Acad. Sci. Ser. C.*, 226:627.
108. Leprohon, C. E., Woodger, T. L., Ashley, D. V. M., and Anderson, G. H. (1979): Effect of mineral mixture in diet on protein intake regulation in the weanling rat. *J. Nutr.*, 109:827–831.
109. Leshner, A. I., and Collier, G. (1973): The effect of gonadectomy on the sex differences in the dietary self-selection patterns and carcass composition of rats. *Physiol. Behav.*, 11:671–676.
110. Leshner, A. J., Collier, G. H., and Squibb, R. L. (1971): Dietary self-selection at cold temperatures. *Physiol. Behav.*, 6:1–3.
111. Leshner, A. I., Siegel, H. I., and Collier, G. (1972): Dietary self-selection by pregnant and lactating rats. *Physiol. Behav.*, 8:151–154.
112. Leshner, A. I., and Walker, W. A. (1973): Dietary self-selection, activity and carcass composition of rats fed Thiouracil. *Physiol. Behav.*, 10:373–378.
113. Leung, P., Larson, D., and Rogers, Q. (1972): Food intake and preference of olfacto bulbectomized rats fed amino acid imbalanced or deficient diets. *Physiol. Behav.*, 9:553–555.
114. Leung, P. M. B., and Rogers, Q. R. (1971): Importance of prepyriform cortex in food intake response of rats to amino acids. *Am. J. Physiol.*, 221:929–935.
115. Logue, A. W., Ophir, I., and Strauss, K. E. (1981): The acquisition of taste aversions in humans. *Behav. Res. Ther.*, 19:319–333.
116. Lytle, L. D. (1977): Control of Eating Behaviour. In: *Nutrition and the Brain, Vol. 2. Control of Feeding Behaviour and Biology of the Brain in Protein-Calorie Malnutrition*, edited by R. J. Wurtman and J. J. Wurtman. Raven Press, New York.
117. Marks-Kaufman, R., and Kanarek, R. (1983): Modification of nutrient selection induced by naloxone in rats. *Psychopharmacology (In press)*.
118. Marks-Kaufman, R., and Kanarek, R. B. (1980): Morphine selectively influences macronutrient intake in the rat. *Pharmac. Biochem. Behav.*, 12:427–430.
119. Mauron, C., Wurtman, J. J., and Wurtman, R. J. (1980): Clonidine increases food and protein consumption in rats. *Life Sci.*, 27:781–791.
120. McArthur, R. A., and Blundell, J. E. (1982): Effects of age and feeding regime on self-selection of protein and carbohydrate. *Appetite: J. Intake Res.*, 3:153–162.
121. McArthur, R. A., and Blundell, J. E. (1982): Effect of dietary form on the self-selection of protein and carbohydrate. *Paper presented to meeting of the British Feeding Group. London*, May 11.
122. McDonald, D. G., Stern, J. A., and Hahn, W. W. (1963):Effects of differential housing and stress on diet selection, water intake and body weight in the rat. *J. Appl. Physiol.*, 18:937–942.
123. Mellinkoff, S. (1957): Digestive System. *Annu. Rev. Physiol.*, 19:175.
124. Morgan, R. (1977): Three weeks in isolation with two schizophrenic patients. *Br. J. Psychiatry*, 131:504–513.
125. Morgane, P. J. (1980): Historical and modern concepts of hypothalamic organisation and function. In: *Handbook of the Hypothalamus, Vol. 1: Anatomy of the Hypothalamus*, edited by P. J. Morgane and J. Panksepp, pp. 1–64. Marcel Dekker, New York.
126. Morley, J. E. (1980): The neuroendocrine control of appetite: The role of the endogenous opiates, cholecystokinin, TRH, gamma-amino-butyric acid and the diazepam receptor. *Life Sci.*, 27:355–368.
127. Mrosovsky, N., and Powley, T. L. (1977): Set points for body weight and fat. *Behav. Biol.*, 20:205–223.
128. Musten, B., Peace, D., and Anderson, G. H. (1974): Food intake regulation in the weanling rat: Self-selection of protein and energy. *J. Nutr.*, 104:563–572.
129. Myers, R. D. (1975): Brain mechanisms in the control of feeding: A new neurochemical profile theory. *Pharmac. Biochem, Behav.* (Suppl. 1), 3:75–83.
130. Nance, D. M. (1976): Sex differences in the hypothalamic regulation of feeding behaviour in the rat. In: *Advances in Psychobiology*, edited by A. H. Rieser and R. F. Thompson, pp. 75–123. John Wiley, New York.
131. Neuringer, M., and Mayer, J. (1970): Absence of protein intake regulation in rats with lesions of the ventromedial nuclei of the hypothalamus. *Fed. Proc.*, 29:657.
132. Orthen-Gambill, N., and Kanarek, R. B. (1982): Differential effects of amphetamine and fenfluramine on dietary self-selection in rats. *Pharmac. Biochem. Behav.*, 16:303–309.
133. Overmann, S. R. (1976): Dietary self-selection by animals. *Psychol. Bull.*, 83:218–235.
134. Overmann, S. R., and Yang, M. G. (1973): Adaptation to water restriction through dietary selection in weanling rats. *Physiol. Behav.*, 11:781–786.

135. Panksepp, J. (1975): Central metabolic and humoral factors involved in the neural regulation of feeding. *Pharmac. Biochem. Behav.* (Suppl. 1), 3:107–119.

136. Panksepp, J. (1978): Dietary constituents and self-selection procedures: Solid foods. In: *Handbook of Psychobiology*, edited by R. D. Myers. Academic Press, New York.

137. Panksepp, J., and Booth, D. A. (1971): Decreased feeding after injections of amino acids into the hypothalamus. *Nature*, 233:341–342.

138. Paykel, E. S., Mueller, P. S., and De La Vergne, P. M. (1973): Amitriptyline, weight gain and carbohydrate craving: a side effect. *Br. J. Psychiatry*, 123:501–507.

139. Peng, Y., Meliza, L. L., Vavich, M. G., and Kemmerer, A. R. (1975): Effects of amino acid imbalance and protein content of diets on food intake and preference of young, adult and diabetic rats. *J. Nutr.*, 105:1395–1404.

140. Peng, Y., Tews, J. K., and Harper, A. E. (1972): Amino acid imbalance, protein intake and changes in rat brain and plasma amino acids. *Am. J. Physiol.*, 222:314–322.

141. Perez-Cruet, J., Tagliamonte, A., Tagliamonte, P., and Gessa, G. L. (1972): Changes in brain serotonin metabolism associated with fasting and satiation in rats. *Life Sci.*, 11:31–39.

142. Pilgrim, F., and Patton, R. (1947): Patterns of self-selection of purified dietary components by the rat. *J. Comp. Physiol. Psychol.*, 40:343–348.

143. Piquard, F., Schaefer, A., and Haberey, P. (1978): Influence of fasting and protein deprivation on food self-selection in the rat. *Physiol. Behav.*, 20:771–778.

144. Powley, T. (1977): The ventromedial hypothalamic syndrome, satiety and a cephalic phase hypothesis. *Psychol. Rev.*, 84:89–126.

145. Reddingius, J. (1980): Control theory and the dynamics of body weight. *Physiol. Behav.*, 24:27–32.

146. Revusky, S. H., and Bedarf, E. W. (1967): Association of illness with prior ingestion of novel foods. *Science*, 155:219–220.

146a. Reynolds, V. (1976): *The Biology of Human Action*, p. 269. Freeman, San Francisco.

147. Richter, C. P. (1942): Increased dextrose appetite of normal rats treated with insulin. *Am. J. Physiol.*, 35:781–787.

148. Richter, C. P. (1943): Total self-regulatory functions in animals and human beings. *Harvey Lecture Series*, 38:63–103.

149. Richter, C. P., and Barelare, B. (1938): Nutritional requirements of pregnant and lactating rats studied by the self-selection method. *Endocrinology*, 23:15–24.

150. Richter, C., Holt, L., and Barelare, B. (1938): Nutritional requirements for normal growth and reproduction in rats studied by the self-selection method. *Am. J. Physiol.*, 122:734–744.

151. Rodin, J. (1978): Has the distinction between internal versus external control of feeding outlived its usefulness? In: *Recent Advances in Obesity Research Vol. II*, edited by G. Bray. Newman, London.

152. Rodin, J. (1981): The current status of the internal-external obesity hypothesis: What went wrong? *Am. Psychologist*, 36:361–372.

153. Rogers, P. J., and Blundell, J. E. (1980): Investigation of food selection and meal parameters during the development of dietary-induced obesity. *Appetite*, 1:85.

154. Rogers, Q. R., and Leung, P. (1973): The influence of amino acids on the neuroregulation of food intake. *Fed. Proc.*, 32:1709–1719.

155. Romsos, D. R., and Ferguson, D. (1982): Self-selected intake of carbohydrate, fat and protein by obese (ob/ob) and lean mice. *Physiol. Behav.*, 28:302–305.

156. Rozin, P. (1968): Are carbohydrate and protein intake separately regulated? *J. Comp. Physiol. Psychol.*, 65:23–29.

157. Rozin, P. (1976): The selection of foods by rats, humans and other animals. In: *Advances in the Study of Behaviour VI*, edited by J. Rosenblatt, R. Hinde, C. Beer, and E. Shaw, pp. 21–76. Academic Press, New York.

158. Rozin, P., and Kalat, J. W. (1971): Specific hungers and poison avoidance as adaptive specialisations of learning. *Psychol. Rev.*, 78:459–486.

159. Russell, G. R. M. (1972): Pre-menstrual tension and 'psychogenic' amenorrhea: Psychophysical interactions. *J. Psychosom. Res.*, 16:279–287.

160. Sanger, D. (1981): Endorphinergic mechanisms in the control of food and water intake. *Appetite*, 2:193–208.

161. Schoenfeld, T. A., and Hamilton, L. W. (1976): Multiple factors in short-term behavioural control of protein intake in rats. *J. Comp. Physiol. Psychol.*, 90:1092–1104.

162. Schutz, H. G., and Pilgrim, F. J. (1954): Changes in the self-selection pattern for purified dietary components by rats after starvation. *J. Comp. Physiol. Psychol.*, 47:444–449.
163. Sclafani, A. (1978): Dietary obesity. In: *Recent Advances in Obesity Research II*, edited by G. Bray, pp. 123–132. Newman, London.
164. Scott, E. (1946): Self-selection of diet I: Selection of purified components. *J. Nutr.*, 31:397–406.
165. Scott, E. M., Smith, S. J., and Verney, E. L. (1948): Self-selection of diet VII: The effect of age and pregnancy on selection. *J. Nutr.*, 35:281–286.
166. Seligman, M. E. P. (1970): On the generality of the laws of learning. *Psychol. Rev.*, 69:379–399.
167. Seligman, M. E. P., and Hager, J. (1972): *Biological Boundaries of Learning*. Appleton-Century-Crofts, New York.
168. Smith, G. P., and Gibbs, J. (1981): Brain—gut peptides and the control of food intake. In: *Neurosecretion and Brain Peptides*, edited by J. B. Martin, S. Reichlin, and K. L. Bick, pp. 389–395. Raven Press, New York.
169. Smith, S. L., and Sander, C. (1969): Food cravings, depression, and pre-menstrual problems. *Psychosom. Med.*, 31:281–287.
170. Stellar, E. (1954): The physiology of motivation. *Psychol. Rev.*, 61:5–22.
171. Stunkard, A. J. (1975): Satiety is a conditioned reflex. *Psychosom. Med.*, 37:383–387.
172. Szepesi, B., and Freedland, R. A. (1968): Dietary effects on rat liver enzymes in meal fed rats. *J. Nutr.*, 96:382–390.
173. Tretter, J. R., and Leibowitz, S. F. (1980): Specific increase in carbohydrate consumption after norepinephrine (NE) injection into the paraventricular nucleus (PVN). In: *Proceedings of the Society for Neuroscience 10th Annual Meeting*, Cincinnati, Nov. 9–14, Abstracts, Vol. 6, p. 532.
174. Tribe, D. E. (1955): Choice of diets by rats. 4. The choice of purified food constituents during growth, pregnancy and lactation. *Br. J. Nutr.*, 9:103–109.
175. Valenstein, E. S. (1966): The anatomical locus of reinforcement. In: *Progress in Physiological Psychology*, edited by E. Stellar and J. Sprague. Academic Press, New York.
176. Vanderweele, D. A., and Geiselman, P. J. (1977): Dietary self-selection following destruction of the lateral hypothalamus. In: *Proceedings of the Society for Neuroscience, 7th Annual Meeting*.
177. Wade, G. N. (1975): Some effects of ovarian hormones on food intake and body weight in female rats. *J. Comp. Physiol. Psychol.*, 88:183–193.
178. Wade, G. N. (1976): Sex hormones, regulatory behaviours and body weight. In: *Advances in the Study of Behaviour, Vol. 6*, edited by V. S. Rosenblatt, R. A. Hinde, E. Shaw, and C. Beer, pp. 201–279. Academic Press, New York.
179. Watson, P. J., and Cox, J. S. (1976): An analysis of barbiturate-induced eating and drinking in the rat. *Physiol. Psychol.*, 4:325–332.
180. Wiepkema, P. R. (1971): Positive feedbacks at work during feeding. *Behaviour*, 39:266–273.
181. Wiepkema, P. R. (1971): Behavioural factors in the regulation of food intake. *Proc. Nutr. Soc.*, 30:142–149.
182. Wirtshafter, D., and Davis, J. D. (1977): Set points, settling points, and the control of body weight. *Physiol. Behav.*, 19:75–78.
183. Woodger, T. L., Sirek, A., and Anderson, G. B. Diabetes, dietary tryptophan and protein intake and regulation in weanling rats. *Am. J. Physiol.*, 236:R307–R311.
184. Wooley, S. C. (1972): Physiological versus cognitive factors in short term food regulation in the obese and non-obese. *Psychosom. Med.*, 34:62–68.
185. Wright, P., and Crow, R. (1973): Menstrual cycle: Effect on sweetness preference in women. *Horm. Behav.*, 4:387–391.
186. Wurtman, J. J., and Baum, M. J. (1980): Estrogen reduces total food intake and carbohydrate intake, but not protein intake, in female rats. *Physiol. Behav.*, 24:823–827.
187. Wurtman, J. J., and Wurtman, R. J. (1977): Fenfluramine and fluoxetine spare protein consumption while suppressing caloric intake by rats. *Science*, 198:1178–1180.
188. Wurtman, J. J., and Wurtman, R. J. (1979): Drugs that enhance central serotoninergic transmission diminish elective carbohydrate consumption by rats. *Life Sci.*, 24:895–904.
189. Wurtman, J. J., and Wurtman, R. J. (1981): Suppression of carbohydrate consumption as snacks and at mealtime by DL-fenfluramine or tryptophan. In: *Anorectic Agents—Mechanisms of Action and Tolerance*, edited by S. Garattini and R. Samanin, pp. 169–182. Raven Press, New York.
190. Wurtman, J. J., Wurtman, R. J., Growdon, J. H., Henry, P., Lipscomb, A., and Zeisel, S. H. (1982): Carbohydrate craving in obese people: suppression by treatments affecting serotoninergic transmission. *Int. J. Eating Disorders*, 1:2–15.

191. Wurtman, R. J., Heftl, F., and Melamed, E. (1981): Precursor control of neurotransmitter synthesis. *Pharmacol. Rev.*, 32:315–335.
192. Wynn, P., and Redgrave, P. (1979): Feeding following microinjection of cholinergic substances into substantia nigra. *Life Sci.*, 25:333–338.
193. Wynn, V. T. (1972): Measurements of small variations in absolute pitch. *J. Physiol. (Lond.)*, 220:627–637.
194. Young, P. (1948): Appetite, palatability and feeding habit: A critical review. *Psychol. Bull.*, 45:289–320.
195. Zelger, J. L., and Carlini, E. A. (1980): Anorexigenic effects of two amines obtained from *Catha edulis* Forsk. (Khat) in rats. *Pharmacol. Biochem. Behav.*, 12:701–705.

Nutrition and the Brain, Vol. 6 edited by
R. J. Wurtman and J. J. Wurtman.
Raven Press, New York © 1983.

Precursor Control of the Function of Monoaminergic Neurons

Alan F. Sved

Department of Neuroscience, New Jersey Medical School, University of Medicine and Dentistry of New Jersey, Newark, New Jersey 07103

I. INTRODUCTION

Serotonin and the catecholamines dopamine (DA) and norepinephrine (NE) function as neurotransmitters at certain synapses within the mammalian central nervous system (CNS). These compounds are synthesized from the amino acids tryptophan and tyrosine, respectively. This chapter examines the thesis that neurotransmission mediated by these monoamines can be affected by the availability of their precursor amino acids. Since these precursors are supplied to the body via the diet, the possibility is also considered that diet-induced alterations in plasma composition can affect serotonin and catecholamine synthesis. Clinical evidence of this relationship has been reviewed previously in this series (116); hence the present chapter focuses on data from laboratory animals. Similarly, the substantial evidence relating choline availability to synthesis and release of acetylcholine was discussed in detail in *Nutrition and the Brain, Vol. 5* (23) and in other recent reviews (287), and so is not covered here.

For precursor availability to affect the synthesis of a neurotransmitter, two conditions must exist. First, brain levels of the precursor must not be so tightly regulated that they are not subject to change. Such regulation could take place in the periphery (i.e., if mechanisms existed that kept plasma levels more or less constant); at the level of the blood–brain barrier; or within the CNS itself. Second, changes in the concentration or amount of the precursor available to the neuron must affect the rate of synthesis of the transmitter. This implies that the enzyme catalyzing the rate-limiting step in the synthesis of the neurotransmitter must not be saturated with its substrate. Although these two criteria may seem obvious or simplistic, they are worth pointing out because of the number of neurotransmitter candidates for which they are not satisfied. For example, the transmitter γ-aminobutyric acid (GABA) is synthesized from the amino acid glutamate, but brain glutamate levels are generally regulated within narrow limits (170,216). However, even if brain glutamate levels could vary over a wide range, the rate of GABA synthesis still probably would not be altered, given the kinetic properties of the enzyme that converts glutamate to GABA (282). Synthesis of the various CNS peptides that may function as neurotransmitters probably also would not be affected by precursor control, since brain protein synthesis is not affected by physiologic variations in amino acid availability (24,138).

Precursor regulation of transmitter synthesis might be demonstrable in either or both of two types of studies, i.e., "pharmacological" experiments, in which the investigator alters precursor levels (e.g., by administering a large dose of the precursor) or "physiological" experiments, in which the investigator simply allows precursor levels to change (e.g., after a meal), and observes whether transmitter synthesis does or does not vary in parallel. If a relationship between precursor levels and transmitter synthesis exists physiologically, then this raises intriguing questions as to whether it might serve some particular function, e.g., to inform the brain about peripheral metabolic state. However, if precursor dependence is demonstrable only pharmacologically, it still becomes important to determine whether the precursor—which is a nutrient—can be used as though it were a drug to treat a disease characterized by a neurotransmitter deficit, or to modify synaptic events in experimental animals.

II. PRECURSOR CONTROL OF SEROTONINERGIC FUNCTION

A. Effect of Tryptophan Availability on Serotonin Synthesis

The biosynthesis of serotonin (5-hydroxytryptamine) is accomplished by a two-step process: First, 5-hydroxytryptophan is formed by the 5' hydroxylation of tryptophan. Next, this amino acid is decarboxylated to form the amine. The enzymes that catalyze these reactions are tryptophan hydroxylase (TpOH) and aromatic amino acid decarboxylase (AAAD), respectively (see Fig. 1). 5-Hydroxyindole acetic acid (5-HIAA), the major metabolite of serotonin, is formed by the actions of monoamine oxidase (MAO) and aldehyde dehydrogenase.

The hydroxylation of tryptophan to 5-hydroxytryptophan (5-HTP) is the rate-limiting step in the synthesis of serotonin. The enzyme that catalyzes this reaction, TpOH, is a mixed-function oxygenase that requires a reduced pterin cofactor (tetrahydrobiopterin) and molecular oxygen in addition to tryptophan. The factors regulating the activity of TpOH are not fully understood, but in addition to the availability of tryptophan, other processes or compounds that may influence this reaction include nerve impulse activity, activation of the enzyme by phosphorylation, and the availability of the cofactor (53,120,129,160,161,182,241). End-product inhibition does not appear to operate, at least with physiological levels of serotonin (53).

For tryptophan availability to affect the rate of tryptophan hydroxylation (and thus serotonin synthesis), TpOH must not be fully saturated with tryptophan *in vivo*. The K_m of TpOH for tryptophan (estimated *in vitro* by using a partially purified enzyme preparation) is approximately 50 μM (147), which means that at this concentration of tryptophan the enzyme would be only half-saturated with substrate, and, if tryptophan were the sole determinant regulating the rate of this reaction, it would proceed at 50% of its maximal rate (V_{max}). (It should be noted that the reported values for the K_m of TpOH for tryptophan vary greatly depending on the cofactor used in the assay; 50 μM is the K_m determined by using the natural cofactor, tetrahydrobiopterin.) Since brain tryptophan levels are about 20 μM, well below the K_m of TpOH, it would appear that TpOH is not normally saturated with tryptophan *in vivo*, suggesting that increasing tryptophan availability could increase the rate of serotonin synthesis. In fact, the initial observations that increasing brain

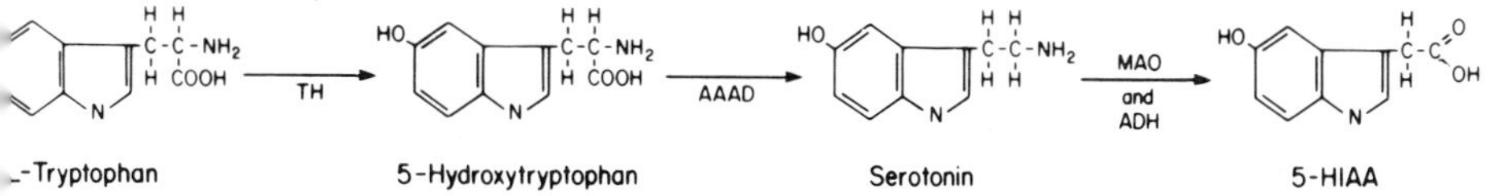

FIG. 1. Biosynthesis and metabolism of serotonin in brain.

tryptophan levels does increase brain serotonin levels (17,272) preceded kinetic characterization of the enzyme.

It is now well established that elevating brain tryptophan levels increases brain levels of serotonin and its major metabolite, 5-HIAA (59,83,112,201). As would be expected, decreasing tryptophan availability has the opposite effect (80). Brain serotonin and 5-HIAA levels are very sensitive to alterations in tryptophan availability, such that even small changes in brain tryptophan levels produce significant effects on serotonin levels (Fig. 2). As would be expected from the K_m of TpOH for tryptophan, as brain tryptophan levels approach 200 μM (40 μg/g), TpOH becomes saturated with substrate, so that further increases in brain tryptophan beyond this range fail to cause further increases in serotonin levels (83).

Although many laboratories have observed that tryptophan administration to laboratory animals increases brain tryptophan and serotonin levels, one negative report warrants comment. All the early publications demonstrating that tryptophan injection increased serotonin and 5-HIAA levels used fluorometric methods to measure the hydroxyindoles. In contrast, when Gal et al. (94) used a highly specific gas chromatographic method to measure brain hydroxyindoles, they found tryptophan administration to have no effect on serotonin levels. They thus suggested that conclusions based on the fluorometric assays were in error as a consequence of interfering fluorescence in the assay from the elevated tryptophan levels. Recent studies using high performance liquid chromatography (HPLC) with electrochemical

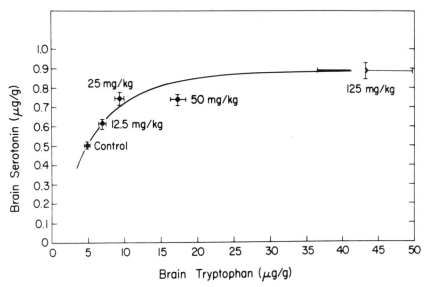

FIG. 2. Dose–response relationship of brain tryptophan and serotonin. Groups of 10 rats received injections of L-tryptophan (0, 12.5, 25, 50, or 125 mg/kg i.p.) at noon and were killed 1 hr later. Brains were removed and assayed for tryptophan and serotonin. *Horizontal bars* represent SEM for brain tryptophan and *vertical bars* represent SEM for brain serotonin. All brain tryptophan and serotonin levels were significantly higher than controls, $p < 0.01$. From Fernstrom and Wurtman (83).

detection to measure serotonin and 5-HIAA confirm the original conclusion that tryptophan injection does indeed increase brain serotonin and 5-HIAA levels (183,225).

The increases in serotonin and 5-HIAA levels produced by tryptophan administration reflect an increased rate of serotonin synthesis. This is clearly demonstrated by studies measuring the rate of 5-HTP accumulation following AAAD inhibition (43,44), a technique that assesses the *in vivo* rate of tryptophan hydroxylation. Since this is the rate-limiting step in serotonin synthesis, the method provides a good estimate of the rate at which serotonin would otherwise be formed *in vivo* (i.e., if AAAD were not inhibited) (43,44). Using this approach, Carlsson and co-workers (43,44) examined the effects on 5-HTP formation of varying brain tryptophan concentrations over a wide range, and concluded that increases or decreases in brain tryptophan levels strongly influence the rate of serotonin synthesis. From their data it is possible to calculate the *in vivo* K_m of TpOH for tryptophan, and thereby to estimate the degree of saturation of the enzyme with substrate *in vivo*. Such calculations (43,44) agree closely with the values predicted from the *in vitro* studies. The rate at which brain serotonin accumulates after inhibition of MAO (the intracellular enzyme that breaks down the indolamine) also provides a useful index of serotonin synthesis *in vivo* (209). Studies using this method have also provided evidence that the rate of serotonin synthesis varies directly with brain tryptophan levels (88,108). Perhaps surprisingly, Neckers et al. (208) found that treatments that decreased brain tryptophan levels also increased the activity (V_{max}) of TpOH as measured *in vitro*. They proposed that low tryptophan concentrations exposed additional catalytic sites on the enzyme. If such changes in the kinetics of TpOH do occur, they would tend to buffer the effects of changing tryptophan availability on serotonin synthesis. However, overwhelming evidence supports the conclusion that changes in brain tryptophan availability do cause parallel alterations in the rate of serotonin synthesis *in vivo*.

Studies examining the effect of tryptophan availability on serotonin synthesis within discrete brain regions have found that tryptophan availability affects serotonin synthesis both in regions containing primarily serotoninergic cell bodies and in regions containing only terminals of serotoninergic neurons (50,152), with no obvious differences between the two. However, differences in the responses of certain terminal field regions have been noted (50,152). For instance, some investigators report that increased tryptophan levels do not affect serotonin synthesis in the hypothalamus, cerebellum, and striatum (50,152). Such differences could reflect differences in serotonin turnover within various terminal fields, perhaps deriving from variations in neuronal firing frequencies or serotonin pool sizes. Also, normal tryptophan levels in the hypothalamus are about two-fold higher than in other brain regions (152), so the failure to observe changes in serotonin levels in response to small increases in tryptophan may result from TpOH in this region being more fully saturated with tryptophan.

As would be expected from the specific localization of TpOH to serotoninergic neurons (137), the increase in brain serotonin following tryptophan administration occurs only in such neurons. This has been demonstrated experimentally (4) by means of a histochemical fluorescence technique to visualize the serotonin. In contrast, the increase in serotonin following the administration of 5-HTP is not restricted to serotoninergic neurons (which is not surprising, given the widespread distribution of AAAD).

Serotonin is not confined to neurons within the CNS. In fact, more than 95% of all the serotonin in the body is located outside the brain, primarily in the gut. Serotonin synthesis in the gut, as in the brain, is dependent on tryptophan availability (51).

B. Tryptophan Availability and Serotoninergic Neurotransmission

Increased serotonin levels and synthesis in response to increased tryptophan availability do not necessarily indicate a proportionate increase in the release of serotonin into synapses (or, as might occur, into the brain extracellular space). For this to occur, the number of serotonin molecules released per nerve impulse must increase (with no concurrent decrease in the neuronal firing frequency), or the amount of transmitter that "leaks" out of the terminal must increase. Although 5-HIAA levels increase in response to increased tryptophan availability, 5-HIAA is an intracellular metabolite and thus can be reflective of serotonin's synthesis as well as of its rate of release (225a). Two regulatory mechanisms have been proposed that could maintain serotonin release at a constant level, despite increased serotonin synthesis. First, Grahame-Smith (108,109) suggested that the "extra" serotonin synthesized in response to increased tryptophan availability is metabolized intracellularly and is therefore not functionally active. Alternatively, small increases in tryptophan levels might, by increasing serotonin synthesis, decrease the firing frequencies of serotoninergic neurons (95,262). This latter mechanism would imply that at least some of the "extra" serotonin synthesized is functionally active (i.e., is released into synapses, with effects on neurotransmission), but that its ultimate effects on serotoninergic neurotransmission are small. For example, a 50 mg/kg dose of tryptophan in rats roughly doubles the rate of serotonin synthesis (108) but reduces the firing frequencies of serotoninergic neurons by approximately one-half (262); the end result would thus appear to be approximately the same amount of serotonin released into the synapse.

To determine whether changes in tryptophan availability actually alter the release of serotonin into synapses, one would need a method capable of monitoring such release. Although the techniques of push–pull perfusion (25) or *in vivo* electrochemistry (46) could provide useful information bearing on this issue, the techniques have not yet been systematically applied to this question. Electrical recording from cells postsynaptic to serotoninergic cells before and after tryptophan administration would also address this question, but again the experiments have yet to be done.

Another strategy for examining the relationship between tryptophan availability and serotoninergic neurotransmission involves examining brain outputs thought to depend on serotoninergic neurotransmission. This strategy is, of course, complicated by the fact that any brain output involves very many more transmitters than just serotonin alone, and the likelihood that complex regulatory mechanisms characteristic of all brain functions will counteract any effect that tryptophan might produce. Further, it is difficult to prove the involvement of serotoninergic neurons in any brain output. Still, this approach has proven extremely useful. The effects of altering tryptophan availability on some brain outputs thought to involve serotonin-mediated neurotransmission are discussed below. A summary of some of these effects is presented in Table 1.

1. Effects of Tryptophan Availability on Behavioral Activity

Although tryptophan administration to rats consistently increases brain serotonin and 5-HIAA levels, no gross behavioral responses (e.g., hyperactivity, sedation, abnormal movement or posture) result from such treatment (108,136,185). The lack of an effect of tryptophan administration on locomotion or activity noted by many investigators is, however, contradicted by several reports (38,198,259) that tryptophan administration reduces activity level. Modigh (198) showed that a large dose of tryptophan (800 mg/kg) decreased activity in mice; however, on the basis of further pharmacological study of this response, it was concluded that the de-

TABLE 1. *Effect of altering tryptophan availability on brain outputs dependent on serotoninergic neurons*

Brain output	Tryptophan availability	Response	Inferred change in serotonin	Response
Response to pain	↓	Hyperalgesia (175,192)	↓	Hyperalgesia (87,126,172)
	↑	No effect (132,175,192)	↑	Analgesia (194,232)
Aggression	↓	Enhanced aggression in rats (100,144)	↓	Enhanced aggression (99,110,196)
Sleep	↑	Reduced sleep latency or increased sleep time (115,122,123,279,290)	↓	Insomnia (141)
Sexual behavior	↓	Increased sexual behavior (45)	↓	Increased sexual behavior (61,240,242,257)
Startle response	↓	Exaggerated response (267)	↓	Exaggerated response (63,64)
Abnormal locomotion in Scottish Terrier dogs	↑	Increased latency of response (222)	↑	Increased latency of response (195)
Blood pressure in hypertensive rats	↑	Fall in blood pressure (254)	↑	Fall in blood pressure (90,92)
Growth hormone	↑	Increased release (15)	↑	Increased release (16,186)
Prolactin	↑	Increased release (176,206)	↑	Increased release (3,97,142)
Renin	↑	Increased release (301)	↑	Increased release (301)
β-Endorphin	↑	Increased release (235)	↑	Increased release (235)

creased activity was produced by tryptophan itself rather than some metabolite (e.g., serotonin). Since the other studies noting a decrease in activity following tryptophan administration used much smaller doses (20–150 mg/kg), it remains difficult to fit all the data together. Hingtgen and Aprison (130), using a very different paradigm, also concluded that tryptophan injection produced behavioral depression; they demonstrated that tryptophan reduced the response rate of pigeons in an operant conditioned situation of bar-pressing for food.

In contrast to the effect on activity of tryptophan administered alone, tryptophan given together with an MAO inhibitor causes hyperactivity (88,108,136). Actually, the hyperactivity is just one component of a whole spectrum of behaviors observed after tryptophan plus MAO inhibition. This syndrome, first described by Grahame-Smith (108), is characterized by marked increases in activity and rectal temperature, accompanied by piloerection, salivation, proptosis, and head weaving.

That this syndrome is produced by increased serotonin synthesis (resulting from the tryptophan injection) plus slowed serotonin metabolism (resulting from the action of the MAO inhibitor) is indicated by (a) a strong positive correlation between the rate of accumulation of serotonin and the development of hyperactivity or hyperpyrexia (108); (b) the inhibition of the hyperactivity or hyperpyrexia by drugs that interfere with the conversion of tryptophan to serotonin (e.g., p-chlorophenylalanine, NSD-1055) (108); (c) the dissimilarity in certain instances of the responses to tryptophan plus MAO inhibition and to tryptamine plus MAO inhibition (108,114).

Since MAO inhibition does not markedly alter the rate of serotonin synthesis (209) or block the capacity of tryptophan to enhance serotonin synthesis (136a), the amount of serotonin produced in brains of rats given tryptophan with or without MAO inhibition should be the same. However, only in conjunction with MAO inhibition does tryptophan produce the characteristic syndrome. This led Grahame-Smith (108,109) and Green and Grahame-Smith (112,113) to hypothesize that following the injection of tryptophan alone, the "extra" serotonin produced is functionally inactivated by deamination within the presynaptic terminal. Following MAO inhibition, this "extra" serotonin is not metabolized presynaptically, and therefore remains "functionally active" and capable of enhancing serotoninergic neurotransmission. This hypothesis implies that precursor regulation of serotonin synthesis does not normally affect serotonin-mediated neurotransmission (i.e., in the absence of MAO inhibition).

The hypothesis of Grahame-Smith and Green is not universally accepted, and other explanations of their data have been proposed. Foldes and Costa (88) noted that the hyperactivity produced by injection of tryptophan plus an MAO inhibitor was prevented by treatments that interfere with catecholaminergic neurotransmission (i.e., 6-hydroxydopamine, α-methyl-p-tyrosine); this was compatible with an earlier report by Green and Grahame-Smith (111) that the syndrome is inhibited by depletion of brain dopamine. Foldes and Costa suggested that an indole metabolite other than serotonin could trigger the motor activation by an effect on catecholaminergic neurons. However, another possibility is that enhanced serotonin release increases activity only when it occurs in conjunction with increased catecholaminergic neurotransmission, such as produced by MAO inhibition. Whatever the actual explanation, the observations described below suggesting that tryptophan administration can, by itself, produce responses indicative of enhanced serotoninergic neurotransmission, argue against the view presented by Grahame-Smith and Green (108,109,112,113).

2. Effect of Tryptophan Availability on Responses to Pain

There is good evidence that serotoninergic neurons are involved in nociceptive responses (for review, see ref. 193). Drugs and other treatments that reduce serotoninergic transmission generally produce hyperalgesia (87,126,172) whereas drugs that increase such neurotransmission are often analgesic (194,234). Therefore, if tryptophan availability affects serotonin release, it should also affect responsiveness to pain.

Acute reduction of brain tryptophan levels by injection of valine decreased brain serotonin synthesis and pain threshold (192). Reduction of serotonin levels by maintaining rats on a low-tryptophan diet also increased the animals' sensitivity to pain (175,192); this hyperalgesia was reversed by tryptophan administration (175,192). Tryptophan administration has also been reported to reverse the hyperalgesia produced by lesions of the ascending serotonin projections (54). However, tryptophan administration to otherwise untreated rats apparently does not alter pain responsivity (132,175,192).

Serotonin-releasing neurons also may participate in the analgesic effect of morphine. Morphine accelerates serotonin turnover (127,293), and drugs that increase serotoninergic neurotransmission potentiate morphine analgesia (107,263,291). Tryptophan injection, however, was reported to antagonize rather than potentiate the action of morphine (131).

3. Effect of Tryptophan Availability on Aggression

Serotoninergic neurons are thought to be involved in inhibiting aggressive behavior in rats. Numerous studies (e.g., 99,110,196) show that reducing brain serotonin pharmacologically or by lesions increases muricide (predatory mouse killing) and shock-induced fighting, two commonly used measures of aggression in rats. Gibbons et al. (100) reported that feeding rats a tryptophan-free diet for 4 to 6 days, which reduced 5-hydroxyindole levels by about 30%, induced mouse killing in nonkiller rats and decreased the attack latency of "killers." (Killers were rats that attacked mice under baseline testing conditions, whereas nonkillers did not display predatory behavior during baseline testing.) Supplementation of this diet with tryptophan reversed the effects on both brain serotonin and aggression. Kantak et al. (144) confirmed and extended these results, finding that a tryptophan-free diet increased both muricide and shock-induced fighting. However, these authors raised the possibility that the increase in muricide is solely the result of inadequate food intake, as evidenced by a decrease in body weight among rats fed the tryptophan-free diet. When rats were food-deprived to produce a decrease in body weight similar to that of rats eating the tryptophan-free diet, muricide was increased to a degree similar to that produced by the tryptophan-free diet, although brain serotonin levels increased rather than decreased. Kantak et al. (144) also noted that supplementing the control diet with tryptophan, which increased brain serotonin, did not modify either shock-induced fighting or the incidence of muricide.

Aggression in mice, as measured by isolation-induced fighting, is decreased by lesions and drug treatments that diminish serotoninergic transmission (158,180,187). Kantak et al. (143) found that isolation-induced fighting also was reduced by feeding mice a tryptophan-free diet. Supplementing this diet with 0.15% tryptophan reversed this effect. Predatory cricket killing, another measure of aggression in mice, was increased in mice fed a tryptophan-free diet (143); this behavior also can be enhanced by drugs that interfere with serotoninergic neurotransmission (188). However, similar to the observations of Kantak et al. on muricidal rats (144), this effect may be caused by inadequate food intake rather than by a specific decrease in tryptophan availability. Thurmond et al. (260,261) found that supplementing a normal diet with 0.25% or 0.5% tryptophan increased aggression (fighting) in mice fed the diet for 2 weeks. In mice fed the diets for longer periods of time, or fed diets containing more tryptophan (1% or 4%), the increased aggression was not observed.

Taken together, these studies suggest that decreasing tryptophan availability, by reducing the tryptophan content of the diet, alters aggression in a manner similar to that observed with drugs that decrease serotoninergic neurotransmission. Conversely, increasing tryptophan availability by supplementing the diet with tryptophan may alter aggression in the opposite direction, although this effect is less clear and may depend on the level of dietary supplementation and the length of time the animals are fed the diet. Further, the studies of Kantak et al. (143,144) highlight the importance of controlling for weight loss (adequate nutrition) in studies on the effects of tryptophan-free diets. Data on the effects on aggression of acute alterations in tryptophan availability would be interesting, but are not available at present.

4. Effects of Tryptophan Availability on Sleep

Abundant evidence supports a role for serotoninergic neurons in the sleep–wake cycle (for review, see ref. 141). Treatments that decrease serotoninergic neurotransmission, such as *p*-chlorophenylalanine or lesions of the raphe nuclei, produce insomnia in laboratory animals (141). Therefore, if tryptophan administration increases serotonin release, it might be expected to enhance sleep, perhaps by accelerating sleep onset. Several studies, mostly by Hartmann and co-workers (122–125), have examined this possibility. In rats, initial findings suggested that only very high doses of tryptophan (450–600 mg/kg i.p.) significantly altered sleep (123); the only effect noted was reduced sleep latency (the time it takes to fall asleep). A more recent study in rats (279) also described a reduction in sleep latency in response to tryptophan, but occurring after a much lower dose (30 mg/kg). These authors suggest that higher doses of tryptophan may fail to reduce sleep latency because of enhanced tryptamine synthesis. (Tryptamine has been shown to increase activity.)

In studies on normal human subjects and patients with insomnia, tryptophan administration consistently reduced sleep latency, and, in some studies, also increased total sleep time (115,122,124,125,290).

Although most investigators seem to agree that tryptophan administration reduces sleep latency and/or increases sleep time, conflicting reports exist (2), and the nature of the effects of tryptophan on different stages of sleep is still controversial.

5. Effect of Tryptophan Availability on Blood Pressure

Central serotonin-releasing neurons are also involved in the regulation of arterial blood pressure, although the nature of this involvement remains a topic of debate (for review, see ref. 162). Pharmacological enhancement of serotoninergic transmission has been found both to increase and to decrease blood pressure (see ref. 162). However, tryptophan administration to normal animals had no effect on blood pressure (14,213). In contrast with this lack of an effect in normotensive rats, tryptophan injection was found by Sved et al. (254) to lower blood pressure in spontaneously hypertensive (SHR) rats (see Table 2). That this antihypertensive action results from increased serotoninergic neurotransmission receives support from the following observations: (a) The action of tryptophan is blocked by a serotonin receptor antagonist (metergoline) or an inhibitor of serotonin synthesis (*p*-chlorophenylalanine); (b) fluoxetine, a serotonin reuptake blocker, potentiates the fall in blood pressure produced by tryptophan; (c) other drugs that enhance serotoninergic neurotransmission lower blood pressure in SHR rats (90,92); and (d) valine, a large neutral amino acid (LNAA) that competes with tryptophan for transport into the brain, attenuates the antihypertensive action of tryptophan (254). Thus, the decrease in blood pressure of SHR rats elicited by tryptophan represents one of the clearest

TABLE 2. *Effect of tryptophan administration on blood pressure in SHR*

Dose of tryptophan (mg/kg)	Change in blood pressure (mm Hg)
0	-6 ± 3
25	-11 ± 3
50	-23 ± 5[a]
100	-28 ± 5[a]

Groups of five SHR rats received an intraperitoneal injection of tryptophan immediately after determination of baseline blood pressure. Blood pressure was measured again 2 hr after the tryptophan injection, the time of maximal antihypertensive action. Data are expressed as change from baseline value, means $\pm$ SEM.
Adapted from Sved et al. (254).
[a]Significant difference from the 0 mg/kg dose, $p < 0.05$.

examples of a change in brain tryptophan levels affecting a brain output by increasing serotonin release.

6. Effect of Tryptophan Availability on Anterior Pituitary Function

Central nervous system serotoninergic neurons participate in the mechanisms regulating the release of several hormones from the anterior pituitary gland. Serotoninergic neurons are thought to stimulate growth hormone release (15,186); Arnold and Fernstrom (16) have shown that tryptophan injection enhances the secretion of this hormone. Serotonin also appears to stimulate prolactin release (cf. refs. 3,97,142); however, although a few studies have reported prolactin release to be increased by tryptophan administration (176,206), most studies find tryptophan to have no such effect (74,105,133,278). Recently, Sapun et al. (235) provided evidence that β-endorphin release from the pituitary is increased by the administration of tryptophan, as well as by drugs that enhance serotoninergic neurotransmission.

The pituitary–adrenal axis also is influenced by serotoninergic neurons, although there is debate as to whether these neurons are stimulatory or inhibitory (cf. refs. 159,266). Most serotonin agonists seem to raise serum corticosteroid levels, presumably by an action on cells in the hypothalamus that release corticotropin-releasing factor (40,91,139). Data on the effects of tryptophan administration on blood ACTH or corticosterone levels are conflicting, with some laboratories reporting decreases with tryptophan injection and others reporting increases (199, 200,266,281).

Kennett and Joseph (149) examined the effect of valine injection on the stress-induced elevation of serum corticosterone levels. They found that valine injection blunts the stress-induced rises in serum corticosterone and in brain 5-HIAA. Since stress raises brain tryptophan levels (153), they argue that valine produces these effects by blocking this rise in tryptophan levels, thereby preventing the increase in serotonin synthesis. If such an interpretation proves to be correct, this set of relationships would provide an interesting example of the physiological consequences of the precursor control of serotonin synthesis.

7. Tryptophan Availability and Behavioral Responses to Drugs

Tryptophan availability also affects the behavioral responses to drugs thought to act on serotoninergic neurons. Some of the behavioral effects of drugs that cause the release of serotonin (i.e., fenfluramine, p-chloroamphetamine, high doses of amphetamine) are potentiated by tryptophan administration (39,56,77,166). For example, some of the abnormal motor movements (i.e., circling, backward walking) produced by high doses of amphetamine (15 mg/kg) are thought to be mediated via serotoninergic neurons (78), and are increased after tryptophan administration (166). Likewise, certain effects of p-chloroamphetamine (e.g., tremor) are potentiated by tryptophan injection (39,77), whereas others (e.g., rearing, forward walking) are unaffected. In addition, some, but not all, behaviors elicited by fenfluramine injection are potentiated by tryptophan administration. Decreasing brain tryptophan levels by the injection of valine did not affect any of these behavioral responses to amphetamine, fenfluramine, or *p*-chloroamphetamine (77).

Tryptophan availability can also affect the actions of drugs that do not work directly on serotoninergic neurons. For example, Sahakian et al. (232) showed that two effects of DA agonists (stereotypy and hypothermia) were attenuated in rats fed a low-tryptophan diet. Also, the circling behavior elicited by DA agonists in animals with unilateral nigrostriatal lesions was attenuated by tryptophan administration (197). Other serotonin agonists produce similar responses.

C. Tryptophan Availability and Serotoninergic Transmission: Summary and Conclusions

Clearly, serotonin synthesis varies with changes in tryptophan availability. Further, it appears obvious from the preceding discussion that altered availability of tryptophan can affect brain outputs that are dependent on serotoninergic neurotransmission. The observations that tryptophan administration alone (i.e., without an MAO inhibitor) can elicit responses via enhanced serotoninergic neurotransmission (e.g., a decrease in blood pressure in SHR rats; enhanced growth hormone release) argue against the hypothesis that the additional serotonin synthesized following a tryptophan load is metabolized before reaching the synapse.

Still, the lack of an effect of tryptophan administration in many test situations that respond to other serotoninergic manipulations is difficult to explain. It may be that the complex regulation of many of these brain systems prevents the output from being altered by a modest increase in serotonin release. Another possible explanation is a relationship between the activity of serotoninergic neurons and the amount of this "additional" serotonin that is released. That is, in a normal resting animal, tryptophan administration would lead to enhanced serotonin synthesis but not to enhanced release (i.e., if the firing frequencies of serotoninergic neurons decreased in parallel); however, if the tryptophan load coincides with the enhanced activity in particular serotoninergic neurons, then the increase in serotonin synthesis would cause increases in the release of the transmitter.

III. PRECURSOR CONTROL OF CATECHOLAMINERGIC FUNCTION

A. Regulation of Catecholamine Synthesis

The catecholamine neurotransmitters DA and NE are synthesized by the pathway outlined in Fig. 3. DA neurons contain the enzymes tyrosine hydroxylase (TOH) and aromatic amino acid decarboxylase (AAAD), but lack the enzyme dopamine-β-hydroxylase (DBH); therefore, DA is the final catecholamine product in these neurons. Noradrenergic neurons contain DBH in addition to TOH and AAAD, and thus the DA formed in these cells is rapidly β-hydroxylated to form NE.

The initial reaction in the biosyntheses of DA and NE is the hydroxylation of tyrosine to form dihydroxyphenylalanine (DOPA). This is the rate-limiting step in

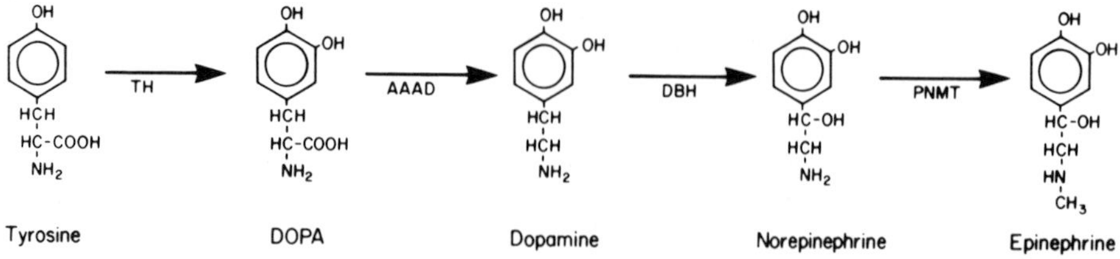

FIG. 3. Catecholamine biosynthetic pathway.

catecholamine biosynthesis, a conclusion based on observations that: (a) the activity of TOH, assayed *in vitro*, is much less than the activities of the other enzymes involved in catecholamine synthesis (207); (b) inhibitors of TOH severely deplete tissues of catecholamines (248), whereas a similar degree of catecholamine depletion does not occur following inhibition of the other enzymes in the catecholamine biosynthetic pathway (212); (c) the apparent K_m of the overall reaction (tyrosine $\rightarrow$ NE) is comparable to the K_m for the conversion of tyrosine to DOPA by partially purified TOH (169); and (d) with tyrosine as substrate, a maximal rate of NE synthesis is achieved with a concentration below 10^{-4}M, whereas with DOPA or DA as substrate much higher concentrations are required (169).

Tyrosine hydroxylase, the enzyme responsible for catalyzing this reaction, is relatively specific for L-tyrosine as its amino acid substrate (207). In addition to the substrates tyrosine and molecular oxygen, the enzyme requires a reduced pterin cofactor (135,207), the natural cofactor being tetrahydrobiopterin (see refs. 147,148).

Several mechanisms have been proposed as regulating the rate at which tyrosine is hydroxylated, and thus catecholamines synthesized. These include end-product inhibition (247), nerve impulse activity (55,173,229,230,274), enzyme activation (173,274), enzyme induction (55), presynaptic receptors (229,230), cofactor availability (150,168,219), and, as discussed below, the availability of the substrate tyrosine. Experimental data suggest that each of these mechanisms can affect the rate of catecholamine synthesis under certain conditions.

B. Effect of Tyrosine Availability on Catecholamine Synthesis

For the availability of tyrosine to be a factor in the regulation of tyrosine hydroxylation (and thus catecholamine synthesis), TOH must not be fully saturated with tyrosine *in vivo*. The K_m of partially purified rat brain TOH for tyrosine (i.e., the concentration of tyrosine at which the reaction proceeds at 50% of the maximal rate), determined using a saturating concentration of tetrahydrobiopterin, is approximately 10 μM (147,148). Brain tyrosine levels normally range from 5 to 10 times this value (e.g., 50 to 100 μM), suggesting that TOH is mostly, but not fully, saturated with tyrosine *in vivo*. By substituting these values (K_m = 10 μM; tyrosine concentration = 75 μM) into the Michaelis-Menten equation (which describes the relationship between substrate concentration and reaction velocity), it can be calculated that the hydroxylation of tyrosine would proceed at 88% of the maximal rate. Thus, if tyrosine alone controlled catecholamine synthesis, even large increases in its availability would increase synthesis by only about 14%.

Working with a peripheral tissue preparation (guinea pig heart) *in vitro*, Levitt et al. (169) examined the relationship between the tyrosine concentration of the medium and the rate of catecholamine synthesis. These investigators showed that the half-maximal rate of NE synthesis (analogous to the K_m of the overall reaction) occurred when the heart was perfused with approximately 20 μM tyrosine. The maximal rate of NE synthesis occurred with tyrosine concentrations of about 50 to 100 μM, similar to physiological levels. These values are in good agreement with the results of experiments on partially purified TOH, and suggest that TOH is mostly, if not fully, saturated with tyrosine *in vivo*. (Of course, in these experiments, the catecholaminergic neurons containing the enzyme are not firing; as described below, firing frequency markedly affects the responsiveness of the neuron to added tyrosine.)

Carlsson and Lindqvist (44) attempted to measure directly the saturation of brain TOH *in vivo* by looking at the rate of DOPA production in rat brain, following treatments that increased (tyrosine injection) or decreased (injection of LNAAs) brain tyrosine concentrations. They determined the *in vivo* K_m for tyrosine to be approximately 25 μM, and estimated that TOH would be 70 to 80% saturated with tyrosine *in vivo*. These results are roughly comparable to the observations described above. (Here too, it must be appreciated that the firing frequencies of catecholaminergic neurons may be altered, because the decarboxylase inhibitor would likely perturb normal synaptic dynamics.)

On the basis of this information on the degree of saturation of TOH with tyrosine, it would appear that (a) TOH is not fully saturated with tyrosine *in vivo*, and thus catecholamine synthesis may be affected by tyrosine availability; (b) the maximum increase in catecholamine synthesis resulting from increased tyrosine availability would not exceed about 20 to 30% of the normal rate; and (c) decreasing brain tyrosine availability may more profoundly affect catecholamine synthesis than increasing tyrosine levels.

Studies on the effect of increasing brain tyrosine levels by the injection of tyrosine on catecholamine levels have repeatedly shown that DA and NE levels are not altered by tyrosine administration (60,77,245). However, since catecholamine levels do not reflect the rates of catecholamine synthesis or release (e.g., 276), such results do not really provide useful information about the effects of tyrosine.

Initial studies on the effect of tyrosine administration on the rate of catecholamine synthesis produced conflicting results (42,288; see Table 3). In experiments designed to examine the effect of tyrosine injection on catecholamine synthesis (by measuring the rate of DOPA accumulation following inhibition of brain AAAD) Wurtman et al. (288) found that increasing brain tyrosine levels twofold, by intraperitoneal injection of tyrosine, produced an approximately 13% increase in DOPA accumulation in whole rat brain. However, in an almost identical experiment, Carlsson et al. (42) observed that similar increases in brain tyrosine levels had no effect on DOPA accumulation. In subsequent studies examining brain regions rather than whole brain, Carlsson and Lindqvist (44) noted that tyrosine injection had no effect on DOPA accumulation in striatum or limbic forebrain, although a 25%

TABLE 3. *Effect of tyrosine administration on catecholamine synthesis in otherwise untreated rats*

Reference	Parameter measured	Brain region	Effect of tyrosine injection on parameter
Wurtman et al. (288)	DOPA accumulation	Whole brain	+13%
Carlsson et al. (42)	DOPA accumulation	Whole brain	None
Carlsson and Lindqvist (44)	DOPA accumulation	Limbic forebrain, caudate, hemispheres	None
Gibson and Wurtman (103)	MOPEG-SO$_4$ (after probenecid)	Whole brain	+15%
Scally et al. (236)	HVA	Striatum	None
Sved et al. (251)	DOPAC, HVA	Striatum, hypothalamus	None
Melamed et al. (191)	DOPAC, HVA	Striatum	None
Sved and Fernstrom (249)	DOPAC, HVA, DOPA accumulation	Striatum	None
Sved and Fernstrom (250)	DOPA accumulation	Striatum, median eminence	None

increase in DOPA accumulation was noted in the cerebral hemispheres after a dose of tyrosine that increased brain tyrosine levels more than 10-fold. Sved and Fernstrom (249,250) also reported the absence of an effect of tyrosine administration on DOPA accumulation in striatum and median eminence.

Perhaps a better index of changes in the rate of catecholamine synthesis (when catecholamine levels remain unchanged) is changes in brain levels of particular catecholamine metabolites (156,157,228). In untreated rats, tyrosine administration did not alter levels of either the NE metabolite methoxyhydroxyphenylethylene glycol sulfate (MOPEG-SO$_4$) (103) or the DA metabolites dihydroxyphenylacetic acid (DOPAC) and homovanillic acid (HVA) (191,236,249,251). Gibson and Wurtman (103) did note, however, that following treatment with probenecid (to block MOPEG-SO$_4$ efflux from brain) tyrosine injection caused a small increase in whole-brain MOPEG-SO$_4$ levels. In analogous experiments on effects of tyrosine on DA metabolites in brains of probenecid-pretreated rats, no effect of tyrosine treatment was found (236). Thus, the overall picture that emerges from these experiments is that increasing tyrosine availability has little effect overall on catecholamine synthesis in, or release from, CNS catecholamine neurons in otherwise untreated rats.

On the other hand, reductions in brain tyrosine levels (e.g., by injections of LNAAs) clearly slowed brain catecholamine synthesis (44,288). A large decrease in brain tyrosine concentration (approximately 70%) has also been reported to produce a sizable fall in brain DOPAC and HVA levels (32b).

Although much of the available data suggests that increasing the availability of tyrosine does not alter catecholamine synthesis in otherwise untreated rats, numerous experimental situations have been described in which tyrosine administration enhanced catecholamine synthesis when given in conjunction with some other treatment (see Table 4). Thus, following the administration of haloperidol (44,236), reserpine (251), γ-butyrolactone (249), yohimbine (101), or prolactin (250) some

TABLE 4. *Effect of tyrosine administration in conjunction with other treatment on catecholamine synthesis*

Reference	Treatment	Parameter measured	Brain region	Effect of tyrosine on parameter
Scalley et al. (236)	Haloperidol	HVA	Striatum	+60%
Carlsson and Lindqvist (44)	Haloperidol	DOPA accumulation	Striatum, limbic forebrain hemispheres	+15%
Gibson and Wurtman (103)	Cold-stress	MOPEG-SO$_4$	Whole brain	+70%
Gibson (101)	Yohimbine	MOPEG-SO$_4$	Whole brain	+35%
Melamed et al. (191)	Nigrostriatal lesion	DOPAC, HVA	Striatum	+60%
Sved et al. (251)	Reserpine	DOPAC, HVA	Striatum, hypothalamus	+40%
Sved and Fernstrom (249)	GBL	DOPA accumulation	Striatum	+25%
Sved and Fernstrom (250)	Prolactin	DOPA accumulation	Median eminence	+30%
Sved et al. (252)	SHR rats	MOPEG-SO$_4$	Whole brain	+40%
Yamori et al. (292)	SHR rats	MOPEG-SO$_4$	Brain stem, forebrain	+15%

index of DA or NE synthesis has been found to be increased by tyrosine administration. The amino acid also enhanced DA synthesis in rats with partial lesions of the nigrostriatal pathway (191) and NE synthesis in cold-stressed rats (103) and SHR rats (252,292). The increases in catecholamine synthesis range from 15 to 70%, i.e., often greater than the maximum effect of increased tyrosine availability predicted from *in vitro* studies on TOH.

In each of the instances in which tyrosine administration has been shown to enhance catecholamine synthesis following some pretreatment, the pretreatment is thought to increase the rate of catecholamine synthesis in certain catecholaminergic neurons (which become tyrosine-responsive) but not in others. This relationship suggests that the capacity of a catecholaminergic neuron to respond to additional tyrosine requires some biochemical consequence of its "activation." [A similar relationship between neuronal activity and precursor control has also been demonstrated in the case of acetylcholine (30,31).] Another possibility is that it is easier to detect increases in catecholamine synthesis among neurons that are already rapidly synthesizing catecholamines; a 25% increase in catecholamine synthesis is large when the basal rate of catecholamine synthesis is large and small when basal synthesis is low. However, the results of an experiment comparing the effects of tyrosine availability on DA synthesis in median eminences of male versus female rats (250) seem to rule out this possibility. This study showed that the rate of DOPA formation in the median eminence of male rats was not affected by increased tyrosine availability unless rats were pretreated with prolactin to activate these DA neurons. Tyrosine administration also failed to affect DOPA accumulation in the median eminence of female rats even though DOPA formation in the median eminence of female rats is about equal to that in male rats injected with prolactin. As in male rats, DOPA production was increased if females were treated with prolactin before injection with tyrosine. Thus, the effect of increased tyrosine availability on DA synthesis appears to be independent of the actual rate of catecholamine synthesis. Instead, what seems to be important is an increase in the activity of the DA neuron above its basal level.

The hypothesis that only activated catecholaminergic neurons are influenced by tyrosine availability receives strong support from several other observations. Sved and Fernstrom (250) showed that although tyrosine injection does not normally alter DA synthesis in the striatum or median eminence, following the intracerebral injection of ovine prolactin—a treatment that selectively activates tuberoinfundibular DA neurons projecting to the median eminence (12,13,202)—tyrosine injection does increase DA synthesis in the median eminence, but not in the striatum (see Table 5). [That striatal DA synthesis can be affected by tyrosine administration is demonstrated in experiments in which these neurons are activated by other treatments (44,191,236,249).] Thus, in the same animal, increased tyrosine availability can selectively affect different populations of DA neurons, depending on which have been activated. A differential effect of increased tyrosine availability on particular populations of catecholaminergic neurons has also been noted in SHR rats (see Table 6): Tyrosine injection increased brain stem and forebrain MOPEG-SO$_4$ levels, indicating increased NE synthesis, but not MOPEG-SO$_4$ levels in the spinal cord. Further, tyrosine administration failed to alter DA metabolite levels in any brain region examined in SHR rats (Table 6). Similar conclusions were drawn from a

TABLE 5. *Effects of tyrosine and ovine prolactin (OPrl) on DOPA accumulation in the median eminences and striata of male rats*

	DOPA	
Treatment	Median eminence (ng/mg protein)	Striatum (μg/g)
Vehicle–vehicle	5.2 ± 0.2[a]	1.57 ± 0.15
Vehicle–tyrosine	5.5 ± 0.5[a]	1.56 ± 0.08
OPrl–vehicle	7.1 ± 0.5[b]	1.42 ± 0.09
OPrl–tyrosine	8.8 ± 0.3[c]	1.62 ± 0.07

Groups of eight rats were injected with OPrl (1 μg/rat i.c.v. in 10 μl of saline) or vehicle followed 20 hr later by an injection of tyrosine (200 mg/kg i.p.) or vehicle. Thirty minutes later, rats received 100 mg/kg of *m*-hydroxbenzylhydrazine (NSD-1015) and the rats were killed 30 min thereafter. Median eminences and striata were dissected out and assayed for DOPA.

Numbers followed by different letters are significantly different ($p < 0.05$), determined by one-way analysis of variance and the Newman-Keuls test.

From Sved and Fernstrom (250).

TABLE 6. *Effect of tyrosine administration on catecholamine metabolite levels in SHR rats*

Region Treatment	Catecholamine metabolite (ng/g)	
Experiment 1	MOPEG-SO$_4$	
Brain		
Vehicle	138 ± 8	
Tyrosine	183 ± 12[a]	
Spinal cord		
Vehicle	118 ± 8	
Tyrosine	112 ± 4	
Experiment 2	DOPAC	HVA
Hypothalamus		
Vehicle	27 ± 5	26 ± 2
Tyrosine	72 ± 7	30 ± 2
Striatum		
Vehicle	860 ± 40	425 ± 25
Tyrosine	835 ± 50	430 ± 25
Limbic forebrain		
Vehicle	490 ± 40	165 ± 10
Tyrosine	520 ± 50	150 ± 15

Groups of six SHR rats were injected with tyrosine (200 mg/kg i.p.) or vehicle and killed 1 hr later. Brain regions were dissected out and assayed for MOPEG-SO$_4$ or DOPAC and HVA. Data are expressed as means ± SEM.
[a]Significant difference from the vehicle-treated group, $p < 0.05$. In the brain stems from the animals in experiment 2, MOPEG-SO$_4$ levels were elevated by approximately 40% compared with the vehicle-treated rats ($p < 0.05$).
From Sved and Fernstrom, *unpublished observations.*

very elegant study by Melamed et al. (191), in which partial lesions of the nigro-striatal pathway, which increased the firing frequencies of remaining nigrostriatal DA neurons ipsilateral to the lesion (8,191), rendered these neurons responsive to increased tyrosine availability, but not the normal nigrostriatal neurons on the unlesioned contralateral side. All these findings support the hypothesis that only activated catecholaminergic neurons respond to increases in tyrosine availability. [Korf et al. (157) noted that during direct electrical stimulation of the nigrostriatal neurons, tyrosine administration had no effect on striatal HVA levels, a finding inconsistent with the hypothesis that activated DA neurons are affected by precursor availability. However, this study involved only three rats, and the tyrosine levels were not measured.]

If increased tyrosine availability does affect catecholamine synthesis only in activated catecholaminergic neurons, what mechanism could account for this relationship? The most likely mechanism coupling tyrosine responsiveness to neuronal firing frequency would involve the activation of TOH known to occur when catecholaminergic neurons fire more frequently (173,229,230,274). This interpretation receives experimental support from studies using γ-butyrolactone (GBL). This drug both inhibits the firing of nigrostriatal DA neurons and concurrently activates the TOH in these neurons (203,268–270). The increase that GBL produces in striatal DA synthesis is significantly correlated with striatal tyrosine levels over a wide range (249; see Table 7). Thus, the activation of TOH per se, in the absence of any increase in neuronal activity or catecholamine release, is sufficient to make a catecholaminergic neuron responsive to changes in tyrosine availability.

The activation of TOH by GBL (173) or other treatments that increase the activity of DA neurons (173,229,230,274) appears to reflect an increase in the affinity of the enzyme for its cofactor, tetrahydrobiopterin. Although it is difficult to determine the tetrahydrobiopterin concentration at the site of catecholamine biosynthesis, it has been estimated that the concentration of this cofactor in striatal DA nerve terminals is roughly 100 μM (168). Accurate measurements of the K_m of TOH for tetrahydrobiopterin are also problematic, since this K_m varies depending on pH (1,224). However, it appears that the K_m of the activated (phosphorylated) enzyme (approximately 30 μM for adrenal TOH assayed at pH 6.8) is well below the cofactor concentration (and so the enzyme is saturated with cofactor) whereas in the non-activated state the K_m (approximately 600 μM for adrenal TOH assayed at pH 6.8 [see ref. 168]) exceeds the tetrahydrobiopterin concentration (and thus the enzyme is unsaturated with cofactor). Thus, the extent to which the enzyme is saturated with this cofactor is probably the rate-limiting factor controlling catecholamine synthesis under most conditions (150,168,219), and the failure of tyrosine administration to affect catecholamine synthesis in nonactivated neurons may reflect the fact that, in such neurons, the enzyme is much less saturated with cofactor than with its substrate. Following activation of TOH and the resulting increase in the

TABLE 7. *Effect of γ-butyrolactone and tyrosine on striatal DOPA accumulation in rats*

Treatment	DOPA (μg/g)	Tyrosine (μg/g)
Vehicle–vehicle	1.51 ± 0.08[a]	26.6 ± 0.9[a]
Tyrosine–vehicle	1.52 ± 0.09[a]	38.5 ± 1.3[b]
Vehicle–GBL	4.73 ± 0.46[b]	25.4 ± 1.0[a]
Tyrosine–GBL	5.96 ± 0.34[c]	37.5 ± 2.2[b]

Groups of eight rats were injected with tyrosine (200 mg/kg i.p.) or vehicle (4 ml/kg). Fifteen minutes later the rats received γ-butyrolactone (GBL, 750 mg/kg i.p.) or vehicle (2 ml/kg), and after another 5 min were injected with the decarboxylase inhibitor, NSD-1015, (100 mg/kg). Rats were killed 30 min after administration of the decarboxylase inhibitor.

Numbers in each column followed by different superscript letters are significantly different, $p < 0.05$, by analysis of variance and Newman-Keuls test.

From Sved and Fernstrom (249).

affinity of the enzyme for its cofactor, the TOH may no longer be limited by the availability of the tetrahydrobiopterin, and may thus become dependent on tyrosine. Of course, another explanation is that when TOH becomes activated, tyrosine gets hydroxylated at such a rate that the tyrosine concentration in catecholaminergic nerve terminals actually falls—in which case tyrosine administration could enhance CA synthesis by preventing its own depletion.

C. Tyrosine Availability and Peripheral Catecholaminergic Cells

Catecholamine-synthesizing cells in the periphery (i.e., postganglionic sympathetic neurons and adrenal chromaffin cells) are also affected by tyrosine availability (5,6,7,9; see Table 8). In rats given a water load sufficient to induce diuresis, tyrosine administration increases urinary NE and epinephrine levels (6,9), indicative of increased catecholamine release from peripheral catecholaminergic cells (154). In rats placed in a cold environment, a treatment that enhances sympathetic nervous activity and thus raises urinary catecholamine levels, the effect of tyrosine administration is more dramatic. It is interesting that although tyrosine injection increases the levels of all three catecholamines in the urine, the increase in urinary DA is by far the greatest; the source of DA in the urine is at present unknown, but possibly arises from the kidneys (165). Pretreatment with carbidopa, an inhibitor of AAAD in the periphery but not in the brain, blocks the rise in urinary catecholamine levels in response to tyrosine injection (9). However, urinary DOPA levels are greatly increased, suggesting an increase in catecholamine synthesis in response to the tyrosine load. Plasma catecholamine levels, another index of peripheral catecholamine release, have also been reported to be increased by tyrosine administration (37). Tyrosine administration has also been shown to increase urinary catecholamine levels in human subjects (5).

It is unclear whether these observations are compatible with the hypothesis that only activated catecholaminergic neurons are affected by increases in tyrosine avail-

TABLE 8. *Effect of tyrosine administration on urinary catecholamine levels*

Treament	Urinary catecholamine (ng/3 hr/100 g body weight)		
	NE	EPI	DA
Control	190 ± 15	51 ± 4	104 ± 19
Tyrosine	290 ± 34[a]	70 ± 5[a]	290 ± 34[a]

Groups of six rats were placed in a cold environment (4°C) and were injected with tyrosine (200 mg/kg i.p.) and given 7 ml of water to induce diuresis. Urine was collected for 3 hr and assayed for catecholamines. Data are expressed as means ± SEM.
Adapted from Alonso et al. (9).
[a]$p < 0.01$ from vehicle-treated group.

ability. The effect of tyrosine on urinary catecholamine excretion in cold-stressed rats is clearly consistent with the hypothesis, but data obtained from water-loaded rats maintained at room temperature and from rats treated with tyrosine for several days during continuous urine collection seem to be inconsistent with this idea. One explanation of these findings is that increased tyrosine availability enhances catecholamine synthesis and release only during periods of increased sympathetic activity that normally occur during the course of the day. This explanation remains to be tested. It is also possible that the mechanisms by which tyrosine availability affects catecholamine synthesis differ in the CNS and peripheral cells, e.g., because the latter are not controlled by multisynaptic feedback loops.

D. Comparison of the Effects of Precursor Availability on DA and NE Neurons

Although no published studies have specifically dealt with comparing the effects of tyrosine availability on DA versus NE neurons, several reports comment on possible differences between responses of NE and DA neurons to a tyrosine load. Carlsson and Lindqvist (44) noted that tyrosine administration enhanced DOPA production to a greater extent in the cerebral hemispheres (primarily noradrenergic) than in the striatum or limbic forebrain (primarily dopaminergic). They comment that maybe "tyrosine hydroxylase is less saturated with tyrosine in noradrenaline than in dopamine neurons." Wurtman and co-workers (103,236,286) noted that in rats treated with probenecid to block the efflux of catecholamine metabolites from the brain, tyrosine administration increases the levels of the NE metabolite MOPEG-SO_4 but not the DA metabolite HVA. They suggest the possibility (286) that "in the basal state, dopaminergic brain neurons may be less dependent on tyrosine levels than neurons that form norepinephrine." In addition, Yamori et al. (292) wrote that "recent unpublished experiments from our laboratory (Juskevich et al., to be published) show that tyrosine hydroxylation in synaptosomes from dopamine rich brain regions is less dependent upon the medium concentration of tyrosine than hydroxylation in synaptosomes from noradrenergic regions." Thus, although several laboratories hint that NE neurons may be more responsive to changes in precursor availability, this intriguing hypothesis remains to be tested.

As mentioned above, the relationship between tyrosine availability and catecholamine synthesis seems to be dependent on neuronal firing rate and the activation of TOH. In general, DA neurons are more active than NE neurons and DA synthesis is more rapid than NE synthesis (e.g., ref. 66). This would imply that DA neurons should be more responsive to changes in tyrosine availability—which does not seem to be the case. This discrepancy may reflect some basic difference in the manner in which catecholamine synthesis is regulated in DA and NE neurons.

E. Phenylalanine as a Catecholamine Precursor

Although the initial report on the properties of TOH described the enzyme as being absolutely specific for L-tyrosine (207), it was later shown that when tetrahydrobiopterin is used in the assay, TOH hydroxylates phenylalanine at least as well as tyrosine (243). That catecholaminergic neurons can synthesize catecholamines from phenylalanine has now been convincingly demonstrated (20–22,145,146). It appears that the phenylalanine hydroxylated by TOH does not mix with the free tyrosine pool, but is further hydroxylated to DOPA (20,21,145). However, physiologically the majority of brain catecholamine molecules (90%) appear to be synthesized from tyrosine (275).

Very few data are available on the relationship between phenylalanine levels and the rate of catecholamine synthesis. Carlsson and Lindqvist (44) reported that phenylalanine injection enhanced brain DOPA accumulation in AAAD-inhibited rats more effectively than did tyrosine. However, Wurtman et al. (288) observed that similar doses of phenylalanine slightly decreased the rate of DOPA production. In interpreting these experiments, it must be kept in mind that exogenous phenylalanine can interact with catecholamine synthesis at three loci, i.e., a portion of the administered amino acid is converted to tyrosine in the liver (72); unchanged phenylalanine competes with circulating tyrosine for uptake into the brain (215); and some of the phenylalanine entering the brain is converted to tyrosine and DOPA by TOH (20–22,145,146,275). High phenylalanine concentrations can inhibit TOH activity.

F. Tyrosine Availability and Catecholaminergic Neurotransmission

As described above for tryptophan and serotonin, increased synthesis of a neurotransmitter does not necessarily mean that more transmitter is released into the synapse. If tyrosine availability does influence catecholamine synthesis and release, then tyrosine availability should also influence brain outputs (i.e., behaviors, physiological processes, and responses to drugs) that are dependent on catecholaminergic neurotransmission. Such a relationship has been demonstrated in several instances, as described below.

1. Interaction of Tyrosine Availability and Responses to Drugs

The first evidence that tyrosine availability might alter brain outputs involving catecholaminergic neurotransmission was provided by Chiel and Wurtman (48). They demonstrated that L-valine injection, which reduces brain tyrosine levels, attenuated the hypothermic response to amphetamine treatment. The reduction in brain tyrosine levels was significantly correlated to the attenuation of the hypothermic response. Since amphetamine presumably reduces body temperature by increasing DA release at some site in the brain (294,295), it was suggested that L-valine antagonizes this action of amphetamine by reducing the availability of tyrosine, thereby decreasing the rate at which DA can be synthesized and released. Subsequently, Beaton and co-workers (26,27) have shown that L-valine and other LNAAs attenuate another response to amphetamine that is mediated via increased DA release—rotational behavior induced by amphetamine in rats with unilateral lesions of the nigrostriatal pathway (264). Recently, Fernando and Curzon (77) reported that valine did not alter several other behavioral responses to amphetamine (e.g., rearing, gnawing/licking, forward walking) thought to be mediated by increased DA release. However, in these experiments valine injection did not decrease brain tyrosine levels, leaving the results inconclusive. Fernando and Curzon (77) also observed that the responses to amphetamine were not affected by tyrosine injection. Unfortunately, the earlier studies did not examine the effects of increased tyrosine availability.

2. Effects of Tyrosine Availability on Blood Pressure

Since the regulation of blood pressure is very dependent on catecholaminergic neurons in both the brain and periphery (cf. refs. 47,265), Sved et al. (252) examined the effects of tyrosine administration on blood pressure in rats. In normotensive rats, the administration of a large dose of tyrosine (400 mg/kg i.p.) produced a slight but significant fall in blood pressure, a response also noted after the intravenous infusion of tyrosine (37). On the other hand, in SHR rats, tyrosine injection produced a marked fall in blood pressure (252) (see Fig. 4). This antihypertensive action of tyrosine in SHR rats is thought to be mediated by an increase in NE synthesis and release within the brain because (a) the response is blocked by the

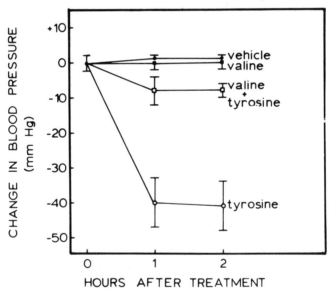

FIG. 4. Effect of valine on the antihypertensive action of L-tyrosine in SHR rats. Tyrosine (100 mg/kg; 0.55 mmoles/kg; ○), valine (0.55 mmoles/kg; ■), tyrosine plus valine (0.55 mmoles/kg of each; □), or vehicle (●) was administered to groups of four SHR rats. Blood pressures were determined just before treatment and then at 1-hr intervals thereafter. Data are expressed as the change in blood pressure from baseline values (mean ± SEM). Tyrosine injection caused a significant fall in blood pressure ($p < 0.01$); treatment with tyrosine plus valine produced a slight decrease in blood pressure ($p < 0.05$), but this effect was less than that produced by tyrosine alone ($p < 0.01$). Valine injection had no effect on blood pressure. Data were analyzed by analysis of variance and the Newman-Keuls test. From Sved et al. (252).

coadministration of LNAAs (Fig. 4), suggesting a central action of tyrosine; (b) tyrosine administered into the cerebral ventricles is also antihypertensive (292); (c) the antihypertensive response to tyrosine is accompanied by an increase in brain MOPEG-SO$_4$ levels, indicating increased NE release in the brain (252,292; Table 6); (d) NE at certain sites in the brain is known to lower blood pressure (47,265). Administration of several other amino acids (e.g., valine, leucine, alanine, aspartate, arginine) did not alter blood pressure in SHR rats (252). However, it should be noted that larger doses of valine (400 mg/kg i.p.) that decrease brain tyrosine levels increased blood pressure in SHR rats (Sved and Fernstrom, *unpublished data*). Tyrosine administration also decreases blood pressure in other forms of experimental hypertension, i.e., DOCA-salt hypertension (163,238,239) and renal hypertension (37), and is currently being tested in humans with essential hypertension.

Recently, Conlay et al. (52) reported that tyrosine administration increased arterial pressure in hypotensive rats. Following controlled hemorrhage that decreased blood pressure to about one-half of normal values, tyrosine administration significantly raised blood pressure. The action of tyrosine was antagonized by adrenalectomy, suggesting that it is at least partly mediated via increased synthesis and release of catecholamines from the adrenal medulla.

These data on the effects of tyrosine administration on blood pressure are consistent with the hypothesis presented above that tyrosine administration increases catecholamine synthesis only in activated catecholaminergic neurons. In the hypotensive rats, presumably the sympathoadrenal cells are the activated "neurons" and thus tyrosine acts in these cells to increase catecholamine release, resulting in vasoconstriction and an increase in blood pressure. In normotensive animals, where no population of catecholaminergic neurons would be expected to be activated, tyrosine administration produces only minor effects on blood pressure. On the other hand, in hypertensive rats a population of central sympathoinhibitory neurons may be activated (223), and therefore tyrosine acts within the CNS to decrease sympathetic outflow, producing a fall in blood pressure. This would suggest that in SHR rats only certain catecholaminergic neurons are affected by the increased tyrosine availability, a notion supported by the observations that although tyrosine administration increases forebrain and brain stem levels of MOPEG-SO$_4$, it fails to alter spinal cord MOPEG-SO$_4$ levels and levels of DA metabolites in the striatum, hypothalamus, and limbic forebrain (see Table 6).

The sympathetic nervous system also influences the susceptibility of the heart to ventricular arrhythmias (174). Thus, if tyrosine administration, by enhancing NE release at certain loci in the CNS, can decrease sympathetic outflow (as suggested by the studies in hypertensive rats), it should also protect the heart against ventricular arrhythmias. Just such an effect has been demonstrated by Scott et al. (237). They showed that intravenous administration of tyrosine (2 to 6 mg/kg) significantly raised the ventricular fibrillation threshold (the minimum amount of electrical current applied to the heart that induces arrhythmia) in dogs. It is interesting that tyrosine presumably acted within the CNS to decrease sympathetic outflow rather than at the sympathetic nerve terminals to enhance NE release, which would have increased ventricular fibrillation. One explanation, which is consistent with the idea that tyrosine selectively affects rapidly firing neurons, is that by acting in the brain to enhance NE release and suppress sympathetic neuron activity, tyrosine decreased the sensitivity of the sympathetic neurons to changes in tyrosine availability.

3. Effects of Tyrosine Availability on Prolactin Release

The release of prolactin from the anterior pituitary gland is controlled, in large part, by DA neurons of the tuberoinfundibular system (177,210). DA released from nerve terminals in the median eminence into the portal blood acts directly on the mammotrophs of the anterior pituitary to inhibit tonically the release of prolactin. Thus, this system provides an ideal model to examine the effects of treatments on the release of DA.

Tyrosine injection does not alter serum prolactin levels in normal male rats (69,251), which is not surprising considering that tyrosine injection does not appear to increase DA synthesis in normal rats. However, after activation of the tuberoinfundibular DA neurons by the administration of reserpine, tyrosine injection does decrease serum prolactin levels (251) (Table 9). The hypothesis that this effect is mediated via increased DA synthesis and release is supported by the observation that tyrosine increased the levels of the DA metabolites in brain regions from reserpine-treated rats (251; Table 9). In further support of this hypothesis, Sved and Fernstrom (250) have shown that tyrosine injection increased DOPA production in the median eminence following the intracerebral administration of ovine prolactin, a treatment that selectively activates tuberoinfundibular DA neurons (11,12,202).

TABLE 9. Effect of tyrosine injection on serum prolactin
levels and hypothalamic levels of DA metabolites in
reserpine-treated rats

Treatment	Serum prolactin (ng/ml)	Hypothalamic	
		DOPAC	HVA
		(ng/g)	
No reserpine			
Vehicle	52 ± 13	56 ± 18	187 ± 20
Tyrosine	49 ± 9	85 ± 21	243 ± 35
Chronic reserpine			
Vehicle	156 ± 14	78 ± 8	386 ± 29
Tyrosine	80 ± 8[a]	336 ± 126[a]	595 ± 109[a]

Groups of five rats received tyrosine (200 mg/kg) or vehicle and were killed 1 hr later; animals had been pretreated with either reserpine (2.5 mg/kg i.p. twice daily for 4 days: chronic reserpine) or vehicle (no reserpine). Sera were collected and assayed from prolactin and hypothalami were removed and assayed for DOPAC and HVA. Data are expressed as means ± SEM.
Adapted from Sved et al. (251).
[a]$p < 0.05$ compared with vehicle-treated animals of the same pretreatment group.

Thus, studies on the relationship between tyrosine availability, DA synthesis and release, and prolactin release again support the hypothesis that tyrosine administration enhances DA release only from activated DA neurons.

Recently, Reymond and Porter (226) noted that tyrosine injection did not affect basal DA release into the pituitary portal circulation in aged female rats. Unfortunately, the effect of tyrosine was not examined under circumstances where tuberoinfundibular DA neurons would be activated.

4. Other Brain Outputs Affected by Tyrosine Administration

Although tyrosine administration has been reported to restore estrous cycling in aged, anestrous female rats (an action that it shares with L-DOPA and other DA agonists) (171), the effects of tyrosine availability on other brain outputs dependent on catecholaminergic neurotransmission have not been studied in any detail. This remains an interesting area for future research.

A few studies have also examined the effects of tyrosine administration on brain processes in human subjects. The administration of tyrosine to patients with Parkinson's disease, which is characterized by loss of nigrostriatal DA neurons, alleviated some of the symptoms in patients with mild forms of the disease (117,118). That tyrosine produced this effect by enhancing DA synthesis and release is supported by an increase in cerebrospinal fluid (CSF) levels of HVA produced by administration of tyrosine in these patients (117,118). Tyrosine administration has also been reported to be beneficial in the treatment of some cases of depression (98,106). Since some forms of depression may result from inadequate release of NE at some site in the brain, and drugs that enhance noradrenergic neurotransmission are often used in the treatment of depression, it is possible that tyrosine produces its antidepressant action by enhancing NE synthesis and release. If the administration of tyrosine turns out to be efficacious in treating disease states characterized by insufficient catecholaminergic transmission in some area in the brain, it might be expected to produce less side effects than more conventional drugs, since tyrosine appears to accelerate catecholamine synthesis only in activated catecholaminergic neurons.

G. Tyramine and Tyrosine

Although all the data presented above are consistent with the hypothesis that tyrosine administration affects certain brain outputs by enhancing catecholamine synthesis and release as a consequence of increased availability of precursor, the possibility that tyrosine may produce these effects by increasing tyramine (or octopamine) formation must also be considered. (Tyramine and octopamine are the decarboxylated and decarboxylated plus β-hydroxylated metabolites of tyrosine, respectively.) Tyrosine administration does accelerate the syntheses of these amines in brain, as evidenced by (a) the greater increase in octopamine levels in brains of animals treated with tyrosine and an MAO inhibitor than in animals treated with the MAO inhibitor alone (36,121) and (b) the increase in deaminated metabolites of tyramine and octopamine in brain following tyrosine administration (70,71). Further, these amines administered into the CSF have been shown to produce at least one effect similar to tyrosine administration, i.e., a decrease in blood pressure (65,128).

But tyrosine administration *does* enhance catecholamine synthesis in some instances. Conceivably, tyramine (or octopamine) formation in response to increased tyrosine availability could displace catecholamines from nerve terminals, thereby increasing catecholamine synthesis. However, tyramine and octopamine actually *decrease* catecholamine synthesis (155,277). Also, since this sequence of events would be expected to occur whenever tyramine formation is enhanced, such a mechanism does not appear to explain the selective increase in catecholamine synthesis in activated catecholaminergic neurons. For example, tyrosine administration to otherwise untreated rats increases brain tyramine and octopamine synthesis, but not catecholamine synthesis. Further, following depletion of catecholamines with reserpine, the increase in DA synthesis produced by tyrosine administration is difficult to explain as being secondary to an increase in tyramine formation. It is equally difficult to explain the increase in DA synthesis produced by tyrosine injection in rats treated with GBL as a result of tyramine formation.

Thus, although tyrosine administration may increase the syntheses of the trace amines tyramine and octopamine, it also enhances catecholamine synthesis under certain conditions. Since the effects of tyrosine administration on catecholamine synthesis cannot be explained by increased formation of tyramine or octopamine, the observations that the synthesis of tyramine and octopamine are enhanced by tyrosine administration do not detract from the hypothesis that tyrosine administration, by increasing the degree of saturation of TOH, can increase the synthesis of catecholamines. Further, the behavioral and physiological consequences of tyrosine administration can be explained by increased tyrosine availability increasing catecholamine synthesis and release; a role for tyramine or octopamine is not necessary. The roles of tyramine and octopamine in the behavioral and physiological effects of tyrosine administration warrant further investigation.

H. Tyrosine Availability and Catecholaminergic Transmission: Summary and Conclusions

The relationship between tyrosine availability and catecholamine synthesis appears more complex than that between tryptophan and serotonin: For a neuron to respond to additional tyrosine, it must be physiologically activated. Tyrosine administration does affect brain outputs dependent on catecholaminergic neurotransmission (e.g., blood pressure, prolactin release), suggesting that tyrosine availability is one factor controlling catecholamine synthesis and release.

IV. REGULATION OF BRAIN TRYPTOPHAN AND TYROSINE LEVELS

The collective evidence presented in the preceding discussion indicates that tryptophan and tyrosine levels in brain do affect the output of serotonin and catecholamines from neurons. Thus, it becomes important to consider factors that normally determine these levels. Tissue amino acid levels reflect their influx and efflux from the body's total amino acid pool. Sources of free amino acids in the brain include transport from blood, liberation from protein, and, in some cases, net synthesis. On the other hand, incorporation into protein, catabolism, efflux into circulating fluids, and synthesis of specialized molecules (e.g., neurotransmitters) are processes that draw from free amino acid pools. The roles these processes may play in controlling the availability of neuronal tryptophan and tyrosine are discussed below. [A more complete review of the regulation of brain amino acid levels is provided by Pardridge (215) in *Nutrition and the Brain*, Vol. 1.]

A. Brain Tryptophan

Whole-brain tryptophan levels are normally in the range of 10 to 30 nmoles/g. Variations among different brain regions have been noted; tryptophan levels in the hypothalamus are twice as high as in other regions (152), possibly a reflection of greater uptake in this region (68). Some portion of tryptophan uptake into brain may result specifically from uptake into terminals of serotoninergic neurons, since destruction of these neurons reduces tryptophan uptake in brain regions receiving rich serotoninergic innervation (68).

Since whole-brain tryptophan uptake is approximately 300 nmoles/g/hr and whole-brain serotonin turnover is estimated at only 2 nmoles/g/hr, less than 1% of the tryptophan entering the brain is actually used for neurotransmitter synthesis. A rapid elevation of tryptophan levels following intracerebral injection of the protein synthesis inhibitors puromycin or cycloheximide is an indication that the fate of most of the tryptophan taken up is incorporation into protein (32).

Although the brain is capable of breaking down tryptophan, the absence of a measurable arteriovenous difference across the brain (29) suggests that metabolism does not occur to any great extent. Tryptophan pyrrolase activity has been demonstrated in brain (93,94), and product formation (as indicated by brain kynurenine levels) reportedly is enhanced by tryptophan administration (94). Thus, this pathway may serve to blunt increases in brain tryptophan. Decarboxylation to tryptamine [subsequently metabolized to indoleacetic acid (IAA)] also occurs in brain (184,231,297), primarily in monoaminergic neurons (184). Tryptamine formation as reflected by tryptamine accumulation following MAO inhibition or by IAA levels also appears to be dependent on brain tryptophan levels (184,297). A brain enzyme capable of transaminating tryptophan has also been described (28); however, the K_m of this enzyme for tryptophan is extremely high (167) and thus it is probably not physiologically relevant.

B. Brain Tyrosine

Normal whole-brain tyrosine levels in the rat are about 15 μg/g or, roughly, 75 μM. The level of tyrosine throughout the brain is not constant, but varies almost twofold from the area with the highest level (medulla) to the region with the lowest level (cortex) (204). There may also be a difference in the distribution of tyrosine between extracellular fluid and intracellular compartments. Synaptosomes appear to possess a high-affinity (K_m approximately 8 μM) uptake system for tyrosine (205), suggesting that nerve terminals concentrate tyrosine whereas other cell compartments may not. It is not clear whether regional variations in high-affinity uptake (or tyrosine levels) are directly attributable to catecholaminergic neurons. However, it should be noted that the synaptosomal uptake mechanism for tyrosine is not specific for tyrosine, but rather for all LNAAs (205). The free brain tyrosine pool is derived both from tyrosine transported into the brain from blood and from tyrosine released from proteins. Garlick and Marshall (96) have estimated that about 60% of the free tyrosine pool comes directly from blood, whereas the remaining 40% results from protein catabolism. Nonetheless, since proteins do not readily penetrate the blood–brain barrier, all brain tyrosine ultimately comes from the blood. Phenylalanine hydroxylase activity is lacking in brain, although tyrosine hydroxylase may act on phenylalanine to a small extent (20,145,146) and, in any case, tyrosine synthesized in this way does not equilibrate with the free tyrosine pool, but is instead rapidly converted to catecholamines (20,21,145).

Tyrosine in brain is utilized in the synthesis of protein or catecholamines, metabolized, or transported back into blood. The conversion of tyrosine to catecholamines is actually a very minor pathway. The influx of tyrosine into brain (as calculated from plasma amino acid levels and the kinetics of the transport system) is about 44 nmoles/g/hr. Since the synthesis rate for catecholamines is on the order of 1 nmole/g/hr, less than 2.5% of the tyrosine entering the brain is converted to catecholamines. Also, since there is no measurable arteriovenous difference of tyrosine across the brain (29), metabolism of tyrosine by brain tyrosine aminotransferase (181) must also be a very minor pathway.

C. Transport of Tryptophan and Tyrosine into Brain

Circulating amino acids are transported across the blood–brain barrier into brain by one of three carrier-mediated transport systems (215,218). These transport systems are each specific for one class of amino acids (i.e., basic, acidic, or large neutral) and are energy-dependent, saturable, and highly stereospecific (215,218). Because the transport systems are saturable and specific for groups of amino acids, the individual amino acids in each group compete with each other for uptake into brain.

Tryptophan and tyrosine share the transport system for LNAAs together with the other LNAAs (phenylalanine, valine, leucine, isoleucine, methionine, histidine and threonine). Because of the competitive mechanisms at work, the amount of a given amino acid that is transported does not depend on its level in blood, but rather on its level in blood relative to that of the other amino acids in its class. An example of this is illustrated in Fig. 5. Brain levels of α-methyldopa, a synthetic LNAA, after administration to rats consuming diets designed to alter blood LNAA levels within the physiological range, are correlated to a ratio of serum levels of α-

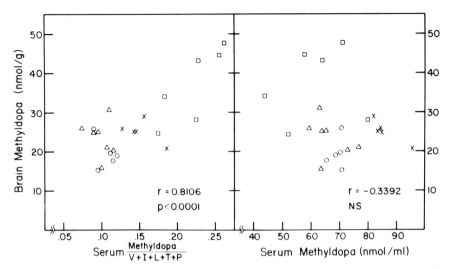

FIG. 5. Correlations relating brain α-methyldopa level with serum methyldopa and to the serum ratio of α-methyldopa to LNAAs. Rats were fasted overnight and then given access to one of the experimental diets for 90 min. Rats were then injected with the synthetic LNAA α-methyldopa (MD; 25 mg/kg i.p.) and sacrificed 30 min later. Brains were removed and assayed for MD and sera were assayed for MD and LNAA. Each point represents the data from a single animal. X, Fasted control; ○, total mix containing free amino acids to simulate 18% casein hydrolysate; □, total mix minus LNAAs; Δ, total mix minus acidic amino acids. The **right panel** shows the correlation of brain MD levels with serum MD levels and the **left panel** shows the correlation of brain MD levels with the ratio of serum MD levels to the sum of the serum levels of valine (V), isoleucine (I), leucine (L), tyrosine (T), and phenylalanine (P). From Sved et al. (253).

methyldopa to the LNAAs, but not to the serum levels of α-methyldopa alone. This same type of relationship has been demonstrated for each of the natural LNAAs (79). Since the affinity of the transport carrier for each LNAA is not the same, the use of this ratio is a simplification; however, when the different K_ms are included in the calculations the same relationship results (79).

The transport of tryptophan into brain is somewhat different from that of the other LNAAs because only tryptophan circulates bound to protein (189,190). Thus, blood tryptophan represents two pools: a free pool (10 to 20% of total) and an albumin-bound pool (80 to 90% of total) (189,190). The nature of the pool available for transport into brain has been an area of controversy. In 1972, Knott and Curzon (151) reported that in food-deprived rats, both free tryptophan in serum and brain tryptophan were elevated but total serum tryptophan (free plus bound) was not. They concluded that free serum tryptophan levels control brain tryptophan levels, a conclusion also reached by Tagliamonte et al. (255). These investigators showed that while fasting lowered total serum tryptophan, it elevated free serum tryptophan and brain tryptophan. Further, the rise in brain tryptophan following the administration of the amino acid to fasted rats correlated better with the rise in free serum tryptophan than with the rise in total serum tryptophan. [However, in none of these studies were the decreases in other LNAAs attributable to fasting (75) considered.]

Studies using drugs (e.g., acetylsalicyclic acid) that displace tryptophan from albumin and thus increase the free serum pool also increase brain tryptophan levels (58,256).

In marked contrast, insulin administration or carbohydrate-induced insulin secretion elevates total serum and brain tryptophan but depresses free serum tryptophan levels (178). Further, diets containing a high fat content raise serum levels of nonesterified fatty acids (NEFAs), which, in turn, displace tryptophan from albumin (190), thereby raising free serum tryptophan while lowering brain and total serum tryptophan (82,179). In these experiments, the ratio of total serum tryptophan to the other LNAAs correlated better with brain levels of tryptophan than did free tryptophan levels.

To try to resolve this conflict, Yuwiler et al. (300) and Etienne et al. (73) studied the effects of albumin binding and LNAAs on the transport of tryptophan into brain using the Oldendorf technique (214). This method involves injecting into the carotid artery of an anesthetized rat a bolus of buffer containing ^{14}C-labeled test substance (e.g., tryptophan), [^{3}H]water (used as a freely diffusible reference), and the substances to be studied for effect on transport. After 15 sec, the rat is decapitated and the amount of ^{14}C relative to ^{3}H in brain is determined. This ratio reflects the fraction of the test substance transported into brain. Both studies (73,300) found that although albumin slightly retarded the transport of tryptophan into brain, competition with other LNAAs within the physiological range was quantitatively more important. The results of these studies also suggest that a considerable fraction of the albumin-bound tryptophan is stripped from the albumin during passage through the brain.

However, Bloxam et al. (33), using a similar technique but examining transport of [^{14}C]tryptophan from a bolus of rat plasma rather than buffer, concluded that binding to albumin is a significant factor, since the transport of tryptophan correlated best with the free tryptophan pool. In a recent study by Gillman et al. (104), the increase in cortical tryptophan levels resulting from an infusion of the amino acid correlated almost perfectly with the plasma pool of free tryptophan. Surprisingly, the correlation coefficients for both free and total plasma tryptophan were decreased when expressed as the ratio to other LNAAs.

Pardridge (217) has applied the principles of competitive ligand binding to a theoretical examination of this issue. Because of the high capacity of the transport system for tryptophan, it can compete with albumin for tryptophan binding. Thus, the amount of transportable tryptophan available *in vivo* is underestimated by measurements made on the free pool *in vitro*. Because the apparent affinities for tryptophan of both albumin and the transport carrier are affected by concentrations of compounds that compete for binding (e.g., NEFAs in the case of albumin, LNAAs in the case of the transport system) the extent of the relative tryptophan binding, and thus the amount of transportable tryptophan, will vary. Therefore, depending on physiological changes in blood levels of LNAAs and NEFAs, the transportable pool *in vivo* may approach either the free or total pools as measured *in vitro*. According to Pardridge's calculations, under conditions where NEFAs are low and/

or LNAAs are high (e.g., fasting or a high-protein–low-fat meal) the transportable pool will approximate the *in vitro* free pool. Conversely, when NEFAs are high and/or LNAAs are low (e.g., high-fat–low-protein meal) the total serum tryptophan pool better approximates the transportable fraction. Pardridge's analysis helps to reconcile much of the earlier data.

D. Peripheral Factors in the Regulation of Brain Tryptophan and Tyrosine Levels

The peripheral factors that affect circulating levels of any of the LNAAs may ultimately influence the brain levels of tyrosine and tryptophan as a result of a common transport system into brain. These peripheral factors include amino acid metabolism, excretion of amino acids, and the action of certain hormones, especially insulin. Diet, the major modifier of blood amino acid composition, is considered in a later section.

1. Metabolism

Tryptophan is catabolized in the liver by a pathway beginning with the cleavage of the indole ring by the enzyme tryptophan pyrrolase. On the basis of studies of pharmacological enhancement of tryptophan pyrrolase activity (by the administration of corticosterone and α-methyltryptophan), it was suggested that hepatic tryptophan pyrrolase activity controls blood (and therefore brain) tryptophan levels (57,246). However, physiologically, this does not appear to be the case. Rather, the relationship between the normal diurnal variation in hepatic tryptophan pyrrolase activity (89) and the diurnal changes in blood tryptophan (227) suggests that tryptophan pyrrolase may function to blunt the increase in circulating tryptophan following food ingestion. Decarboxylation of tryptophan to tryptamine by AAAD also occurs in the periphery (298), but this represents a minor pathway.

The liver is also the major site of tyrosine metabolism. Transamination to *p*-hydroxyphenylpyruvate catalyzed by tyrosine aminotransferase represents the major metabolic pathway. Tyrosine aminotransferase activity exhibits dramatic daily variations, with peak activity often exceeding nadir levels by more than fivefold (227,285,289). The variations in tyrosine aminotransferase activity seem to be entrained to the cyclic ingestion of food, specifically protein (227,289). The physiological significance of these marked variations in hepatic tyrosine aminotransferase activity probably lies in the capacity of the enzyme to act as a gating mechanism, limiting the passage of tyrosine from the hepatic portal blood into the systemic circulation (285). Thus, following the ingestion of protein, when tyrosine absorption into portal blood would be high, the activity of hepatic tyrosine aminotransferase would be at its peak. Strangely, tryptophan, not tyrosine, appears to be the protein component responsible for the stimulation of tyrosine aminotransferase activity (285,289). That the activity of the enzyme is regulated by tryptophan rather than tyrosine itself is interesting and may reflect the fact that tryptophan is the most limiting amino acid in protein and the amino acid most effective in causing the *in vivo* aggregation of hepatic polyribosomes (244).

Although it was reported that significant amounts of tyrosine are decarboxylated to tyramine (62), this pathway was subsequently shown to be extremely minor (76,258). Tyrosine is also converted to the pigment melanin, although this also represents an extremely minor pathway.

As discussed above, peripheral metabolism of phenylalanine is important in the regulation of brain tyrosine levels for two reasons: Phenylalanine is an LNAA and thus competes with tyrosine for uptake into brain and phenylalanine can also be converted to tyrosine, thereby increasing tyrosine availability (72). The liver is the main site of phenylalanine metabolism, and the major pathway is *p*-hydroxylation to tyrosine by the enzyme phenylalanine hydroxylase.

Unlike the aromatic amino acids, the branched-chain amino acids (leucine, isoleucine, and valine) are not metabolized in the liver (although the liver does remove these amino acids from the circulation for incorporation into protein). Instead, these amino acids are transaminated in skeletal muscle, kidney, and heart (72,134).

2. Excretion

Amino acids, with the exception of albumin-bound tryptophan, are freely filtered by the kidney. However, since almost all (97 to 99%) of each amino acid is normally reabsorbed (296), only small quantities of amino acids are excreted. Like the brain amino acid transport systems, the kidney reabsorption systems in the proximal tubule are specific for classes of amino acids, and competition among members of each class operates. As clearly demonstrated by Webber (271), infusion of one LNAA substantially increases the excretion of the other LNAAs, but not basic or acidic amino acids. Thus, it is not surprising that the administration of a large dose of one LNAA (e.g., valine) decreases the blood levels of another LNAA (e.g., tyrosine) (see, e.g., ref. 6).

V. DIET, PRECURSOR AVAILABILITY, AND NEUROTRANSMITTER SYNTHESIS

Physiologically, diet is the major determinant of blood (and therefore brain) amino acid levels. Typical laboratory chows contain about 250 mg tryptophan, 900 mg tyrosine, and 1,200 mg phenylalanine per 100 g of food. Thus, an intake of 15 g of food per day, which is normal for an adult rat, corresponds to about 40 mg of tryptophan, 135 mg of tyrosine, and 180 mg of phenylalanine per day, or expressed on a milligram per kilogram weight basis, 150, 550, and 720, respectively. Thus doses of a few hundred milligrams per kilogram generally used in studies where the amino acids are injected are not unreasonable, but represent doses of these amino acids within the physiological range.

A. Acute Diet Studies

Single meals alter the serum amino acid profile, thereby affecting brain amino acid levels. As described above, the major factor determining the transport of an amino acid from blood into brain is the concentration of that amino acid in blood relative to the concentrations of the amino acids with which it competes for uptake into the brain. Fernstrom and Faller (79) demonstrated that the brain levels of each LNAA (including tryptophan and tyrosine) following the consumption of meals containing 0, 18, or 40% protein correlates very well with the ratio of the blood level of that amino acid to the sum of the blood levels of all the other LNAAs (Fig. 6). The brain level of each LNAA does not, however, reflect the amount of that amino acid consumed. For example, the consumption of a 0% protein meal raises the brain levels of the aromatic amino acids (tryptophan, tyrosine, phenylalanine) because insulin, released in response to this meal, markedly decreases the blood levels of the branched-chain amino acids (valine, leucine, and isoleucine), resulting in an increase in the ratios of tryptophan, tyrosine, or phenylalanine to the other LNAAs. On the other hand, a high-protein meal, although it contains a substantial amount of tryptophan, does not raise brain tryptophan levels because blood levels of the other LNAAs increase more.

If precursor availability is a physiological factor regulating serotonin and catecholamine synthesis, then the synthesis of these monoamines should reflect changes in brain amino acid levels following the ingestion of single meals. This has been clearly demonstrated in the case of serotonin. The ingestion of a carbohydrate meal (0% protein) increases brain tryptophan levels and also the levels of serotonin and

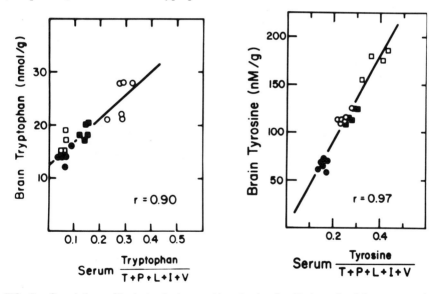

FIG. 6. Correlations of brain tryptophan and tyrosine levels with the ratio of the serum amino acid level to the serum levels of the other LNAAs. Groups of rats were fasted overnight and then allowed access to a 0% protein diet (○), an 18% protein diet (■), or a 40% protein diet (□) for 2 hr before sacrifice. Control animals continued to fast during this period (●). Each point represents data from an individual animal. The **right panel** shows the correlation of brain tyrosine with the ratio of serum tyrosine to the sum of the levels of the other LNAAs and the **left panel** shows the same relationship for brain tryptophan. From Fernstrom and Faller (79).

5-HIAA (80,84,86). A high-protein (40%) meal, which has little effect on brain tryptophan levels, has little effect on the levels of serotonin and 5-HIAA (80,84,86). In fact, 5-hydroxyindole levels in brain correlate extremely well with brain tryptophan levels following ingestion of any of a variety of single meals that alter brain tryptophan levels over a wide range (Fig. 7).

Similar data are available for the effects of single meals on catecholamine synthesis. Gibson and Wurtman (102) found that changes in brain tyrosine levels produced by the ingestion of single meals altered the rate of DOPA production in whole rat brain in the predicted manner (Table 10). They also demonstrated a similar effect of diet on brain MOPEG-SO$_4$ levels in cold-stressed rats (103). The clear increase in brain DOPA formation following the ingestion of either 0 or 40% protein (102) is somewhat surprising in view of the lack of an effect of tyrosine injection on DOPA accumulation usually noted in normal animals. One explanation is that feeding, independent of changes in tyrosine, activates some population of

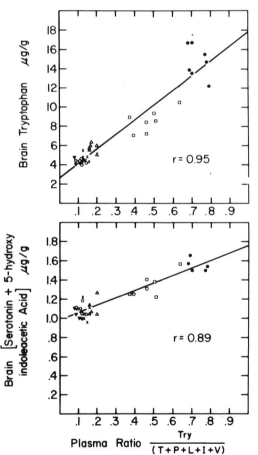

FIG. 7. Correlations of brain tryptophan levels and brain 5-hydroxyindole levels with the ratio of plasma tryptophan levels to the sum of the levels of the other LNAAs in plasma. Groups of rats were fasted overnight and then given access to diets containing either free amino acids to simulate 18% casein hydrolysate (total diet) or total diet lacking tyrosine (T), phenylalanine (P), valine (V), leucine (L), and isoleucine (I) (diet minus LNAAs). Rats were killed 1 or 2 hr later. Brains were removed and assayed for tryptophan, serotonin, and 5-hydroxyindoleacetic acid. ○, Controls after 1 hr; ▼, controls after 2 hr; X, total diet after 1 hr; △, total diet after 2 hr; □, diet minus LNAAs after 1 hr; ●, diet minus LNAAs after 2 hr. From Fernstrom and Wurtman (86).

TABLE 10. *Brain DOPA accumulation
after ingestion of single meals containing
0% or 40% protein*

Treatment	Tyrosine (μg/g)	DOPA (ng/g)
Fasted	12.9 ± 0.6	66.5 ± 4.2
0% Casein	18.8 ± 0.6[a]	116.5 ± 6.0[a]
40% Casein	29.9 ± 0.7[a]	108.0 ± 5.3[a]

Groups of six to eight rats were fasted overnight and then allowed access to one of the diets. One hour later they were injected with Ro4-4602 (800 mg/kg i.p.) and they were sacrificed 30 min thereafter. Brains were removed and assayed for tyrosine and DOPA. Data are presented as means ± SEM.
From Gibson and Wurtman (102).
[a]Difference from fasted group, $p < 0.01$.

TABLE 11. *DA metabolite levels in the striatum after ingestion of single meals*

Diet	Serum tyrosine (μg/ml)	Brain tyrosine (μg/g)	DA metabolites (nmoles/g)
Fasted	12.7 ± 1.3[a]	10.4 ± 0.8[a]	4.82 ± 0.78[a]
Nonnutritive	10.7 ± 0.6[b]	10.5 ± 0.5[a]	6.54 ± 0.68[b]
0% Casein	7.1 ± 0.4[c]	13.6 ± 1.7[b]	6.93 ± 0.46[b]
40% Casein	45.5 ± 2.7[d]	17.4 ± 1.0[c]	8.90 ± 0.62[c]

Groups of six rats were fasted overnight and then allowed access to one of the diets for 2 hr. Rats were then sacrificed and the striata dissected out and assayed for tyrosine and DA metabolites (DOPAC plus HVA). Numbers followed by different symbols are significantly different from each other, $p < 0.01$ by analysis of variance.
From Sved and Fernstrom, *unpublished observations.*

brain catecholaminergic neurons. The literature provides some support for this notion. Biggio et al. (32a) reported that brain DA metabolite levels increase during eating, even if tyrosine levels do not change. Further, glucose administration may affect the firing rates of nigrostriatal DA neurons (233). Thus, it may be that eating per se activates certain DA neurons. Therefore, if the diet also elevates brain tyrosine levels, DA synthesis in the activated neurons may be further enhanced. Such a possibility is supported by preliminary data presented in Table 11. Ingestion of a nonnutritive agar block increased DA metabolite levels in the striatum, although tyrosine levels actually fell. A carbohydrate meal, which slightly increased striatal tyrosine levels, increased DA metabolite levels to about the same degree as did the agar block. A high-protein diet further increased tyrosine and DA metabolite levels. Similar increases in striatal tyrosine levels produced by the injection of tyrosine do not alter levels of the DA metabolites in the striatum (191,249,251). Whatever the explanation, it appears that physiological, diet-induced changes in brain tyrosine concentration *do* effect catecholamine synthesis and release.

B. Chronic Diet Studies

Chronic ingestion of diets that alter brain tryptophan levels also alters brain serotonin levels (85,100,144,175). This has been studied using synthetic, tryptophan-free diets or diets in which corn meal is the sole source of protein. (Corn contains very little tryptophan.) As early as 2 days after rats are placed on a tryptophan-free diet, brain tryptophan and hydroxyindole levels are reduced (302), and they reach their minimum levels within 1 week (302). Injection of tryptophan or addition of tryptophan to the diet rapidly restores brain tryptophan and hydroxyindole levels to normal (81,100).

Rats consuming these tryptophan-deficient diets show behavioral signs of depressed serotoninergic neurotransmission; they are more aggressive, exhibit more sexual behavior, and are hyperalgesic (45,100,144,175). Another sign that serotonin neurotransmission is reduced is that receptor supersensitivity develops (49).

A few studies have also examined the effects of supplementing diets with tryptophan; supplementation of a 12% protein diet with 0.5 to 1% tryptophan elevates brain tryptophan and serotonin levels for as long as the animals remain on the diets (260,261).

Similar experiments have also tested the effects of tyrosine and phenylalanine supplements on catecholaminergic neurons (260,261). No consistent effects on catecholamine levels were observed, and unfortunately no indices of catecholamine synthesis were measured. However, behavioral changes were noted in animals on the high-tyrosine diet; these rats were more aggressive. Studies on the effects of tyrosine-deficient diets are not available.

VI. PRECURSOR REGULATION OF MONOAMINE FUNCTION: IMPLICATIONS

A. Physiological

As described above, it appears that the diet, by its effects on circulating amino acid levels and therefore brain amino acid levels, can alter the function of serotoninergic and catecholaminergic neurons. Such a system seems ideally designed to function in the regulation of food intake or food selection. Studies examining this possibility have provided interesting results. Wurtman and Wurtman (283,284) have reported that drugs that enhance serotoninergic neurotransmission (i.e., fenfluramine, fluoxetine, MK-212) decrease carbohydrate intake while sparing protein intake. Similar results with fenfluramine have also been reported by others (34). Furthermore, impairment of serotoninergic neurotransmission within the CNS (i.e., with administration of para-chlorophenylalanine or 5,7-dihydroxytryptamine or lesions of the raphe nuclei) produces a preference for carbohydrate consumption in rats (19a). Since carbohydrate meals increase brain tryptophan levels, and thus serotoninergic neurotransmission, this would comprise a negative feedback system for carbohydrate intake, which has recently been described (282a).

Although this is an especially attractive hypothesis, it is not totally supported by the literature. For example, the hypothesis would predict that tryptophan administration would selectively reduce carbohydrate consumption relative to protein intake; however, this has not yet been clearly demonstrated. Woodger et al. (280) reported an increase in carbohydrate intake relative to protein intake in rats when the diet was supplemented with tryptophan. On the other hand, tryptophan has also been reported to have no effect on nutrient selection (221). Two other studies found tryptophan administration to decrease (164) or have no effect on (243) food intake. However, these studies gave rats access to only a single diet, so possible alterations in nutrient selection produced by tryptophan (like a selective decrease in carbohydrate consumption) could not be assessed.

In longer term food selection experiments (2 weeks as opposed to acute, 24-hr experiments) Ashley and Anderson (10,11,18,19) have demonstrated an inverse correlation between protein intake and the plasma tryptophan to LNAA ratio. Since brain serotonin varies directly with the plasma tryptophan to LNAA ratio, this relationship would suggest that increased serotoninergic neurotransmission inhibits protein intake. This contrasts with results of acute studies which show that serotonin decreases carbohydrate intake relative to protein intake.

B. Pharmacological

Pharmacological manipulation of precursor availability offers a useful strategy for altering catecholaminergic or serotoninergic neurotransmission. By administering tryptophan, tyrosine, or other LNAAs, it is possible to increase or decrease the availability of the monoamine precursors to the brain, thereby altering the level of monoaminergic neurotransmission.

One major problem with the use of these precursors as drugs is the limited magnitude of their effect. Since they do not bypass the rate-limiting step in the neurotransmitter synthetic pathways, their maximal effect depends on the maximum velocity of that reaction. In the case of catecholamines, this reaction normally proceeds at close to the maximal rate (with respect to tyrosine), and therefore tyrosine administration cannot be expected to produce more than a 25 to 30% increase in catecholamine synthesis; the magnitude of the effect of tryptophan on serotonin synthesis is somewhat larger. This problem can be remedied in part by administering the precursor in combination with another drug (e.g., a reuptake blocker) to enhance the effect of the additional transmitter molecules synthesized in response to increased precursor availability.

The major advantage of using these precursors as drugs to manipulate the serotonin and catecholamine release is that this approach appears to be more specific than the use of other pharmacological agents. For example, as a result of the specific localization of TpOH, tryptophan is converted to serotonin only in neurons that normally synthesize and release serotonin, limiting its action to sites that normally receive serotonin input. In contrast, 5-HTP is taken up by catecholaminergic neurons in addition to serotoninergic neurons and causes the release of catecholamines as well as serotonin. In fact, many effects produced by 5-HTP administration are actually the result of its actions on catecholaminergic neurons (e.g., 41,211,299). Direct-acting serotonin agonists are also of limited selectivity, since, even if they are specific for serotonin receptors, serotonin receptors may be present at sites not normally receiving serotonin input (119).

In a similar fashion, administration of tyrosine would be more specific than DOPA in affecting catecholaminergic neurons. The use of tyrosine seems to provide an additional dimension in selectivity; it enhances catecholamine synthesis only in activated catecholaminergic neurons. Tyrosine appears to be the only compound with such specificity.

The one problem with the specificity of monoamine precursors is that both tryptophan and tyrosine are LNAAs, and so they compete with each other for uptake into the brain. Thus, when tryptophan is administered to increase serotonin synthesis, at the same time it is decreasing the availability of the catecholamine precursor. When another LNAA is given to decrease the availability of either tryptophan or tyrosine, it will decrease the availability of the other in addition. It is conceivable that mixing appropriate amounts of amino acids together could eliminate this problem, but such a level of sophistication has not yet been reached.

Clinically, the use of tyrosine and tryptophan to treat neurological and psychiatric disorders thought to involve deficits in catecholamine or serotonin appears promising, and has already received some attention (see refs. 116,287). This remains an exciting area for futher investigation.

REFERENCES

1. Acheson, A. L., Kapatos, G., and Zigmond, M. J. (1981): The effects of phosphorylating conditions on tyrosine hydroxylase activity are influenced by assay conditions and brain region. *Life Sci.*, 28:1407–1420.
2. Adams, K., and Oswald, I. (1979): One gram of L-tryptophan fails to alter the time taken to fall asleep. *Neuropharmacology*, 18:1025–1027.
3. Advis, J. P., Simpkins, J. W., Bennett, J., and Meites, J. (1979): Serotonergic control of prolactin release in male rats. *Life Sci.*, 24:359–366.
4. Aghajanian, G. K., and Asher, I. M. (1971): Histochemical fluorescence of raphe neurons: Selective enhancement by tryptophan. *Science*, 172:1159–1161.
5. Agharanya, J. C., Alonso, R., and Wurtman, R. J. (1981): Changes in catecholamine excretion after short-term tyrosine ingestion in normally fed human subjects. *Am. J. Clin. Nutr.*, 34:82–87.
6. Agharanya, J. C., and Wurtman, R. J. (1982): Effect of acute administration of large neutral and other amino acids on urinary excretion of catecholamines. *Life Sci.*, 30:739–746.
7. Agharanya, J. C., and Wurtman, R. J. (1982): Studies on the mechanism by which tyrosine raises urinary catecholamines. *Biochem. Pharmacol.*, 31:3577–3580.
8. Agid, Y., Javoy, F., and Glowinski, J. (1973): Hyperactivity of remaining dopaminergic neurons after partial destruction of the nigro-striatal dopaminergic system in the rat. *Nature (New Biol.)*, 245:150–151.
9. Alonso, R., Agharanya, J. C., and Wurtman, R. J. (1980): Tyrosine loading enhances catecholamine excretion by rats. *J. Neural Transm.*, 49:31–43.
10. Anderson, G. H. (1977): Regulation of protein intake by plasma amino acids. In: *Advances in Nutritional Research, Vol. 1*, edited by H. H. Draper, pp. 145–166. Plenum Press, New York.

11. Anderson, G. H. (1979): Control of protein and energy intake: Role of plasma amino acids and brain neurotransmitters. *Can. J. Physiol. Pharmacol.*, 57:1043–1057.
12. Annunziato, L. (1979): Regulation of the tuberoinfundibular and nigrostriatal systems. *Neuroendocrinology*, 29:66–76.
13. Annunziato, L., and Moore, K. E. (1978): Prolactin in CSF selectively increases dopamine turnover in the median eminence. *Life Sci.*, 22:2037–2042.
14. Antonaccio, M. J., and Robson, R. D. (1973): Cardiovascular effects of 5-hydroxytryptophan in anesthetized dogs. *J. Pharm. Pharmacol.*, 25:495–497.
15. Arnold, M. A., and Fernstrom, J. D. (1978): Serotonin receptor antagonists block a natural, short term surge in serum growth hormone levels. *Endocrinology*, 103:1159–1163.
16. Arnold, M. A., and Fernstrom, J. D. (1981): L-Tryptophan injection enhances pulsatile growth hormone secretion in the rat. *Endocrinology*, 108:331–335.
17. Ashcroft, G. W., Eccleston, D., and Crawford, T. B. B. (1965): 5-Hydroxyindole metabolism in rat brain: A study of intermediary metabolism using a technique of tryptophan loading. *J. Neurochem.*, 12:483–492.
18. Ashley, D. V. M., and Anderson, G. H. (1975): Food intake regulation in the weanling rat: Effects of the most limiting essential amino acids of gluten, casein, and zein on the self-selection of protein and energy. *J. Nutr.*, 105:405–411.
19. Ashley, D. V. M., and Anderson, G. H. (1975): Correlation between the plasma tryptophan to neutral amino acid ratio and protein intake in the self-selecting weanling rat. *J. Nutr.*, 105:412–421.
19a. Ashley, D. V. M., Cosina, D. V., and Anderson, G. H. (1979): Selective decrease in protein intake following brain serotonin depletion. *Life Sci.*, 24:973–984.
20. Bagchi, S. P., and Zarycki, E. P. (1972): Hydroxylation of phenylalanine by various areas of brain *in vitro*. *Biochem. Pharmacol.*, 21:584–589.
21. Bagchi, S. P., and Zarycki, E. P. (1973): Formation of catecholamines from phenylalanine in brain—effects of chlorpromazine and catron. *Biochem. Pharmacol.*, 22:1353–1368.
22. Bagchi, S. P., and Zarycki, E. P. (1975): Catecholamine formation in brain from phenylalanine and tyrosine: Effects of psychotropic drugs and other agents. *Biochem. Pharmacol.*, 24:1381–1390.
23. Barbeau, A., Growdon, J. H., and Wurtman, R. J. (Eds.) (1979): *Nutrition and the Brain, Vol. 5.* Raven Press, New York.
24. Barra, H. S., Unates, L. E., Sayavedra, M. S., and Capputto, R. (1972): Capacities of binding amino acids by tRNAs from rat brain and their changes during development. *J. Neurochem.*, 19:2287–2297.
25. Bartholini, G., Stadler, H., Gadea Ciria, M., and Lloyd, K. G. (1976): The use of the push-pull cannula to estimate the dynamics of acetylcholine and catecholamines within various brain regions. *Neuropharmacology*, 15:515–519.
26. Beaton, J. M., and Bradley, R. H. (1978): The suppression of amphetamine-induced circling by L-valine in rats with substantia-nigral lesions. *Pharmacologist*, 20:222.
27. Beaton, J. M., and Humaideh, I. H. (1979): The effects of several neutral amino acids on D-amphetamine and apomorphine induced circling in rats with lesions in the substantia nigra. *Neurosci. Abstr.*, 5:396.
28. Benuck, M., Stern, F., and Lajtha, A. (1971): Transamination of amino acids in homogenates of rat brain. *J. Neurochem.*, 18:1555–1567.
29. Betz, A. L., and Gilboe, D. D. (1973): Effect of pentobarbital on amino acid and urea flux in the isolated dog brain. *Am. J. Physiol.*, 224:580–587.
30. Bierkamper, G. G., and Goldberg, A. M. (1979): Effect of choline on the release of acetylcholine from the neuromuscular junction. In: *Nutrition and the Brain, Vol. 5*, edited by A. Barbeau, J. H. Growdon, and R. J. Wurtman, pp. 243–252. Raven Press, New York.
31. Bierkamper, G. G., and Goldberg, A. M. (1980): Release of acetylcholine from the vascular perfused rat phrenic nerve–hemidiaphragm. *Brain Res.*, 202:234–237.
32. Biggio, G., Mereu, G., Vargiu, L., and Tagliamonte, A. (1972): Effect of protein synthesis inhibition on tryptophan level and serotonin in the rat brain. *Rivista Farmacol. Ther.*, 111:229–236.
32a. Biggio, G., Porceddu, M. L., Fratta, W., and Gessa, G. L. (1977): Changes in dopamine metabolism associated with fasting and satiation. *Adv. Biochem. Psychopharmacol.*, 16:377–380.
32b. Biggio, G., Porceddu, M. L., and Gessa, G. L. (1976): Decrease of homovanillic acid, dihy-

droxyphenylacetic acid and cyclic-adenosine-3',5'-monophosphate content in the rat caudate nucleus induced by the acute administration of an amino acid mixture lacking tyrosine and phenylalanine. *J. Neurochem.*, 26:1253–1255.

33. Bloxam, D. L., Tricklebank, M. D., Patel, A. J., and Curzon, G. (1980): Effects of albumin, amino acids, and clofibrate on the uptake of tryptophan by the rat brain. *J. Neurochem.*, 34:43–49.

34. Blundell, J. E., and McArthur, R. A. (1981): Behavioral flux and feeding: Continuous monitoring of food intake and food selection, and the video-recording of appetitive and satiety sequences for the analysis of drug action. In: *Anorectic Agents: Mechanism of Action and Tolerance*, edited by S. Garattini and R. Samanin, pp. 19–43. Raven Press, New York.

35. Blundell, J. E., Tombros, E., Rogers, P. J., and Latham, C. J. (1980): Behavioural analysis of feeding: Implications for the pharmacological manipulation of food intake in animals and man. *Prog. Neuropsychopharmacol.*, 4:319–326.

36. Brandau, K., and Axelrod, J. (1972): The biosynthesis of octopamine. *Naunyn Schmiedebergs Arch. Pharmacol.*, 273:123–133.

37. Breshnahan, M. R., Hatzinikolaou, P., Brunner, H. R., and Gavras, H. (1980): Effects of tyrosine infusion in normotensive and hypertensive rats. *Am. J. Physiol.*, 239:H201–H211.

38. Brown, B. B. (1960): CNS drug actions and interactions in mice. *Arch. Int. Pharmacodyn.*, 128:391–414.

39. Brown, D. R., and Growdon, J. H. (1980): L-Tryptophan administration potentiates serotonin-dependent myoclonic behavior in the rat. *Neuropharmacology*, 19:343–347.

40. Buckingham, J. C., and Hodges, J. R. (1979): Hypothalamic receptors influencing the secretion of corticotrophin releasing hormone in the rat. *J. Physiol. (Lond.)*, 290:421–431.

41. Butcher, L. L., Engel, J., and Fuxe, K. (1974): Behavioral, biochemical and histochemical analysis of the central effects of monoamine precursors after peripheral decarboxylase inhibition. *Brain Res.*, 41:387–411.

42. Carlsson, A., Davis, J. N., Kehr, W., Lindqvist, M., and Atack, C. V. (1972): Simultaneous measurement of tyrosine and tryptophan hydroxylase activities in brain *in vivo* using an inhibitor of the aromatic amino acid decarboxylase. *Naunyn Schmiedebergs Arch. Pharmacol.*, 275:153–168.

43. Carlsson, A., and Lindqvist, M. (1972): The effect of L-tryptophan and some psychotropic drugs on the formation of 5-hydroxytryptophan in the mouse brain *in vivo*. *J. Neural Transm.*, 33:23–43.

44. Carlsson, A., and Lindqvist, M. (1978): Dependence of 5-HT and catecholamine synthesis on precursor amino acid levels in rat brain. *Naunyn Schmiedebergs Arch. Pharmacol.*, 303:157–164.

45. Carruba, M. O., Picotti, G. B., Genovese, E., and Mantegazza, P. (1977): Stimulatory effect of a maize diet on sexual behavior of male rats. *Life Sci.*, 20:159–164.

46. Cespuglio, R., Faradji, H., Ponchon, J., Buda, M., Riou, F., Gonon, F., Pujol, J. E., and Jouvet, M. (1981): Differential pulse voltametry in brain tissue. I. Detection of 5-hydroxyindoles in the rat striatum. *Brain Res.*, 223:287–298.

47. Chalmers, J. P. (1975): Brain amines and models of experimental hypertension. *Circ. Res.*, 36:469–480.

48. Chiel, H. J., and Wurtman, R. J. (1976): Suppression of amphetamine-induced hypothermia by the neutral amino acid valine. *Psychopharmacol. Commun.*, 2:207–217.

49. Clemens, J. A., Bennett, D. R., and Fuller, R. W. (1980): The effect of tryptophan free diet on prolactin and corticosterone release by serotoninergic stimuli. *Horm. Metab. Res.*, 12:35–38.

50. Colmenares, J. L., Wurtman, R. J., and Fernstrom, J. D. (1975): Effects of ingestion of a carbohydrate-fat meal on the levels and synthesis of 5-hydroxyindoles in various regions of the rat central nervous system. *J. Neurochem.*, 25:825–829.

51. Colmenares, J. L., and Wurtman, R. J. (1979): The relation between urinary 5-hydroxyindolacetic acid levels and the ratio of tryptophan to other large neutral amino acids in the stomach. *Metabolism*, 28:820–827.

52. Conlay, L. A., Maher, T. J., and Wurtman, R. J. (1981): Tyrosine increases blood pressure in hypotensive rats. *Science*, 212:559–560.

53. Cooper, J. R., Bloom, F. E., and Roth, R. H. (1978): *The Biochemical Basis of Neuropharmacology*. Oxford University Press, New York.

54. Coscina, D. V., Watt, V., Godse, D. D., and Stancer, H. C. (1975): L-Tryptophan normalizes

hyperalgesia but not forebrain serotonin loss induced by unilateral lesions of the medial forebrain bundle in rats. *Neurosci. Abstr.*, 1:151.
55. Costa, E., and Guidotti, A. (1978): Molecular mechanisms mediating the transsynaptic regulation of gene expression in adrenal medulla. In: *Psychopharmacology: A Generation of Progress*, edited by M. A. Lipton, A. DiMascio, and K. F. Killam, pp. 235–246. Raven Press, New York.
56. Curzon, G., Fernando, J. C. R., and Marsden, C. A. (1978): 5-Hydroxytryptamine: The effects of impaired synthesis on its metabolism and release in rat. *Br. J. Pharmacol.*, 63:627–634.
57. Curzon, G., and Green, A. R. (1968): Effect of hydroxycortisone on rat brain 5-hydroxytryptamine. *Life Sci.*, 7:657–663.
58. Curzon, G., and Knott, P. J. (1974): Effects on plasma and brain tryptophan in the rat of drugs and hormones that influence the concentration of unesterified fatty acid in the plasma. *Br. J. Pharmacol.*, 50:197–204.
59. Curzon, G., and Marsden, C. A. (1975): Metabolism of a tryptophan load in the hypothalamus and other brain regions. *J. Neurochem.*, 25:251–256.
60. Dairman, W. (1979): Catecholamine concentrations and the activity of tyrosine hydroxylase after an increase in the concentration of tyrosine in rat tissues. *Br. J. Pharmacol.*, 44:307–310.
61. DaPrada, M., Carruba, M., O'Brien, R. A., Saner, A., and Pletscher, A. (1972): The effect of 5,6-dihydroxytryptamine on sexual behavior of male rats. *Eur. J. Pharmacol.*, 19:288–290.
62. David, J.-C., Dairman, W., and Udenfriend, S. (1974): Decarboxylation to tyramine: A major route of tyrosine metabolism in mammals. *Proc. Natl. Acad. Sci. USA*, 71:1771–1775.
63. Davis, M., and Sheard, M. H. (1974): Habituation and sensitization of the rat startle response: Effects of raphe lesions. *Physiol. Behav.*, 12:425–431.
64. Davis, M., and Sheard, M. H. (1976): *p*-Chloroamphetamine: Acute and chronic effects on habituation and sensitization of the acoustic startle response in rats. *Eur. J. Pharmacol.*, 35:261–273.
65. Delbarre, B., Casset-Senon, D., and Delbarre, G. (1980): Central antihypertensive action of octopamine. *IRCS Med. Sci.*, 8:23–24.
66. Demarest, K. T., Alper, R. H., and Moore, K. E. (1979): DOPA accumulation is a measure of dopamine synthesis in the median eminence and posterior pituitary. *J. Neural Transm.*, 46:183–193.
67. Demarest, K. T., McKay, D. W., Riegle, G. D., and Moore, K. E. (1981): Sexual differences in tuberoinfundibular dopamine nerve activity induced by neonatal androgen exposure. *Neuroendocrinology*, 32:108–113.
68. Denizeau, F., and Sourkes, T. L. (1977): Regional transport of tryptophan in rat brain. *J. Neurochem.*, 28:951–959.
69. Donoso, A. O., Bishop, W., Fawcett, C. P., Krulich, L., and McCann, S. M. (1971): Effects of drugs that modify brain monoamine concentrations on plasma gonadotropin and prolactin levels in the rat. *Endocrinology*, 89:774–784.
70. Edwards, D. J. (1982): Possible role of octopamine and tyramine in the antihypertensive and antidepressant effects of tyrosine. *Life Sci.*, 30:1427–1434.
71. Edwards, D. J., and Rizk, M. (1981): Effects of amino acid precursors on catecholamine synthesis in the brain. *Prog. Neuropsychopharmacol.*, 5:569–572.
72. Elwyn, D. H. (1970): The role of the liver in the regulation of amino acid and protein metabolism. In: *Mammalian Protein Metabolism, Vol. 4*, edited by H. N. Munro, pp. 523–557. Academic Press, New York.
73. Etienne, P., Young, S. N., and Sourkes, T. L. (1976): Inhibition by albumin of tryptophan uptake by rat brain. *Nature*, 262:144–145.
74. Faber, J., Hagen, C., Kirkegaard, C., Birk-Lauridsen, U., and Moller, S. E. (1977): Lack of effects of L-tryptophan on basal and TRH-stimulated TSH and prolactin levels. *Psychoneuroendocrinology*, 2:413–415.
75. Felig, P., Owen, O. E., Wahren, J., and Cahill, G. F. (1969): Amino acid metabolism during prolonged starvation. *J. Clin. Invest.*, 48:584–594.
76. Fellman, J. H., Roth, E. S., and Fujita, T. S. (1976): Decarboxylation to tyramine is not a major route of tyrosine metabolism in mammals. *Arch. Biochem. Biophys.*, 174:562–567.
77. Fernando, J. C. R., and Curzon, G. (1981): Behavioral responses to drugs releasing 5-hydroxytryptamine and catecholamines: Effects of treatments altering precursor concentrations in brain. *Neuropharmacology*, 20:115–122.
78. Fernando, J. C. R., Lees, A. J., and Curzon, G. (1980): Differential antagonism by neuroleptics

of backward-walking and other behaviors caused by amphetamine at high dosage. *Neurophar-macology*, 19:549–553.

79. Fernstrom, J. D., and Faller, D. V. (1978): Neutral amino acids in the brain: Changes in response to food ingestion. *J. Neurochem.*, 30:1531–1538.

80. Fernstrom, J. D., Faller, D. V., and Shabshelowitz, H. (1975): Acute reduction of brain serotonin and 5HIAA following food consumption: Correlation with the ratio of serum tryptophan to the sum of competing neutral amino acids. *J. Neural Transm.*, 36:113–121.

81. Fernstrom, J. D., and Hirsch, M. J. (1975): Rapid repletion of brain serotonin in malnourished corn-fed rats following L-tryptophan injection. *Life Sci.*, 17:455–464.

82. Fernstrom, J. D., Hirsch, M. J., Madras, B. K., and Sudarsky, L. (1975): Effect of skim milk, whole milk, and light cream on serum tryptophan binding and brain tryptophan concentrations in rats. *J. Nutr.*, 105:1359–1362.

83. Fernstrom, J. D., and Wurtman, R. J. (1971): Brain serotonin content: Physiological dependence on plasma tryptophan levels. *Science*, 173:149–152.

84. Fernstrom, J. D., and Wurtman, R. J. (1971): Brain serotonin content: Increase following ingestion of carbohydrate diet. *Science*, 174:1023–1025.

85. Fernstrom, J. D., and Wurtman, R. J. (1971): Effect of chronic corn consumption on serotonin content of rat brain. *Nature (New Biol.)*, 234:62–64.

86. Fernstrom, J. D., and Wurtman, R. J. (1972): Brain serotonin content: Physiological regulation by plasma neutral amino acids. *Science*, 178:414–416.

87. Fibiger, H. C., Mertz, P. H., and Campbell, B. A. (1972): The effect of para-chlorophenylalanine on aversion thresholds and reactivity to foot shock. *Physiol. Behav.*, 8:259–263.

88. Foldes, A., and Costa, E. (1975): Relationship of brain monoamines and locomotor activity in rats. *Biochem. Pharmacol.*, 24:1617–1621.

89. Fuller, R. W. (1970): Daily variations in liver tryptophan, tryptophan pyrrolase, and tyrosine transaminase in rats fed *ad libitum* or single daily meals. *Proc. Soc. Exp. Biol. Med.*, 133:620–622.

90. Fuller, R. W., Holland, D. R., Yen, T. T., Bemis, K. G., and Stamm, N. B. (1979): Antihypertensive effects of fluoxetine and L-5-hydroxytryptophan in rats. *Life Sci.*, 25:1237–1242.

91. Fuller, R. W., and Snoddy, H. D. (1980): Effect of serotonin releasing drugs on serum corticosterone concentration in rats. *Neuroendocrinology*, 31:96–100.

92. Fuller, R. W., Yen, T. T., and Stamm, N. B. (1981): Lowering of blood pressure by direct and indirect acting serotonin agonists in spontaneously hypertensive rats. *Clin. Exp. Hypertens.*, 3:497–508.

93. Gal, E. M. (1974): Cerebral tryptophan 2,3 dioxygenase and its induction in rat brain. *J. Neurochem.*, 22:861–863.

94. Gal, E. M., Young, R. B., and Sherman, A. D. (1978): Tryptophan loading: Consequent effects on the synthesis of kynurenine and 5-hydroxyindoles in rat brain. *J. Neurochem.*, 31:237–244.

95. Gallager, D. W., and Aghaganian, G. K. (1976): Inhibition of firing of raphe neurons by tryptophan and 5-hydroxytryptophan: Blockade by inhibiting synthesis with Ro4-4602. *Neuropharmacology*, 15:149–156.

96. Garlick, P. J., and Marshall, I. (1972): A technique for measuring brain protein synthesis. *J. Neurochem.*, 19:577–583.

97. Garthwaite, T. L., and Hagen, T. C. (1979): Evidence that serotonin stimulates a prolactin-releasing factor in the rat. *Neuroendocrinology*, 29:215–220.

98. Gelenberg, A. J., Wojcik, J. D., Growdon, J. H., Sved, A. F., and Wurtman, R. J. (1980): Tyrosine for the treatment of depression. *Am. J. Psychiatry*, 137:622–623.

99. Gibbons, J. L., Barr, G. A., Bridger, W. H., and Leibowitz, S. F. (1978): Effects of parachlorophenylalanine and 5-hydroxytryptophan on mouse killing behavior in killer rats. *Pharmacol. Biochem. Behav.*, 9:91–98.

100. Gibbons, J. L., Barr, G. A., Bridger, W. H., and Leibowitz, S. F. (1979): Manipulation of dietary tryptophan: Effects on mouse killing and brain serotonin in the rat. *Brain Res.*, 169:139–153.

101. Gibson, C. J. (1977): *Factors Controlling Brain Catecholamine Biosynthesis: Effect of Brain Tyrosine*. Ph.D. Thesis, Massachusetts Institute of Technology.

102. Gibson, C. J., and Wurtman, R. J. (1977): Physiological control of brain catechol synthesis by brain tyrosine concentration. *Biochem. Pharmacol.*, 26:1137–1142.

103. Gibson, C. J., and Wurtman, R. J. (1978): Physiological control of brain norepinephrine synthesis by brain tyrosine concentration. *Life Sci.*, 22:1399–1406.

104. Gillman, P. K., Bartlett, J. R., Bridges, P. K., Hunt, A., Patel, A. J., Kantamaneni, B. D., and Curzon, G. (1981): Indolic substances in plasma, cerebrospinal fluid, and frontal cortex of human subjects infused with saline or tryptophan. *J. Neurochem.*, 37:410–417.
105. Glass, A. R., Smallridge, R. C., Schaff, M., and Diamond, R. C. (1980): Absent prolactin response to L-tryptophan in normal and acromegalic subjects. *Psychoneuroendocrinology*, 5:261–265.
106. Goldberg, I. K. (1980): Tyrosine in depression. *Lancet*, 2:364.
107. Gorlitz, B. D., and Frey, H. H. (1972): Central monoamines and antinociceptive drug action. *Eur. J. Pharmacol.*, 20:171–180.
108. Grahame-Smith, D. G. (1971): Studies in vivo on the relationship between brain tryptophan, brain 5-HT synthesis and hyperactivity in rats treated with a monoamine oxidase inhibitor and L-tryptophan. *J. Neurochem.*, 18:1053–1066.
109. Grahame-Smith, D. G. (1973): Does the total turnover of brain 5-HT reflect the functional activity of 5-HT in brain? In: *Serotonin and Behavior*, edited by J. Barchas and E. Usdin, pp. 5–7. Academic Press, New York.
110. Grant, L. D., Coscina, D. V., Grossman, S. P., and Freedman, D. X. (1973): Muricide after serotonin depleting lesions of midbrain raphe nuclei. *Pharmacol. Biochem. Behav.*, 1:77–80.
111. Green, A. R., and Grahame-Smith, D. G. (1974): The role of brain dopamine in the hyperactivity syndrome produced by increased 5-hydroxytryptamine synthesis in rats. *Neuropharmacology*, 13:949–959.
112. Green, A. R., and Grahame-Smith, D. G. (1975): 5-Hydroxytryptamine and other indoles in the central nervous system. In: *Handbook of Psychopharmacology, Vol. 3*, edited by L. L. Iversen, S. D. Iversen, and S. H. Snyder, pp. 169–245. Plenum Press, New York.
113. Green, A. R., and Grahame-Smith, D. G. (1976): Effects of drugs on the processes regulating the functional activity of brain 5-hydroxytryptamine. *Nature*, 260:487–491.
114. Green, A. R., and Youdim, M. B. H. (1975): Effects of monoamine oxidase inhibition by clorgyline, deprenil or tranylcypromine on 5-hydroxytryptamine concentrations in rat brain and hyperactivity following subsequent tryptophan administration. *Br. J. Pharmacol.*, 55:415–422.
115. Griffiths, W. J., Lester, B. K., and Coulter, J. D. (1972): Tryptophan and sleep in young adults. *Psychophysiology*, 9:345–356.
116. Growdon, J. H. (1979): Neurotransmitter precursors in the diet: Their use in the treatment of brain disorders. In: *Nutrition and the Brain, Vol. 3*, edited by R. J. Wurtman and J. J. Wurtman, pp. 117–181. Raven Press, New York.
117. Growdon, J. H., and Melamed, E. (1980): Effects of oral tyrosine administration on CSF tyrosine and HVA levels in patients with Parkinson's Disease. *Neurology (Minn.)*, 3:396.
118. Growdon, J. H., Melamed, E., Logue, M., Hefti, F., and Wurtman, R. J. (1982): Effects of oral L-tyrosine administration on CSF tyrosine and homovanillic acid levels in patients with Parkinson's disease. *Life Sci.*, 30:827–832.
119. Haigler, H. J., and Aghajanian, G. K. (1974): Peripheral serotonin antagonists: Failure to antagonize serotonin in brain areas receiving a prominent serotonergic input. *J. Neural Transm.*, 35:257–273.
120. Hamon, M., Bourgoin, S., Artaud, F., and Glowinski, J. (1979): The role of intraneuronal 5-HT and of tryptophan hydroxylase activation in the control of 5-HT synthesis in rat brain slices incubated in K$^+$ enriched medium. *J. Neurochem.*, 33:1031–1042.
121. Harmar, A. J., and Horn, A. S. (1976): Octopamine in mammalian brain: Rapid post mortem increase and effects of drugs. *J. Neurochem.*, 26:987–993.
122. Hartmann, E. (1977): L-tryptophan: A rational hypnotic with clinical potential. *Am. J. Psychiatry*, 134:366–370.
123. Hartmann, E., and Chung, R. (1972): Sleep-inducing effects of L-tryptophan. *J. Pharm. Pharmacol.*, 24:252–253.
124. Hartmann, E., Chung, R., and Chien, C. P. (1971): L-tryptophan and sleep. *Psychopharmacology*, 19:114–127.
125. Hartmann, E., Cravens, J., and List, S. (1974): Hypnotic effects of L-tryptophan. *Arch. Gen. Psychiatry*, 31:394–397.
126. Harvey, J. A., Schlosberg, A. J., and Yunger, L. M. (1974): The effect of p-chlorophenylalanine and brain lesions on pain sensitivity and morphine analgesia in the rat. *Adv. Biochem. Psychopharmacol.*, 10:232–246.

127. Haubrich, D. R., and Blake, D. E. (1973): Modification of serotonin metabolism in rat brain after acute or chronic administration of morphine. *Biochem. Pharmacol.*, 22:2753–2759.
128. Heise, A. (1975): Hypotensive action by central α-adrenergic and dopaminergic receptor stimulation. In: *New Antihypertensive Drugs*, edited by A. Scriabine and C. S. Sweet, pp. 135–145. Spectrum Press, New York.
129. Herr, B. E., Gallager, D. W., and Roth, R. H. (1975): Tryptophan hydroxylase: Activation *in vivo* following stimulation of central serotonergic neurons. *Biochem. Pharmacol.*, 24:2019–2023.
130. Hingtgen, J. N., and Aprison, M. H. (1975): Behavioral depression in pigeons following L-tryptophan administration. *Life Sci.*, 16:1471–1476.
131. Ho, I. K., Brase, D. A., Loh, H. H., and Way, E. L. (1975): Influence of L-tryptophan on morphine analgesia, tolerance and physical dependence. *J. Pharmacol. Exp. Ther.*, 193:35–43.
132. Hole, K., and Marsden, C. A. (1975): Unchanged sensitivity to electric shocks in L-tryptophan treated rats. *Pharmacol. Biochem. Behav.*, 3:95–102.
133. Hyyppa, M. T., Jolma, T., Liira, J., Langvik, V. A., and Kytomaki, O. (1979): L-tryptophan treatment and the episodic secretion of pituitary hormones and cortisol. *Psychoneuroendocrinology*, 4:29–35.
134. Ichihara, A., and Koyama, E. (1966): Transaminase of branched chain amino acids. I. Branched chain amino acids—α-ketoglutarate transaminase. *J. Biochem.*, 59:160–169.
135. Ikeda, M., Fahien, L. A., and Udenfriend, S. (1966): A kinetic study of bovine adrenal tyrosine hydroxylase. *J. Biol. Chem.*, 241:4452–4456.
136. Jacobs, B. L., Eubanks, E. E., and Wise, W. D. (1974): Effect of indolealkylamine manipulations on locomotor activity in rats. *Neuropharmacology*, 13:575–583.
136a. Jacoby, J., Colmenares, J. L., and Wurtman, R. J. (1975): Failure of decreased serotonin uptake or monoamine oxidase inhibition to block the acceleration in brain 5-hydroxyindole synthesis that follows food consumption. *J. Neur. Trans.*, 37:25-32.
137. Joh, T. H., Shikimi, T., Pickel, V. M., and Reis, D. J. (1975): Brain tryptophan hydroxylase: Purification of, production of antibodies to, and cellular and ultrastructural localization in serotonergic neurons of rat midbrain. *Proc. Natl. Acad. Sci. USA*, 72:3575–3579.
138. Johnson, T. C., and Chou, K. (1973): Level and amino acid acceptor activity of mouse brain tRNA during neuronal development. *J. Neurochem.*, 20:405–414.
139. Jones, M. T., Hillhouse, E. W., and Burden, J. (1976): Effect of various putative neurotransmitters on the secretion of corticotrophin releasing hormone from the rat hypothalamus *in vitro*. A model of the neurotransmitters involved. *J. Endocrinol.*, 69:1–20.
140. Joseph, M. H., Young, S. N., and Curzon, G. (1976): The metabolism of a tryptophan load in rat brain and liver. The influence of hydrocortisone and allopurinol. *Biochem. Pharmacol.*, 25:2599–2604.
141. Jouvet, M. (1978): Neuropharmacology of the sleep-waking cycle. In: *Handbook of Psychopharmacology, Vol. 8*, edited by L. L. Iversen, S. D. Iversen, and S. H. Snyder, pp. 204–249. Plenum Press, New York.
142. Kamberi, I. A., Mical, R. S., and Porter, J. C. (1971): Effects of melatonin and serotonin on the release of FSH and prolactin. *Endocrinology*, 88:1288–1293.
143. Kantak, K. M., Hegstrand, L. R., and Eichelmann, B. (1980): Dietary tryptophan modulation and aggressive behavior in mice. *Pharmacol. Biochem. Behav.*, 12:675–679.
144. Kantak, K. M., Hegstrand, L. R., Whitman, J., and Eichelman, B. (1980): Effects of dietary supplements and tryptophan-free diet on aggressive behavior in rats. *Pharmacol. Biochem. Behav.*, 12:173–179.
145. Kapatos, G., and Zigmond, M. (1977): Dopamine biosynthesis from L-tyrosine and L-phenylalanine in rat brain synaptomsomes: Preferential use of newly accumulated precursors. *J. Neurochem.*, 28:1109–1119.
146. Karobath, M., and Baldessarini, R. J. (1972): Formation of catechol compounds from phenylalanine and tyrosine with isolated nerve endings. *Nature (New Biol.)*, 236:206–208.
147. Kaufman, S. (1974): Properties of pterin-dependent aromatic amino acid hydroxylases. In: *Aromatic Amino Acids in the Brain*, edited by G. E. W. Wolstenholm and D. W. Fitzsimons, pp. 85–108. Associated Scientific Publishers, Amsterdam.
148. Kaufman, S. (1975): Regulatory properties of tyrosine hydroxylase. In: *Neurobiological Mechanisms of Adaptation and Behavior*, edited by A. J. Mandell, pp. 127–136. Raven Press, New York.

149. Kennett, G. A., and Joseph, M. H. (1981): The functional importance of increased brain tryptophan in the serotonergic response to restraint stress. *Neuropharmacology*, 20:39–43.
150. Kettler, R., Bartholinin, G., and Pletscher, A. (1974): *In vivo* enhancement of tyrosine hydroxylation in rat striatum by tetrahydrobiopterin. *Nature*, 249:476–478.
151. Knott, P. J., and Curzon, G. (1972): Free tryptophan in plasma and brain tryptophan metabolism. *Nature*, 239:452–453.
152. Knott, P. J., and Curzon, G. (1974): Effect of increased rat brain tryptophan on 5-hydroxytryptamine and 5-hydroxyindoleacetic acid in the hypothalamus and other brain regions. *J. Neurochem.*, 22:1065–1071.
153. Knott, P. J., Joseph, M. H., and Curzon, G. (1973): Effects of food deprivation and immobilization on tryptophan and other amino acids in rat brain. *J. Neurochem.*, 20:249–251.
154. Kopin, I. J. (1964): Metabolism of catecholamines. *Z. Klin. Chem.*, 4:115–123.
155. Kopin, I. J., Weise, V. K., and Sedvall, G. C. (1969): Effect of false transmitters on norepinephrine synthesis. *J. Pharmacol. Exp. Ther.*, 170:246–252.
156. Korf, J., Aghajanian, G. K., and Roth, R. H. (1973): Stimulation and destruction of the locus coeruleus: Opposite effects on 3-methoxy-4-hydroxyphenylglycol sulfate levels in the rat cerebral cortex. *Eur. J. Pharmacol.*, 21:305–310.
157. Korf, J. L., Grasdijk, L., and Westerink, B. H. C. (1976): Effects of electrical stimulation of the nigrostriatal pathway of the rat on dopamine metabolism. *J. Neurochem.*, 26:579–584.
158. Kostowski, W., and Valzelli, L. (1974): Biochemical and behavioral effects of lesions of the raphe nuclei in aggressive mice. *Pharmacol. Biochem. Behav.*, 2:277–280.
159. Krieger, D. T. (1976): Serotonin regulation of ACTH secretion. *Ann. NY Acad. Sci.*, 297:527–534.
160. Kuhn, D. M., and Lovenberg, W. (1982): Role of calmodulin in the activation of tryptophan hydroxylase. *Fed. Proc.*, 41:2258–2264.
161. Kuhn, D. M., Vogel, R. L., and Lovenberg, W. (1978): Calcium dependent activation of tryptophan hydroxylase by ATP and magnesium. *Biochem. Biophys. Res. Commun.*, 82:759–766.
162. Kuhn, D. M., Wolf, W. A., and Lovenberg, W. (1980): Review of the role of the central serotonergic neuronal system in blood pressure regulation. *Hypertension*, 2:243–255.
163. Laborit, H., and Valette, N. (1974): The action of L-tyrosine and arachidonic acid on the experimental hypertension in rat: Physiopathogenic deductions. *Res. Commun. Chem. Pathol. Pharm.*, 8:489–504.
164. Latham, C. J., and Blundell, J. E. (1979): Evidence for the effect of tryptophan on the pattern of food consumption in free feeding and food deprived rats. *Life Sci.*, 24:1971–1978.
165. Lee, M. R. (1982): Dopamine and the kidney. *Clin. Sci.*, 62:439–448.
166. Lees, A. J., Fernando, J. C. R., and Curzon, G. (1979): Serotonergic involvement in behavioral responses to amphetamine at high dosage. *Neuropharmacology*, 18:153–158.
167. Lees, G. J., and Weiner, N. (1973): Transaminations between amino acids and keto acids elevated in phenylketonuria and maple syrup urine disease. *J. Neurochem.*, 20:389–403.
168. Levine, R. A., Miller, L. P., and Lovenberg, W. (1981): Tetrahydrobiopterin in the striatum: Localization in dopamine nerve terminals and role in catecholamine synthesis. *Science*, 214:919–921.
169. Levitt, M., Spector, S., Sjoerdsma, A., and Udenfriend, S. (1965): Elucidation of the rate-limiting step in norepinephrine biosynthesis in the perfused guinea-pig heart. *J. Pharmacol. Exp. Ther.*, 148:1–9.
170. Liebschutz, J., Airoldi, L., Brownstein, M. J., Chinn, N. G., and Wurtman, R. J. (1977): Regional distribution of endogenous and parenteral glutamate, aspartate and glutamine in rat brain. *Biochem. Pharmacol.*, 26:443–446.
171. Linnoila, M., and Cooper, R. L. (1976): Reinstatement of vaginal cycles in aged female rats. *J. Pharmacol. Exp. Ther.*, 199:477–482.
172. Lints, C. E., and Harvey, J. A. (1969): Altered sensitivity to footshock and decreased brain content of serotonin following brain lesions in the rat. *J. Comp. Physiol. Psychol.*, 67:23–31.
173. Lovenberg, W., Ames, M. M., and Lerner, P. (1978): Mechanism of short-term regulation of tyrosine hydroxylase. In: *Psychopharmacology: A Generation of Progress*, edited by M. A. Lipton, A. DiMascio, and K. F. Killam, pp. 247–259. Raven Press, New York.
174. Lown, B., Verrier, R. L., and Rabinowitz, S. H. (1977): Neural and psychologic mechanisms and the problem of sudden cardiac death. *Am. J. Cardiol.*, 39:890–902.

175. Lytle, L. D., Messing, R. B., Fisher, L., and Phebus, L. (1975): Effects of chronic corn consumption on brain serotonin and the response to electric shock. *Science*, 190:692–694.
176. MacIndoe, J. H., and Turkington, R. W. (1973): Stimulation of human prolactin secretion by intravenous infusion of L-tryptophan. *J. Clin. Invest.*, 52:1972–1978.
177. MacLeod, R. M. (1976): Regulation of Prolactin Secretion. In: *Frontiers in Neuroendocrinology, Vol. 4*, edited by L. Martini and W. F. Ganong, pp. 169–194. Raven Press, New York.
178. Madras, B. K., Cohen, E. L., Fernstrom, J. D., Larin, F., Munro, H. N., and Wurtman, R. J. (1973): Dietary carbohydrate increases brain tryptophan and decreases serum free tryptophan. *Nature*, 244:34–35.
179. Madras, B. K., Cohen, E. L., Messing, R. B., Munro, H. N., and Wurtman, R. J. (1974): Relevance of free tryptophan in serum to tissue tryptophan concentrations. *Metabolism*, 23:1107–1116.
180. Malick, J. B., and Barnett, A. (1976): The role of serotonergic pathways in isolation-induced aggression in mice. *Pharmacol. Biochem. Behav.*, 5:55–61.
181. Mandel, P., and Aunis, D. (1974): Tyrosine aminotransferase in the rat brain. In: *Aromatic Amino Acids in the Brain*, edited by G. E. W. Wolstenholm and D. W. Fitzsimons, pp. 67–79. Associated Scientific Publishers, Amsterdam.
182. Mandell, A. J. (1978): Redundant mechanisms regulating brain tyrosine and tryptophan hydroxylases. *Annu. Rev. Pharmacol. Toxicol.*, 18:461–493.
183. Marsden, C. A. (1981): Effect of L-tryptophan on mouse brain 5-hydroxytryptamine: Comparison of values obtained using a fluorimetric assay and a liquid chromatographic assay with electrochemical detection. *J. Neurochem.*, 36:1621–1626.
184. Marsden, C. A., and Curzon, G. (1974): Effects of lesions and drugs on brain tryptamine. *J. Neurochem.*, 23:1171–1176.
185. Marsden, C. A., and Curzon, G. (1976): Studies on the behavioral effects of tryptophan and *p*-chlorophenylalanine. *Neuropharmacology*, 15:165–171.
186. Martin, J. B., Durand, D., Gurd, W., Faille, G., Audet, J., and Brazeau, P. (1978): Neuropharmacologic regulation of episodic growth hormone and prolactin secretion in the rat. *Endocrinology*, 102:106–112.
187. Matte, A. C. (1979): A method of quantitating aggressive behavior revealing possible dissociation of motor activity and aggression. *Psychopharmacology*, 60:247–251.
188. McCarty, R. C., Whitesides, G. H., and Tomosky, T. K. (1976): Effects of *p*-chlorophenylalanine on the predatory behavior of *Onychomys torridus*. *Pharmacol. Biochem. Behav.*, 4:217–220.
189. McMenamy, R. H., Lund, C. C., and Oncley, J. L. (1957): Unbound amino acid concentrations in human blood plasma. *J. Clin. Invest.*, 36:1672–1697.
190. McMenamy, R. H., and Oncley, J. L. (1958): The specific binding of L-tryptophan to serum albumin. *J. Biol. Chem.*, 233:1436–1440.
191. Melamed, E., Hefti, F., and Wurtman, R. J. (1980): Tyrosine administration increases striatal dopamine release in rats with partial nigrostriatal lesions. *Proc. Natl. Acad. Sci. USA*, 77:4305–4309.
192. Messing, R. B., Fisher, L., Phebus, L., and Lytle, L. D. (1976): Interaction of diet and drugs in the regulation of brain 5-hydroxyindoles and the response to painful electric shock. *Life Sci.*, 18:707–714.
193. Messing, R. B., and Lytle, L. D. (1977): Serotonin-containing neurons: Their possible role in pain and analgesia. *Pain*, 4:1–21.
194. Messing, R. B., Phebus, L., Fisher, L., and Lytle, L. D. (1975): Analgesic effect of fluoxetine HCL (Lilly 110140), a specific uptake inhibitor for serotonin neurons. *Psychopharmacol. Commun.*, 1:511–521.
195. Meyers, K. M., Dickson, W. M., and Schaub, R. G. (1973): Serotonin involvement in a motor disorder of Scottish Terrier dogs. *Life Sci.*, 13:1261–1274.
196. Miczek, K. A., Altman, J. L., Appel, J. B., and Boggan, W. D. (1975): Parachlorophenylalanine, serotonin and killing behavior. *Pharmacol. Biochem. Behav.*, 3:355–361.
197. Milson, J. A., and Pycock, C. J. (1976): Effects of drugs on cerebral 5-hydroxytryptamine mechanisms on dopamine-dependent turning behavior in mice. *Br. J. Pharmacol.*, 56:77–85.
198. Modigh, K. (1973): Effects of L-tryptophan on motor activity in mice. *Psychopharmacology*, 30:123–134.
199. Modlinger, R. S., Schonmuller, J. M., and Arora, S. P. (1979): Stimulation of aldosterone, renin, and cortisol by tryptophan. *J. Clin. Endocrinol. Metab.*, 48:599–604.

200. Modlinger, R. S., Schonmuller, J. M., and Arora, S. P. (1980): Adrenocorticotropin release by tryptophan in man. *J. Clin. Endocrinol. Metab.*, 50:360–363.
201. Moir, A. T. B., and Eccleston, D. (1968): The effects of precursor loading in the cerebral metabolism of 5-hydroxyindoles. *J. Neurochem.*, 15:1093–1108.
202. Moore, K. E., Annunziato, L., and Gudelsky, G. A. (1978): Studies on tuberoinfundibular dopamine neurons. *Adv. Biochem. Psychopharmacol.*, 19:193–204.
203. Morgenroth, V. H. III, Walters J. R., and Roth, R. H. (1976): Dopaminergic neurons—alterations in the kinetic properties of tyrosine hydroxylase after cessation of impulse flow. *Biochem. Pharmacol.*, 25:655–661.
204. Morre, M. C., Hefti, F., and Wurtman, R. J. (1980): Regional tyrosine levels in rat brain after tyrosine administration. *J. Neural Transm.*, 49:45–50.
205. Morre, M. C., and Wurtman, R. J. (1981): Characteristics of synaptosomal tyrosine uptake in various brain regions: Effect of other amino acids. *Life Sci.*, 28:65–75.
206. Mueller, G. P., Twohy, C. P., Chen, H. T., Advis, J. P., and Meites, J. (1976): Effects of L-tryptophan and restraint stress on hypothalamic and brain serotonin turnover, and pituitary TSH and prolactin release in rats. *Life Sci.*, 18:715–724.
207. Nagatsu, T., Levitt, M., and Udenfriend, S. (1964): Tyrosine hydroxylase, the initial step in norepinephrine biosynthesis. *J. Biol. Chem.*, 239:2910–2917.
208. Neckers, L. M., Biggio, G., Moja, E., and Meek, J. L. (1977): Modulation of brain tryptophan hydroxylase activity by brain tryptophan content. *J. Pharmacol. Exp. Ther.*, 201:110–116.
209. Neff, N. H., and Tozer, T. N. (1968): *In vivo* measurement of brain serotonin turnover. *Adv. Pharmacol.*, 6A:97–109.
210. Neill, J. D. (1974): Prolactin: Its secretion and control. In: *Handbook of Physiology, Section 7, Endocrinology, Vol. 4*, pp. 469–488. American Physiological Society, Washington, D.C.
211. Ng, L. K. Y., Chase, T. N., Colburn, R. W., and Kopin, I. J. (1973): Release of [³H]dopamine by L-5-hydroxytryptophan. *Brain Res.*, 59:169–179.
212. Nikodijevic, B., Creveling, C. R., and Udenfriend, S. (1963): Inhibition of dopamine-β-hydroxylase *in vivo* by benzyloxyamine and benzylhydrazine analogs. *J. Pharmacol. Exp. Ther.*, 140:224–228.
213. Nolan, P. L. (1977): The effects of serotonin precursors on the pressor response to intravenous clonidine in conscious rats. *Clin. Exp. Pharmacol. Physiol.*, 4:579–583.
214. Oldendorf, W. H. (1971): Brain uptake of radiolabeled amino acids, amines, and hexoses after arterial injection. *Am. J. Physiol.*, 221:1629–1639.
215. Pardridge, W. M. (1978): Regulation of amino acid availability to the brain. In: *Nutrition and the Brain, Vol. 1*, edited by R. J. Wurtman and J. J. Wurtman, pp. 141–203. Raven Press, New York.
216. Pardridge, W. M. (1979): Regulation of amino acid availability to brain: Selective control mechanisms for glutamate. In: *Glutamic Acid: Advances in Biochemistry and Physiology*, edited by L. J. Filer, M. R. Kare, S. Garattini, W. A. Reynolds, and R. J. Wurtman, pp. 125–137. Raven Press, New York.
217. Pardridge, W. M. (1979): Tryptophan transport through the blood-brain barrier: *in vivo* measurement of free and albumin-bound amino acid. *Life Sci.*, 25:1519–1528.
218. Pardridge, W. M., and Oldendorf, W. H. (1975): Kinetic analysis of blood–brain barrier transport of amino acids. *Biochem. Biophys. Acta*, 401:128–136.
219. Patrick, R. L., and Barchas, J. D. (1976): Dopamine synthesis in rat brain striatal synaptosomes. II. Dibutyryl cyclic adenosine 3′5′ monophosphoric acid and 6-methyltetrahydropterine-induced synthesis increases, without an increase in endogenous dopamine release. *J. Pharmacol. Exp. Ther.*, 197:97–104.
220. Peters, J. C., and Harper, A. E. (1981): Protein and energy consumption, plasma amino acid ratios and brain neurotransmitter concentrations. *Physiol. Behav.*, 27:287–298.
221. Peters, J. C., Tews, J. K., and Harper, A. E. (1981): L-tryptophan injections fails to alter nutrient selection by rats. *Trans. Am. Soc. Neurosci.*, 12:404.
222. Peters, R. I., and Meyers, K. M. (1977): Precursor regulation of serotonergic neuronal function in Scottish Terrier dogs. *J. Neurochem.*, 29:753–755.
223. Philippu, A., Dietl, H., and Sinha, J. N. (1980): Rise in blood pressure increases the release of endogenous catecholamines in the anterior hypothalamus of the cat. *Naunyn Schmiedebergs Arch. Pharmacol.*, 310:237–240.
224. Pradham, S., Alphs, L., and Lovenberg, W. (1981): Characterization of haloperidol-mediated effects on rat striatal tyrosine hydroxylase. *Neuropharmacology*, 20:149–154.

225. Reinhard, J. F., Moskowitz, M. A., Sved, A. F., and Fernstrom, J. D. (1980): A simple, sensitive and reliable assay for serotonin and 5-HIAA in brain tissue using liquid chromatography with electrochemical detection. *Life Sci.*, 27:905–911.

225a. Reinhard, J. F., and Wurtman, R. J. (1977): Relation between brain 5-HIAA levels and the release of serotonin into brain synapses. *Life Sci.*, 21:1741–1746.

226. Reymond, M. J., and Porter, J. C. (1981): Secretion of hypothalamic dopamine into pituitary stalk blood of aged female rats. *Brain Res. Bull.*, 7:69–73.

227. Ross, D. S., Fernstrom, J. D., and Wurtman, R. J. (1973): The role of dietary protein in generating daily rhythms in rat liver tryptophan pyrrolase and tyrosine transaminase. *Metabolism*, 22:1175–1184.

228. Roth, R. H., Murrin, L. C., and Walters, J. R. (1976): Central dopaminergic neurons: Effects of alterations in impulse flow on the accumulation of dihydroxyphenylacetic acid. *Eur. J. Pharmacol.*, 36:163–171.

229. Roth, R. H., Salzman, P. M., and Nowycky, M. (1978): Impulse flow and short-term regulation of transmitter biosynthesis in central catecholaminergic neurons. In: *Psychopharmacology: A Generation of Progress*, edited by M. A. Lipton, A. DiMascio, and K. F. Killam, pp. 185–198. Raven Press, New York.

230. Roth, R. H., Walters, J. R., Murrin, L. C., and Morgenroth, V. H. (1975): Dopamine neurons: Role of impulse flow and pre-synaptic receptors in the regulation of tyrosine hydroxylase. In: *Pre and Post Synaptic Receptors*, edited by E. Usdin and W. E. Bunney, Jr., pp. 5–48. Marcel Dekker, Inc., New York.

231. Saavedra, J. M., and Axelrod, J. (1973): Effect of drugs on the tryptamine content of rat tissues. *J. Pharmacol. Exp. Ther.*, 185:523–529.

232. Sahakian, B. J., Wurtman, R. J., Barr, J. K., Millington, W. R., and Chiel, H. J. (1979): Low tryptophan diet decreases brain serotonin and alters response to apomorphine. *Nature*, 279:731–732.

233. Saller, C. F., and Chido, L. A. (1980): Glucose suppresses basal firing and haloperidol-induced increases in the firing rate of central dopaminergic neurons. *Science*, 210:1269–1271.

234. Samanin, R., Bernasconi, S., and Quattrone, A. (1976): Antinociceptive action of quipazine: Relation to central serotonergic receptor stimulation. *Psychopharmacology*, 46:219–222.

235. Sapun, D. I., Farah, J. M., and Mueller, G. P. (1981): Evidence that a serotonergic mechanism stimulates the secretion of pituitary β-endorphin-like immunoreactivity in the rat. *Endocrinology*, 109:421–426.

236. Scally, M. C., Ulus, I., and Wurtman, R. J. (1977): Brain tyrosine levels control striatal dopamine synthesis in haloperidol-treated rats. *J. Neural Transm.*, 41:1–6.

237. Scott, N. A., DeSilva, R. A., Lown, B., and Wurtman, R. J. (1981): Tyrosine administration decreases vulnerability to ventricular fibrillation in the normal canine heart. *Science*, 211:727–729.

238. Shalita, B., and Dikstein, S. (1977): Central tyramine prevents hypertension in uninephrectomized DOCA-saline treated rats. *Experientia*, 33:1430–1431.

239. Shalita, B., and Dikstein, S. (1979): D-Tyrosine prevents hypertension in DOCA-saline treated uninephrectomized rats. *Pfleugers Arch.*, 379:245–250.

240. Sheard, M. H. (1969): The effect of *p*-chlorophenylalanine on behavior in rats: Relation to brain serotonin and 5-hydroxyindoleacetic acid. *Brain Res.*, 15:524–528.

241. Shields, P. J., and Eccleston, D. (1972): Effects of electrical stimulation of rat midbrain on 5-hydroxytryptamine synthesis as determined by a sensitive radioisotope method. *J. Neurochem.*, 19:265–272.

242. Shillito, E. (1970): The effect of parachlorophenylalanine on social interactions of male rats. *Br. J. Pharmacol.*, 38:305–315.

243. Shiman, R., Akino, M., and Kaufman, S. (1971): Solubilization and partial purification of tyrosine hydroxylase from bovine adrenal medulla. *J. Biol. Chem.*, 246:1330–1340.

244. Sidransky, H., Sarma, D. S. R., Bongiorno, M., and Verney, E. (1968): Effect of dietary tryptophan on hepatic polyribosomes and protein synthesis in fasted mice. *J. Biol. Chem.*, 243:1123–1132.

245. Smith, J. E., Lane, J. D., Shea, P. A., and McBride, W. J. (1977): Neurochemical changes following the administration of precursors of biogenic amines. *Life Sci.*, 21:301–306.

246. Sourkes, T. L., Missala, K., and Oravec, M. (1970): Decrease of cerebral serotonin and 5-hydroxyindoleacetic acid caused by α-methyltryptophan. *J. Neurochem.*, 17:111–115.

247. Spector, S., Gordon, R., Sjoerdsma, A., and Udenfriend, S. (1967): End product inhibition of tyrosine hydroxylase as a possible mechanism for regulation of norepinephrine synthesis. *Mol. Pharmacol.*, 3:549–555.
248. Spector, S., Sjoerdsma, A., and Udenfriend, S. (1965): Blockade of endogenous norepinephrine synthesis by α-methyl-*p*-tyrosine, an inhibitor of tyrosine hydroxylase. *J. Pharmacol. Exp. Ther.*, 147:86–95.
249. Sved, A. F., and Fernstrom, J. D. (1981): Tyrosine availability and dopamine synthesis in the striatum: Studies with gamma-butyrolactone. *Life Sci.*, 29:743–748.
250. Sved, A. F. (1980): The relationship between tyrosine availability and catecholaminergic function: physiological and biochemical studies. Doctoral dissertation, Massachusetts Institute of Technology, Cambridge, Massachusetts.
251. Sved, A. F., Fernstrom, J. D., and Wurtman, R. J. (1979): Tyrosine administration decreases serum prolactin levels in chronically reserpinized rats. *Life Sci.*, 25:1293–1300.
252. Sved, A. F., Fernstrom, J. D., and Wurtman, R. J. (1979): Tyrosine administration reduces blood pressure and enhances brain norepinephrine release in spontaneously hypertensive rats. *Proc. Natl. Acad. Sci. USA*, 76:3511–3514.
253. Sved, A. F., Goldberg, I. M., and Fernstrom, J. D. (1980): Dietary protein intake influences the antihypertensive potency of methyldopa in spontaneously hypertensive rats. *J. Pharmacol. Exp. Ther.*, 214:147–151.
254. Sved, A. F., Van Itallie, C. M., and Fernstrom, J. D. (1982): Studies on the antihypertensive action of L-tryptophan. *J. Pharmacol. Exp. Ther.*, 221:329–333.
255. Tagliamonte, A., Biggio, G., Vargiu, L., and Gessa, G. L. (1973): Free tryptophan in serum controls brain tryptophan level and serotonin synthesis. *Life Sci.*, 12:277–287.
256. Tagliamonte, A., Biggio, G., Vargiu, L., and Gessa, G. L. (1973): Increase in brain tryptophan and stimulation of serotonin synthesis by salicylate. *J. Neurochem.*, 20:909–912.
257. Tagliamonte, A., Tagliamonte, P., Gessa, G. L., and Brodie, B. B. (1969): Compulsive sexual activity induced by *p*-chlorophenylalanine in normal and pinealectomized male rats. *Science*, 166:1433–1435.
258. Tallman, J. F., Saavedra, J. M., and Axelrod, J. (1976): Biosynthesis and metabolism of endogenous tyramine and its normal presence in sympathetic nerves. *J. Pharmacol. Exp. Ther.*, 199:216–221.
259. Taylor, M. (1976): Effects of L-tryptophan and L-methionine on activity in the rat. *Br. J. Pharmacol.*, 58:117–119.
260. Thurmond, J. B., Kramarcy, N. R., Lasley, S. M., and Brown, J. W. (1980): Dietary amino acid precursors: Effect on central monoamines, aggression, and locomotor activity in the mouse. *Pharmacol. Biochem. Behav.*, 12:525–532.
261. Thurmond, J. B., Lasley, S. M., Kramarcy, N. R., and Brown, J. W. (1979): Differential tolerance to dietary amino acid-induced changes in aggressive behavior and locomotor activity in mice. *Psychopharmacology*, 66:301–308.
262. Trulson, M. E., and Jacobs, B. L. (1976): Dose-response relationships between systemically administered L-tryptophan or 5-hydroxytryptophan and raphe unit activity in the rat. *Neuropharmacology*, 15:339–344.
263. Tulanay, F. C., Yano, I., and Takemori, A. E. (1976): The effect of biogenic amine modifiers on morphine analgesia and its antagonism by naloxone. *Eur. J. Pharmacol.*, 35:285–292.
264. Ungerstedt, U. (1971): Postsynaptic supersensitivity after 6-hydroxydopamine induced degeneration of the nigrostriatal dopamine system. *Acta Physiol. Scand. (Suppl. 367)*, 82:69–93.
265. van Zwieten, P. A. (1975): Antihypertensive drugs with a central action. *Prog. Pharmacol.*, 1:1–63.
266. Vernikos-Danellis, J., Kellar, K. J., Kent, D., Gonzales, C., Berger, P. A., and Barchas, J. D. (1977): Serotonin involvement in pituitary-adrenal function. *Ann. NY Acad. Sci.*, 297:518–525.
267. Walters, J. K., Davis, M., and Sheard, M. H. (1979): Tryptophan-free diet: Effects on the acoustic startle reflex in rats. *Psychopharmacology*, 62:103–109.
268. Walters, J. R., Aghajanian, G. K., and Roth, R. H. (1972): Dopaminergic neurons: Inhibition of firing by gamma-hydroxybutyrate. In: *Proceedings of the Fifth International Congress of Pharmacology*, p. 246.
269. Walters, J. R., and Roth, R. H. (1974): Dopaminergic neurons: Drug-induced antagonism of the increase in tyrosine hydroxylase activity produced by cessation of impulse flow. *J. Pharmacol. Exp. Ther.*, 191:82–91.

270. Walters, J. R., and Roth, R. H. (1976): Dopaminergic neurons: An *in vivo* system for measuring drug interactions with presynaptic receptors. *Naunyn Schmiedebergs Arch. Pharmacol.*, 296:5–14.

271. Webber, W. A. (1962): Interactions of neutral and acidic amino acids in renal tubular transport. *Am. J. Physiol.* 202:577–583.

272. Weber, L. J., and Horita, A. (1965): A study of 5-hydroxytryptamine formation from L-tryptophan in the brain and other tissues. *Biochem. Pharmacol.*, 14:1141–1149.

273. Weinberger, S. B., Knapp, S., and Mandell, A. J. (1978): Failure of tryptophan load-induced increases in brain serotonin to alter food intake in the rat. *Life Sci.*, 22:1595–1602.

274. Weiner, N., Lee, F.-L., Dreyer, E., and Barnes, E. (1978): The activation of tyrosine hydroxylase in noradrenergic neurons during acute nerve stimulation. *Life Sci.*, 22:1197–1216.

275. Weiner, N., Lee, F.-L., Waymire, J. C., and Posiviata, M. (1974): The regulation of tyrosine hydroxylase in adrenergic nervous tissue. In: *Aromatic Amino Acids in the Brain*, edited by G. E. W. Wolstenholm and D. W. Fitzsimons, pp. 135–147. Associated Scientific Publishers, Amsterdam.

276. Weiner, N., and Rabadjija, M. (1968): The effect of nerve stimulation on the synthesis and metabolism of norepinephrine in the isolated guinea-pig hypogastric nerve-vas deferens preparation. *J. Pharmacol. Exp. Ther.*, 160:61–71.

277. Weiner, N., and Selvaratnam, I. (1968): The effect of tyramine on the synthesis of norepinephrine. *J. Pharmacol. Exp. Ther.*, 161:21–33.

278. Wiebe, R. H., Handwerger, S., and Hammond, C. B. (1977): Failure of L-tryptophan to stimulate prolactin secretion in man. *J. Clin. Endo. Metab.*, 45:1310–1312.

279. Wojcik, W. J., Fornal, C., and Radulocacki, M. (1980): Effect of tryptophan on sleep in the rat. *Neuropharmacology*, 19:163–167.

280. Woodger, T. L., Sirek, A., and Anderson, G. H. (1979): Diabetes, dietary tryptophan, and protein intake regulation in weanling rats. *Am. J. Physiol.*, 236:R307–R311.

281. Woolf, P. D., and Lee, L. (1977): Effect of the serotonin precursor tryptophan on pituitary hormone secretion. *J. Clin. Endocrinol. Metab.*, 45:123–133.

282. Wu, J.-Y. (1976): Purification, characterization, and kinetic studies of GAD and GABA-T from mouse brain. In: *GABA in Nervous System Function*, edited by E. Roberts, T. N. Chase, and D. B. Tower, pp. 7–55. Raven Press, New York.

282a. Wurtman, J. J., Moses, P. L., and Wurtman, R. J. (1983): Prior carbohydrate consumption affects the amount of carbohydrate that rats choose to eat. *J. Nutr.*, 113:70–78.

283. Wurtman, J. J., and Wurtman, R. J. (1977): Fenfluramine and fluoxetine spare protein consumption while suppressing caloric intake by rats. *Science*, 198:1178–1180.

284. Wurtman, J. J., and Wurtman, R. J. (1979): Drugs that enhance central serotonergic transmission diminish elective carbohydrate consumption by rats. *Life Sci.*, 24:895–904.

285. Wurtman, R. J. (1975): Daily rhythms in tyrosine transaminase and other hepatic enzymes that metabolize amino acids: Mechanisms and possible consequences. *Life Sci.*, 15:827–847.

286. Wurtman, R. J., Scally, M. C., Gibson, C. J., and Hefti, F. (1980): Relation between brain tyrosine and catecholamine synthesis. In: *Catecholamines: Basic and Clinical Frontiers*, edited by E. Usdin, I. J. Kopin, and J. D. Barchas, pp. 64–66. Pergamon Press, New York.

287. Wurtman, R. J., Hefti, F., and Melamed, E. (1981): Precursor control of neurotransmitter synthesis. *Pharmacol. Rev.*, 32:315–335.

288. Wurtman, R. J., Larin, F., Mostafapour, S., and Fernstrom, J. D. (1974): Brain catechol synthesis: Control by brain tyrosine concentration. *Science*, 185:183–184.

289. Wurtman, R. J., Shoemaker, W. J., and Larin, F. (1968): Mechanism of the daily rhythm in hepatic tyrosine transaminase activity: Role of dietary tryptophan. *Proc. Natl. Acad. Sci. USA*, 59:800–807.

290. Wyatt, R. J., Engelman, K., and Kupfer, D. J. (1970): Effects of L-tryptophan (a natural sedative) on human sleep. *Lancet*, 2:842–846.

291. Yaksh, T. L., DuChateau, J. C., and Rudy, T. A. (1976): Antagonism by methysergide and cinanserin of the antinociceptive action of morphine administered into the periaqueductal gray. *Brain Res.*, 104:367–372.

292. Yamori, Y., Fujiwara, M., Horie, R., and Lovenberg, W. (1980): The hypotensive effect of centrally administered tyrosine. *Eur. J. Pharmacol.*, 68:201–204.

293. Yarborough, G. G., Buxbaum, D. M., and Sanders-Bush, E. (1973): Biogenic amines and narcotic

effects. II. Serotonin turnover in the rat after acute and chronic morphine administration. *J. Pharmacol. Exp. Ther.*, 185:328–335.

294. Yehuda, S., and Wurtman, R. J. (1972): Release of brain dopamine as the probable mechanism for the hypothermic effect of D-amphetamine. *Nature*, 240:477–478.

295. Yehuda, S., and Wurtman, R. J. (1972): The effects of D-amphetamine and related drugs on colonic temperatures of rats kept at various ambient temperatures. *Life Sci.*, 11:851–859.

296. Young, J. A., and Freedman, B. S. (1971): Renal tubular transport of amino acids. *Clin. Chem.*, 17:245–266.

297. Young, S. N., Anderson, G. M., and Purdy, W. C. (1980): Indolamine metabolism in rat brain studied through measurements of tryptophan, 5-hydroxyindoleacetic acid, and indoleacetic acid in cerebrospinal fluid. *J. Neurochem.*, 34:309–315.

298. Young, S. N., St. Arnaud-McKenzie, D., and Sourkes, T. L. (1978): Importance of tryptophan pyrrolase and aromatic acid decarboxylase in the catabolism of tryptophan. *Biochem. Pharmacol.*, 27:763–767.

299. Yunger, L. M., and Harvey, J. A. (1976): Behavioral effects of L-5-hydroxytryptophan after destruction of ascending serotonergic pathways in the rat: The role of catecholaminergic neurons. *J. Pharmacol. Exp. Ther.*, 196:307–315.

300. Yuwiler, A., Oldendorf, W. H., Geller, E., and Braun, L. (1977): Effect of albumin binding and amino acid competition on tryptophan uptake into brain. *J. Neurochem.*, 28:1015–1023.

301. Zimmerman, H., and Ganong, W. F. (1980): Pharmacological evidence that stimulation of central serotonergic pathways increases renin secretion. *Neuroendocrinology*, 30:101–107.

302. Zombotti, F., Carruba, M., Vincentini, L., and Mantegazza, P. (1975): Selective effect of a maize diet in reducing serum and brain tryptophan contents and blood and brain serotonin levels. *Life Sci.*, 17:1663–1669.

Subject Index

Subject Index

277